OXFORD MEDICAL PUBLICATIONS

Current Surgical
Guidelines

Specialist Handbooks published and forthcoming

...ral Oxford Specialist Handbooks

A Resuscitation Room Guide
Addiction Medicine
Day Case Surgery
Parkinson's Disease and Other Movement
    Disorders, 2e
Perioperative Medicine, 2e
Pharmaceutical Medicine
Postoperative Complications, 2e
Renal Transplantation
Retrieval Medicine

Oxford Specialist Handbooks in Anaesthesia

Anaesthesia for Medical and Surgical
    Emergencies
Cardiac Anaesthesia
Neuroanaesthesia
Obstetric Anaesthesia
Ophthalmic Anaesthesia
Paediatric Anaesthesia
Regional Anaesthesia, Stimulation
    and Ultrasound Techniques
Thoracic Anaesthesia

Oxford Specialist Handbooks in Cardiology

Adult Congenital Heart Disease
Cardiac Catheterization and Coronary
    Intervention
Cardiac Electrophysiology and Catheter
    Ablation
Cardiovascular Computed Tomography
Cardiovascular Magnetic Resonance
Echocardiography, 2e
Fetal Cardiology
Heart Failure, 2e
Hypertension
Inherited Cardiac Disease
Nuclear Cardiology
Pacemakers and ICDs
Pulmonary Hypertension
Valvular Heart Disease

Oxford Specialist Handbooks in Critical Care

Advanced Respiratory Critical Care
Cardiothoracic Critical Care

Oxford Specialist Handbooks in End of Life Care

End of Life Care in Cardiology
End of Life Care in Dementia
End of Life Care in Nephrology
End of Life Care in Respiratory Disease
End of Life in the Intensive Care Unit

Oxford Specialist Handbooks in Infectious Disease

Infectious Disease Epidemiology
Manual of Childhood Infections, 4e

Oxford Specialist Handbooks in Neurology

Epilepsy
Parkinson's Disease and Other Movement
    Disorders, 2e
Stroke Medicine, 2e

Oxford Specialist Handbooks in Oncology

Practical Management of Complex
    Cancer Pain

Oxford Specialist Handbooks in Paediatrics

Paediatric Dermatology
Paediatric Endocrinology and Diabetes
Paediatric Gastroenterology, Hepatology,
    and Nutrition
Paediatric Haematology and Oncology
Paediatric Intensive Care
Paediatric Nephrology, 2e
Paediatric Neurology, 2e
Paediatric Palliative Medicine, 2e
Paediatric Radiology
Paediatric Respiratory Medicine
Paediatric Rheumatology

Oxford Specialist Handbooks in Pain Medicine

Spinal Interventions in Pain Management

Oxford Specialist Handbooks in Psychiatry

Addiction Medicine, 2e
Child and Adolescent Psychiatry
Forensic Psychiatry
Medical Psychotherapy
Old Age Psychiatry

Oxford Specialist Handbooks in Radiology

Interventional Radiology
Musculoskeletal Imaging
Pulmonary Imaging
Thoracic Imaging

Oxford Specialist Handbooks in Surgery

Cardiothoracic Surgery, 2e
Colorectal Surgery
Gastric and Oesophageal Surgery
Hand Surgery
Hepatopancreatobiliary Surgery
Neurosurgery
Operative Surgery, 2e
Oral and Maxillofacial Surgery, 2e
Otolaryngology and Head and Neck
    Surgery
Paediatric Surgery
Plastic and Reconstructive Surgery
Surgical Oncology
Urological Surgery
Vascular Surgery, 2e

Oxford Specialist Handbooks in Surgery
Current Surgical Guidelines

Second edition

Abdullah Jibawi
Consultant Vascular, Endovascular & General Surgeon
Academic Instructor to the Royal College of Surgeons
Ashford and St. Peter's Hospitals NHS Foundation Trust
UK

Mohamed Baguneid
Consultant Vascular Surgeon
Chair of Surgery, Al Ain Hospital SEHA, UAE
Honorary Professor University of Salford, Manchester, UK
Adjunct Professor - College of Medicine and
Health Science, UAE University

and

Arnab Bhowmick
Consultant Colorectal & General Surgeon
Lancashire Teaching Hospitals NHS Foundation Trust
UK

OXFORD
UNIVERSITY PRESS

OXFORD
UNIVERSITY PRESS

Great Clarendon Street, Oxford, OX2 6DP,
United Kingdom

Oxford University Press is a department of the University of Oxford.
It furthers the University's objective of excellence in research, scholarship,
and education by publishing worldwide. Oxford is a registered trade mark of
Oxford University Press in the UK and in certain other countries

© Oxford University Press 2018

The moral rights of the authors have been asserted

First edition published in 2010
Second Edition published in 2018

Impression: 1

Published in the United States of America by Oxford University Press
198 Madison Avenue, New York, NY 10016, United States of America

British Library Cataloguing in Publication Data
Data available

Library of Congress Control Number: 2018937415

ISBN 978–0–19–879476–9

Printed and bound in China by
C&C Offset Printing Co., Ltd.

Foreword

It is with some trepidation that I began the task of reviewing the contents of this book. My trepidation was based on the fact that, having had a strong interest in guideline production and dissemination myself, I know just how insipid and monotonous guidelines can be. I need not have worried! Indeed, towards the end of my task, I was positively looking forward to reading the next chapter. The authors are to be commended on compiling such a comprehensive collection of contemporary surgical guidelines, and presenting them so clearly that the busy clinician will have no trouble whatsoever in reading and digesting their contents. The sensible use of simple tables makes it straightforward to identify the information relevant to a specific clinical problem.

I particularly enjoyed the first twenty chapters because they deal with everyday clinical issues that are relevant to surgeons practising in all branches of surgery. I have no doubt that junior doctors who base their day-to-day care of surgical patients on these guidelines will greatly improve the care that they offer. Experienced surgeons will not only find guidelines relevant to their specialist area but can rapidly access contemporary information from areas of surgical practice outside their immediate expertise. It is for these reasons that this book will be invaluable to all surgeons, be they Foundation year doctors or experienced consultants.

The guidelines are UK-based if they are available. Thereafter, the hierarchy is European guidelines followed by North American guidelines. This approach is sensible and pragmatic. In summary, the authors are to be congratulated on compiling and presenting contemporary surgical guidelines in such a way that they are interesting and immediately relevant to clinical practice. I am certain that I will be referring to my own copy on a very regular basis!

Professor Nick London
Professor of Surgery
University of Leicester

Preface to the 2nd Edition

This edition of Oxford handbook Current Surgical Guidelines reflects the advancement in scientific research and clinical guidelines that has emerged over the last 5 years. To ensure the contents and breadth of knowledge of this edition remain clinically relevant and up to date, we welcome the contribution of two distinct new authors and educational leaders, MB and AB. This edition has witnessed the addition of new key chapters on trauma, hernias, skin malignancies, and medicolegal aspects of surgical practice. The chapters incorporate the concise and rich-content style of this book, with the most up to date evidence-based information. All chapters have been fully reviewed and matched against new guidelines, with a further in-depth review by specialist Surgeons and Physicians to ensure their practicality and contemporary advices for a safe and modern practice in surgery. Finally, we have introduced new platforms and tools to enrich the book readability and usability. The book has become available online via the OUP web site, and some additional tools were made available via other platforms such as iPhone and iPads. With this level of new changes, we hope that we provide you with a tool that is able to enlighten your practice and deliver the safest and modern clinical decision making when and where needed.

Preface to the 1st Edition

Documents written for guiding decisions in the diagnosis and management of specific diseases have been in use for many thousands of years. Unlike previous approaches that were often based on authority or tradition, modern guidelines reflect a consensus of expert opinion following a thorough and systematic review of currently available scientific evidence.

Clinical guidelines do not aim to replace the clinical judgement, but to support it. Guideline recommendations attempt to define practices that meet the requirement of most patients in most circumstances, but can give no guarantee of a successful outcome in every individual case. Clinical judgement and decision-making should consider the individual patient's condition, circumstances and wishes, as well as the quality and availability of expertise in the area where care is provided.

In recent years, the number of guidelines produced by national bodies, specialist associations, royal colleges, and others has increased enormously and it has become difficult for busy clinicians to keep up to date with rapidly changing fields. The focus of this handbook is to summarize currently available guidelines in general and vascular surgery in a concise, practical, and friendly way. Neither should it be considered that it includes all acceptable methods of management nor as a standard of clinical care. In short, 'we summarize the guidelines, you make the decision'.

We hope that this book will contribute to the implementation of high quality guidelines in surgical practice.

General Outlines

The principles and rules throughout the book are kept limited to provide consistency in presenting the rather scattered guidelines in a uniform manner.

We have used different search engines to find the most relevant and up-to-date guidelines for each topic. National Institute for Health and Clinical Excellence (NICE), National Library for Guidelines (UK-archived), National Guideline Clearinghouse (US), Scottish Intercollegiate Guidelines Network (SIGN), Google Scholars , and other online portals (e.g. the Association of Surgeons of Great Britain and Ireland, the Royal College of Surgeons of England, and BMJ Clinical Evidence, etc.) were accessed and systematically reviewed. Full text guidelines were retrieved, thoroughly evaluated, and summarized. Guidelines written on the same topic and published by different authorities were compared and summary included within the text as appropriate. Relevant chapters were reviewed independently by the authors and then by appropriate experts in each field.

We have integrated friendly statistics within different sections of each chapter to support a realistic decision-making process and allow informed decisions for patients at the point of care. These statistics can be used, for example, to understand the impact of a risk factor on a specific disease and allow for better understanding of any recommended screening programme (e.g. screening for abdominal aortic aneurysm at the age of 65, chapter 46); to realize the limitations of certain investigations in detecting (sensitivity) and confirming (specificity) certain pathology or disease severity (e.g. endoscopic ultrasound scan (EUS) in oesophageal cancer staging, chapter 21); and to provide the clinician with the latest figures on the efficiency and safety of different treatment options, and therefore, allow for better communication with patients and evidence-based sup- ported decision-making (e.g. efficacy of local glyceryl trinitrate (GTN) for anal fissure healing, chapter 34).

Recommendations for a specific investigation, screening, or treatment have been graded as per the original guideline's grading system, which usually follows the main theme of grading as outlined in chapter 1.

Tables have been used extensively within the handbook for summarizing and easy access purposes. The recommended approach for each disease has been outlined using specially designed algorithms which formulate an integral part of each relevant chapter and have to be interpreted within this context. The recommended approach does not include all acceptable methods of diagnosis or management; sound clinical judgment is always required (chapter 1).

Mobile digital platforms have become an integral part of practice by many clinicians and Trusts. As from edition 2, we have provided a new online platform to enhance readability and links to selected tools to provide an in-depth analysis for instant and easy calculation of certain risks and mortality rates (chapter 6).

Finally, we used a quick reference script to allow for rapid and efficient access to information at the point of care. This style has been adopted based on some constructive feedback we have had during the development process; the handbook is not to replace the more traditional surgical textbooks or handbooks, but to provide the reader with consistent, up-to-date, and sound clinical information. We hope the book will stimulate the reader to read the original documents. Any comments or recommendations are welcomed.

Acknowledgements

We would like to record our sincere thanks to our advisors and contributors on specific sections for the first and second editions of this book.

Contributors to the first edition

David Berry
Consultant Surgeon, University Hospitals of Leicester NHS Trust. UK

David Corless
Consultant Surgeon, the Mid Cheshire Hospitals NHS Trust. UK

Linda De Cossart
Vice President of the Royal College of Surgeons of England. UK

Prof Mohan de Silva
University of Sri Jayawardenepura, Colombo, SRI LANKA

Martin Dennis
Consultant Vascular Surgeon, University Hospitals of Leicester NHS Trust. UK

Ashley Dennison
Consultant Surgeon, University Hospitals of Leicester NHS Trust. UK

Magdi Hanafy
Consultant Surgeon, the Mid Cheshire Hospitals NHS Trust. UK

John Jameson
Consultant Surgeon, University Hospitals of Leicester NHS Trust. UK

Lloyd Jenkinson
Consultant Surgeon, The North West Wales NHS Trust.

Michelle Lapworth
Vascular and Wound Specialist Practice Nurse, University Hospitals of Leicester. UK

Prof. Nick London
Professor of Surgery, University of Leicester and Honorary Consultant Vascular and Endocrine Surgeon, University Hospitals of Leicester NHS Trust. UK

Mark McCarthy
Consultant Vascular Surgeon and Honorary Senior Lecturer, University Hospitals of Leicester NHS Trust. UK

Roddy Nash
Consultant Surgeon, Derbyshire Royal Infirmary. UK

Akhtar Nasim
Consultant Vascular Surgeon, University Hospitals of Leicester NHS Trust. UK

Prof. A Ross Naylor
Professor of Vascular Surgery, University Hospitals of Leicester NHS Trust. UK

Sue Povard
Consultant Haematologist and Lecturer at the University of Leicester. UK

Prof. Robert Sayers
Professor of Vascular Surgery,
University Hospitals of Leicester
NHS Trust. UK

Sulaiman Shoaib
Consultant Surgeon, The
North West Wales NHS
Trust, UK

Sukhbir Ubhi
Consultant Surgeon, University
Hospitals of Leicester NHS
Trust; UK

Mr. Chris Sutton
Consultant Surgeon, University
Hospitals of Leicester NHS
Trust; UK

Andrew Swann
Consultant Microbiologist,
University Hospitals of Leicester
NHS Trust. UK

Douglas A. B.
Turner Consultant Anaesthetist and
Critical Care, University Hospitals
of Leicester NHS Trust. UK

Contributors to the second edition

Arsalan Al Wafi
Senior Clinical Fellow. Vascular
Department. Ashford and St
Peter's Hospital. Surrey. UK

Swethan Alagaratnam
SpR North East Thames
Deanery. North Middlesex
University NHS trust. UK (main
co-author for hernia chapter)

Asad Ali
Senior Clinical Fellow. Surgical
Department. Ashford and St
Peter's Hospital. Surrey. UK

Reza Arsalani-Zadeh
International Clinical Fellow
in Surgery. Specialty Trainee
in Surgery, North West
Deanery. UK

Mohammed Ashrafi
Vascular Research Fellow,
University Hospital South
Manchester NHS Foundation
Trust. UK

Abdulla Baguneid
Core Medical Trainee,
Nottingham. UK

Clare Baguneid
Core Medical Trainee,
Nottingham. UK

Tamir Bashir
Associate Consultant
Surgeon, International Medical
Center Hospital, Jeddah,
SAUDI ARABIA

Robert Brown
Senior Clinical Fellow in Surgery.
Salford Royal Hospitals. UK

Liz Clayton
ST8 Oncoplastic breast and gen-
eral surgery registrar, Frimley
Park Hospital, Frimley. UK

Peter O Coe
Clinical Research Fellow
in Surgery. University of
Manchester. UK

Raouf Daoud
Consultant Oncoplastic Breast Surgeon, Frimley Park Hospital, Frimley. UK

Helen Doran
Consultant Endocrine Surgeon, Salford Royal NHS Foundation Trust. UK

Adrain Franklin
Brachytherapy consultant, St Luke's Cancer Centre, Royal Surrey County Hospital. UK

Simon J Gonsalves
International Colorectal Fellow, Royal Prince Alfred Hospital, Sydney. AUSTRALIA

Kamran Haq
Senior Clinical Fellow. Surgical Department. Ashford and St Peter's Hospital. Surrey. UK

Sue Harris
Lead Tissue Viability Nurse. Ashford and St Peter's Hospital NHS Trust. UK

Shameen Jaunoo
Senior Clinical Fellow Oesophagogastric Surgery, Oxford University Hospitals

Muneer A Junejo
Specialty Trainee in Surgery. North West Deanery. UK

Kavitha Kanesalingam
ST7 Oncoplastic breast and general surgery registrar, Frimley Park Hospital, Frimley. UK

Nitya Krishnamohan
Specialty Trainee in Surgery. North West Deanery. UK

Barun Majumder
Consultant Vascular Surgeon. Ashford and St Peter's Hospital NHS Trust. UK

Mark McGregour
Consultant anaesthetist and Vascular Anaesthetic Lead. Ashford and St Peter's Hospital NHS Trust. UK

Magdy Moawad
Consultant Vascular Surgeon. Ashford and St Peter's Hospital NHS Trust. UK

Ary Phaily
Research Fellow in Upper GI and Bariatric Surgery at Ashford and St. Peters Hospital. UK

Salma Rahman
Senior Clinical Fellow. Vascular Department. Ashford and St Peter's Hospital. Surrey. UK

Firas Safadi
Consultant general and trauma surgeon. Department of General, Visceral, and Thoracic Surgery, Klinikum Darmstadt, Darmstadt, GERMANY

Daren Subar
Consultant Hepatobiliary Surgeon. East Lancashire Hospitals. UK

Miss Chloë Wright
Specialty Registrar General Surgery, Royal Bolton Foundation Trust. UK

We would like also to heartedly appreciate the constructive feedback we had from Prof. Nick London, Professor of Surgery at the University of Leicester (UK), Prof. Murray Brennan, Professor of Surgery at the Memorial Sloan Kettering Cancer Centre (USA), and Prof. Jonathan Meakins, Professor of Surgery at the Nuffield Department of Surgery, University of Oxford (UK).

Finally, we would like to thank our families, without their support this work would not have been completed ever, and all our friends and colleagues for their support.

Contents

Symbols and abbreviations *xxi*

Part 1 Principles of evidence-based medicine
1 Principles of evidence-based medicine | 3

Part 2 General care of the surgical patient
2 Principles of good surgical practice | 17
3 Medico-legal aspects of surgical practice | 27
4 Principles of admission management | 41
5 Day case surgery | 45
6 Good consent practice | 51
7 Preoperative assessment | 55
8 Perioperative fasting | 79
9 Perioperative medical complications | 85
10 Principles of wound care | 105
11 Preoperative assessment of bleeding risk | 115
12 Venous thromboembolism (VTE) prophylaxis | 121
13 Prevention of infective endocarditis (IE) | 127
14 Principles of blood transfusion | 131
15 Perioperative anticoagulation management | 137
16 Principles of care of critically ill patients | 143
17 Principles of trauma management | 151
18 Sepsis and septic shock | 161
19 Antibiotic prophylaxis in surgery | 169
20 Principles of infection control | 179
21 Principles of pain management | 191
22 Principles of nutritional support | 199

Part 3   Oesophagus
23 Gastro-oesophageal reflux disease (GORD)   209
24 Ingestion of foreign bodies   221
25 Achalasia   229
26 Oesophageal cancer   237
27 Barrett's oesophagus   251
28 Management of oesophageal
    variceal haemorrhage   259

Part 4   Stomach and duodenum
29 Peptic ulcer disease   269
30 Gastric cancer   279
31 Neuroendocrine tumours (NETs)   295
32 Surgery for obesity   303

Part 5   Small bowel and appendix
33 Acute appendicitis   313

Part 6   Colorectal
34 Constipation in adults   323
35 Diverticular disease   333
36 Anal fissures   341
37 Haemorrhoid disease   349
38 Colorectal cancer   357

Part 7   Pancreas
39 Acute pancreatitis   371
40 Chronic pancreatitis   379
41 Pancreatic cancer   387

Part 8   Hepatobiliary

42   Gallstone disease   401

43   Surgical management of liver metastasis   415

44   Hepatocellular carcinoma (HCC) and
     hepatic hydatid disease (HHD)   421

Part 9   Spleen

45   Prevention of post-splenectomy sepsis (PSS)   433

Part 10   Vascular

46   Chronic limb ischaemia   443

47   Carotid artery stenosis   453

48   Abdominal aortic aneurysm (AAA)   461

49   Chronic venous insufficiency (CVI)   469

Part 11   Breast

50   Breast cancer   481

51   Benign breast diseases   499

Part 12   Endocrine

52   Thyroid nodules and cancer   507

53   Surgery for hyperparathyroidism   519

Part 13   Hernia

54   Abdominal wall hernias   529

Part 14   Skin

55   Principles of skin malignancies management   543

Index   549

Symbols and abbreviations

AC	attenuation correction
ACA	adenocarcinoma
ADP	adenosine diphosphate
ALARA	as low as reasonably achievable
ALS	advanced life support
AMHP	approved mental health professional
AMP	adenosine monophosphate
aPTT	activated prothromboplastin time
ARDS	acute respiratory distress syndrome
ARSAC	Administration of Radioactive Substances Advisory Committee
ATP	adenosine triphosphate
BADS	British Association of Day Surgery
Bckgnd	background counts
BMI	body mass index
BNP	B-type natriuretic peptide
Bq	becquerel
CABG	coronary artery bypass graft surgery
CASS	Coronary Artery Surgery Study
CDR	clinical decision rule
Ci	curie
CMR	cardiac magnetic resonance
COPD	chronic obstructive pulmonary disease
CPAP	continuous positive airway pressure
CQC	Care Quality Commission
CT	computed tomography
CTA	computed tomography angiography
CTO	community treatment orders
CVA	cardiovascular accident
DEFRA	Department for the Environment, Food and Rural Affairs
DH	Department of Health
DIAD	Detection of Ischaemia in Asymptomatic Diabetics
DOAC	direct oral anticoagulant
DPL	diagnostic peritoneal lavage
DVT	deep venous thrombosis
EA	Environment Agency
EBM	evidence-based medicine

ECG	electrocardiogram
EDC	end-diastolic counts within LV ROI
EDT	emergency department thoracotomy
EF	ejection fraction
EMPIRE	Economics of Myocardial Perfusion Imaging in Europe
END	Economics of Noninvasive Diagnosis
ERASE	Emergency Room Assessment of Sestamibi for Evaluation
ERNV	equilibrium radionuclide ventriculography
ESC	end-systolic counts within LV ROI
FFP	fresh frozen plasma
FPRNV	first-pass radionuclide ventriculography
GCS	graduated compression stockings
GOJ	gastro-oesophageal junction
GORD	gastro-oesophageal reflux disease
GTN	glyceryl trinitrate
H/M ratio	heart-to-mediastinum ratio
HCAI	health care-associated infection
HCM	hypertrophic cardiomyopathy
HDU	high dependency unit
HR	heart rate
HSA	human serum albumin
HSE	Health and Safety Executive
HTS	hypertonic saline
ICD	implantable cardioverter-defibrillator
ICP	integrated care pathway
ICRP	International Commission for Radiation Protection
ICU	intensive care unit
IDDM	insulin-dependent diabetes mellitus
IE	infective endocarditis
IL	interleukin
INSPIRE	adenosine sestamibi SPECT post-infarction evaluation
IPC	intermittent pneumatic compression
IRMER	Ionising Radiation (Medical Exposures) Regulations 2000
IRR99	Ionising Radiations Regulations 1999
JVP	jugular venous pressure/pulse
LAD	left anterior descending
LAO	left anterior oblique
LBBB	left bundle branch block
LCx	left circumflex
LMWH	low molecular weight heparin

LOS	lower oesophageal sphincter
LV	left ventricle/ventricular
MAOI	monoamine oxidase inhibitors
MARS	Medicines (Administration of Radioactive Substances) Regulations 1978/1995
MBq	megabecquerels
mCi	millicuries
MHV	mechanical heart valve
MI	myocardial infarction
MINS	myocardial injury after noncardiac surgery
MIRD	medical internal radiation dose
MPS	myocardial perfusion scintigraphy
MUGA	multi-gated acquisition
NSAID	non-steroidal antiinflammatory drug
NSTEMI/UAP	non-STEMI and unstable angina pectoris
OM	obtuse marginal
PAD	pre-deposit autologous donation
PCI	percutaneous coronary intervention
PDA	posterior descending artery
PE	pulmonary embolism
PET	positron emission tomography
PHA	pulse height analyser
PMI	perioperative myocardial infarction
PMTs	photomultiplier tubes
PT	prothrombin time
QC	quality control
RAO	right anterior oblique
RCA	right coronary artery
RNV	radionuclide ventriculography
ROI	region of interest
RPA	Radiation Protection Advisor
RPS	Radiation Protection Supervisor
RR	relative risk
RRR	relative risk reduction
RSA93	Radioactive Substances Act 1993
RV	right ventricle
SAM	S-adenosyl methionine
SC	stroke counts
SCC	squamous cell carcinoma
SDS	summed difference score

SECU	surgical extended care unit
SNM	Society of Nuclear Medicine
SPECT	single photon emission computed tomography
SRS	summed rest score
SSI	surgical site infection
SSS	summed stress score
STEMI	ST-elevation myocardial infarction
Sv	sievert
TAC	time-activity curve
TIA	transient ischaemic attack
TID	transient ischaemic dilatation
TIMI	thrombolysis in myocardial infarction
TNFα	tumour necrosis factor-alpha
VTE	venous thromboembolism
W_R	radiation weighting factor
W_T	tissue weighting factor
μlinear	linear attenuation coefficient

Part 1

Principles of evidence-based medicine

Chapter 1

Principles of evidence-based medicine

Basic facts 4
EBM useful terms and techniques 6
Reading a scientific paper 12
Further reading 13

Key guidelines
- Oxford's Centre for Evidence-Based Medicine.
- The Cochrane collaboration.
- National Institute for Health and Care Excellence (NICE).

Basic facts

- *Definition*—evidence-based medicine (EBM) is a process of systematically reviewing, appraising, and applying clinical research findings to support the optimum delivery of clinical care to patients.
- *EBM process*—formulating appropriate 'answerable' questions (PICO: what is the clinical Problem, what is the Intervention under question, what is the Comparison group, and what is the Outcome to measure), searching for the best scientific evidence (using clinical guidelines, systematic reviews, clinical evidence sources, and even individual quality research), critically appraising the selected evidence (using valid tools), and application of the best acceptable conclusions into one's practice.
- *How important*—EBM has become an essential part of modern surgical practice. Surgeons should apply current clinical guidelines in their field of practice. The unique features of the individual patient in terms of biology, needs, and special circumstances, often have the ultimate effect on decisions and outcome: the evidence is but one part of a rather complex question.

EBM useful terms and definitions

Understanding EBM—requires familiarity with certain terms and definitions. For example, studying the effect of a risk factor requires a good understanding of incidence and prevalence, relative risk, and odds ratios. Studying the effectiveness of a diagnostic test requires familiarity with certain concepts such as sensitivity and specificity. Finally, studying the effect of a treatment requires deep understanding of odds ratios and number needed to treat, among other things. Supporting examples are used herein for better understanding.

Types of research studies

- A case–control study is an observational study where samples are chosen retrospectively based on presence (case) or absence (control) of disease. A cohort study is an observational study where subjects with or without a risk factor are followed prospectively over time for development of disease. A clinical trial is an experimental study where outcome of a therapeutic intervention is compared between two or more treatment (or placebo) groups. Primary studies report research first hand, such as experiments, clinical trials, surveys, and case–control studies. Secondary (or integrative) studies attempts to summarize and draw conclusions from primary studies such as clinical reviews, meta-analyses, guidelines, and decision and economic analysis (Box 1.1).
- Statistical analysis is performed to show correlation, significant difference, or modelling of specific variables.
  - Numerical data (that can be quantified and verified) is best described using averages (mean, mode, median) and dispersion values (ranges, centiles, standard deviation). Correlation between two numerical datasets is described using a correlation coefficient. Significant difference (or lack of) between a dataset and a fixed/reference value is checked using Student's t-test. Significant difference between two paired datasets (i.e. same individuals subject to different tests/treatments) is checked using student t-test when data distribution is Normal (parametric test) or using Wilcoxon signed-rank test when data distribution is skewed/unknown. Significant difference between two unpaired datasets (most cases) is checked using two-sample t-test when data distribution is Normal or Mann–Whitney U test when data distribution is skewed/unknown. Significant difference for three groups (or more) is checked using one-way analysis of variance (ANOVA) when data distribution is normal, and a non-parametric ANOVA (Kruskal–Wallis test) or a chi-square test when data distribution is skewed/unknown.
  - Categorical data (data that can take one of a limited, usually fixed, number of possible values) is best described using summary (frequency) tables. Association in data is quantified using relative risk (RR) and odds ratio (OR). Testing the presence of association of disease with a risk factor/investigation is best performed by testing if null hypothesis is true or not. Null hypothesis, that is hypothesis of no relation between independent (i.e. test/factor) and dependent

(i.e. disease/event) variables, is true when 'observed' vs 'expected' chi-square statistics (S statics calculated from existing data) is indifferent (obtained from standard tables). For small sample sizes, a Fisher's exact test is more appropriate. A type I error occurs when null hypothesis is mistakenly rejected and a correlation between the factor and disease/event is wrongly believed to exist (akin to convicting an innocent man). Study power is the ability to find a statistically significant difference when difference truly exists.

- *Impact factor (IF)*—of a journal is the average number of citations received per paper published in that journal during the preceding 2y. For example, the IF for *British Journal of Surgery* is 5.899 (Sep 2017)
- *Research bias*—examples would be sampling (subjects are not representative of population), selection (such as a non-random assignment to study group), recall (relates to inaccuracy of subject recollection of past events), and/or late-look (information for study collected at inappropriate time), reporting (occurs when some parts of the data are consistently missing), observer (arises when researchers inadvertently influence the study), and attraction bias (occurs when patients are lost for follow-up).

Box 1.1 Types of research studies

Systematic review of randomized controlled trials
Focused on a single question, systematic reviews are a literature review with the aim of identifying, appraising, selecting, and synthesizing high quality research evidence relevant to that question.

Randomized controlled trials (RCTs)
Involve the random allocation of different types of interventions to subjects. This ensures that confounding factors are evenly distributed between treatment groups, provided that the number of subjects is sufficient enough to obtain valid randomization.

Cohort studies
Studies involving a group of people who share common features or exposure within a defined period and compare their outcome to a comparison group (from the general population from which the cohort is drawn, or from another cohort of people thought to have had little or no exposure to the investigated intervention).

Case–control studies
Compare subjects who have a condition (the 'cases') with subjects who do not have the condition, but are otherwise similar (the 'controls').

Case series
Observational studies that track a series of patients who had similar exposure (same operation) or similar disease prospectively or retrospectively.

Prevalence and incidence

- *Prevalence*—is the total number of cases in the population at any one time.
- *Incidence*—is a measure of the number of new cases within a specified period of time. Incidence is calculated by measuring the number of new cases within a specified time period divided by the size of the population initially at risk. For example, if a population initially contains 10,000 non-diseased persons and 580 develop a condition over 2y of observation, the incidence proportion is 58 cases per 1,000 persons, i.e. 5.8%.

Relative risk

Relative risk (RR)—is used to compare the risk of an event occurring between two groups. For example, if the probability of developing oesophageal cancer among smokers was 10% and among non-smokers 1%, then the relative risk of cancer associated with smoking would be 10. Smokers would be ten times as likely as non-smokers to develop oesophageal cancer. We express such relative risk as RR ×10.

- RR can also be defined—as the rate of an event in a treatment group (experimental event rate or EER) divided by the rate of this event in the control group (control event rate or CER), expressed mathematically as EER/CER.
- RR reduction (or increase)—is the difference between the likelihood of an event happening in two groups, expressed as a percentage of the risk of one group. This is calculated using the formula: (EER–CER)/CER. For example, if 55% of patients achieved a satisfactory pain relief on using ibuprofen, compared to 18% on placebo, then the RR would be 3.1 (0.55/0.18). Ibuprofen is theoretically three times more effective than control. The absolute effect of ibuprofen (excluding that from placebo) can be estimated by calculating the RR reduction (55–18)/18, expressed as percentage (206%).
- Absolute risk is the risk of developing a disease over time period. For example, a patient can have a risk of 1 in 10 delete of developing a disease in life time period.
  - Absolute risk reduction (ARR) (or increase)—is used to express the difference in study end-point outcome between two groups. For example, if 55% of patients achieved a satisfactory pain relief using ibuprofen, compared to 18% on placebo, then ARR is 37% (55–18).

Number needed to treat

Number needed to treat (NNT)—is an epidemiological measure used to assess the effectiveness of an intervention by calculating the number of patients who need to be treated in order to achieve one positive effect or to prevent one additional bad outcome. For example, if 55% of patients achieved a satisfactory pain relief on using ibuprofen, com- pared to 18% on placebo, then the number needed to treat to achieve this 'satisfactory' pain relief is 2.7 (1/0.55–0.18), i.e. we have to treat 2.7 patients with ibuprofen for one to benefit 'satisfactorily' from the ibuprofen.

- NNT is calculated using the inverse of ARR (NNT = 1/ARR).

- The ideal NNT is 1, whereby everyone would improve with treatment and no one would do in the control group. The higher the NNT, the less effective the treatment is expected to be.

Odds ratios (OR)

Odds ratios are another way of calculating the risk of an event (or of developing a disease) related to some difference.

- The odds of an event are calculated as the number of events divided by the number of non-events. For example, if 22 out of 40 patients achieved a satisfactory pain relief on using ibuprofen, compared to 7 out of 40 patients (18%) on placebo, then the OR would be 5.7.
- The main difference between OR and RR is that the range that RR can take depends on the baseline event rate; OR does not need a baseline: it gives the risk of the cases relative to the controls, not relative to the baseline absolute value.
- In many situations in medicine, we can understand and interpret the ORs by pretending that they are RRs: when events are rare, risks and odds are very similar; otherwise, ORs will be different.

Sensitivity and specificity

Sensitivity and specificity—are statistical measures of the performance of a test.

- *Sensitivity*—measures the proportion of true positives out of all those who have the condition. Thus, as a rule, a negative result of a highly sensitive test rules out the diagnosis; a positive result **CANNOT** prove the existence of this specific disease.
- *Specificity*—measures the proportion of true negative out of all those who do not have the condition.
- *Accuracy*—is used to refer to both specificity and sensitivity. Accuracy is closely related to precision, reproducibility, or repeatability, whereby further measurements or calculations are expected to show the same or similar results. Accuracy can be determined from sensitivity and specificity if the prevalence is known, using the following equation:

Formulating a research question

- Questions on symptom prevalence or differential diagnosis—are best answered using non-comparative studies (cohort studies, ecological studies, and case series).
- Questions on confirming diagnosis—are best answered by using diagnostic studies (studies that test the quality of a specific diagnostic test (validation studies) or studies that model the data to obtain relevant diagnostic factors (exploratory studies). Other useful types of studies to answer this type of questions include: Clinical decision rule (CDR) studies (scoring systems which lead to diagnostic pathways or prognostic estimations), absolute SpPin studies (studies with diagnostic finding whose Specificity is high enough that a Positive result rules in the diagnosis), and absolute SnNout studies (studies with diagnostic finding whose Sensitivity is high enough that a Negative result rules out the diagnosis).

- Questions on prognosis—best answer can be obtained from cohort studies or CDR studies. Untreated control group in randomized controlled trial (RCT) studies can be used for answering this question. Other types of studies include 'outcome' research and case series studies.
- Questions on treatment, prevention, aetiology, and harm—best answer can be obtained from RCTs and their systematic reviews. Other lower types of studies include cohort, outcome, and case–control studies.

Level of evidence

A ranking system developed to stratify evidence by quality and ability to answer a specific research question. Different systems have been developed (NICE, SIGN, US Preventive Services Task Force, etc.) with a generally similar concept (Box 1.2).

Grading of recommendations

Recommendations for using certain approach/intervention can be classified by grading systems that balance the risks and benefits of the intervention and the level of evidence on which this decision is based. This takes into account the quality of research evidence, clarity of risks and benefits and implications.

- The grading of recommendations outlined by many guideline development groups (NICE, SIGN, American College of Chest Physicians, etc.) follows a similar approach. Box 1.3 outlines a generic recommendation system.
- The Grading of Recommendations Assessment, Development and Evaluation (GRADE) approach is increasingly being adopted by organizations worldwide to provide a more pragmatic and transparent system for rating quality of evidence and strength of recommendations.

Box 1.2 Levels of evidence

1a Evidence from systematic reviews or meta-analyses of RCTs
1b Evidence from at least one RCT
2a Evidence from at least one controlled study without randomization
2b Evidence from at least one other type of quasi experimental study
3 Evidence from non-experimental descriptive studies, such as comparative studies, correlation studies & case–control studies
4 Evidence from expert committee reports, or opinions &/or clinical experience of respected authorities

Box 1.3 Generic grading of recommendations

Grade [A]   Research evidence is strong enough to suggest that the benefits of the clinical service/intervention substantially out-weigh the potential risks.

Grade [B]   Research evidence is fairly convincing to suggest that the benefits of the clinical service/intervention outweigh the potential risks.

Grade [C]   Research evidence suggests that there are clear benefits provided by the clinical service/intervention. Nevertheless, the balance between benefits and risks are too close for making general recommendations.

Grade [D]   Recommendations with evidence level 3 or 4 or those based on a formal consensus approach.

*Good practice [G] has also been used occasionally in a few guidelines to reflect lower level, but convincing supporting evidence to the specific recommendation.

R = Health and safety regulations

CS = consensus statement used by Scottish Intercollegiate Guidelines Network to refer to statements developed from structured discussion and validated using a formal scoring system.

Reading a scientific paper

- Apply principles of EBM when reading a scientific paper using a thorough and systematic approach. Provide thoughtful answers to three main questions—what are the key messages; are methodologies properly designed to support the research question(s); and are results valid and support/justify the paper's conclusions.
- Start with key facts—this is a [type] study of the [title] published in the [journal] with an impact factor of [IF]. This paper provides level of evidence (Box 1.2) to the question [paper hypothesis]. The research institute is [type of institute] based in [city/country].
- Validate the paper's strength based on the presence (or absence) of specific items:
  - Background/introduction—addresses (or not) important scientific issue; builds up a valid and solid argument/flow towards research question; states clearly (or not) relevant studies of high evidence level; uses contemporary relevant references where appropriate;
  - Research question (hypothesis) to be tested is stated clearly (or not).
  - Methods—research hypothesis is approached with (or without) appropriate design that includes [types of research design: case and control subjects/procedures are described properly [give examples]; appropriate matching of cases to controls [give examples]; potential confounding factors and the ability (or not) to control them discussed [give examples]; study population sample size and key features described (or not); sample selection methods detailed; limitations or bias in sampling predicted/described [give examples]; power calculations for sample size to answer the research question performed (or not); inclusion and exclusion criteria explicitly described; methods for statistical testing are used correctly [give details].
  - Results—appropriate descriptive statistics provided; probability level clearly defined and used; tests of significance described and interpreted using appropriate degrees of freedom; tables and figures well organized and easy to understand; and results clearly described.
  - Conclusion and discussion—each result discussed in terms of original hypothesis to which it relates; generalizations are consistent (or not) with results; possible effects of uncontrolled variables on results discussed; theoretical and practical implications of findings discussed; and suggestions for future actions provided.

Further reading

Oxford's Centre for Evidence-Based Medicine (Bandolier). CEBM. "Home - CEBM". N.p., 2016. Web. 23 Feb. 2016. http://www.cebm.net

The Cochrane Collaboration. Uk.cochrane.org. "HOME | Cochrane UK". N.p., 2016. Web. 23 Feb. 2016.

Sackett DL, Straus S, Richardson S, Rosenberg W, Haynes B (2000). Evidence-based medicine: how to practise and teach EBM, 2nd ed. Churchill Livingstone, London.

Sackett DL, Rosenberg WM, Gray JA, Haynes RB, Richardson WS (1996). Evidence-based medicine: what it is and what it isn't. BMJ 312, 71–2.

The Royal College of Surgeons of England (2014). Royal College of Surgeons of England,. "Good Surgical Practice". N.p., 2014. Web. 23 Feb. 2016.

National Institute for Health and Clinical Excellence (2005). Reviewing and grading the evidence. Nice.org.uk. "Methods For Development Of NICE Public Health Guidance". N.p., 2016. Web. 23 Feb. 2016.

EBM glossary (2008). Available from: http://ebm.bmj.com/cgi/reprint/13/4/128.

Goyatt G, Oxman A, Vist GE, Konz R, Falck-Ytter, Alonso-Coello P, Schünemann HJ. GRADE: an emerging consensus on rating quality of evidence and strength of recommendations. BMJ 2008; 336:924–926 (26 April).

Reuters, Thomson. "Journal Citation Reports - IP & Science - Thomson Reuters". Wokinfo.com. N.p., 2016. Web. 23 Feb. 2016.

"About BJS - British Journal Of Surgery". Bjs.co.uk. N.p., 2016. Web. 21 May 2016.

Part 2

General care of the surgical patient

Principles of good surgical practice

By the bedside *19*
Clinical assessment *20*
Record keeping *20*
Performing procedures *21*
Discharge patients and handover practice *22*
Dealing with emergencies *22*
Working with colleagues *22*
Maintaining professional performance *23*
Safety and quality *23*
Other relevant good practice guidelines *24*
Further reading *26*

Key guidelines
- The Royal College of Surgeons of England (2014). Good surgical practice.
- GMC (2013). Good medical practice.

Background

- All doctors are expected to provide a good standard of surgical practice and care. Patients must be able to trust doctors and doctors have to justify that trust. Dignity and confidentiality must be respected. The General Medical Council describes appraisal of surgeons as being based on the seven core headings presented. (Box 2.1).
- Good surgical standards outline the accepted level of surgical practice, provide quality guidance for appraisal and revalidation processes, and set a framework for authorities to make judgements about surgeons' practice. It is for surgeons to reflect on their practice and work to the set standards. Serious or persistent failure to follow the GMC guidance will put one's registration at risk. We highly recommend reviewing the very informative cases provided on the GMC website (case no. 215, for example).

By the bedside

- *Ensure appropriate and safe environment*—accommodate any special needs requirements.
- *Maintain compassionate and clear communication*—with patients, supporters, and, in the case of children, parents or responsible adults.
- *Respect privacy*—this is a natural requirement for patients to disclose problems and concerns.
- *Provide enough time*—discuss with patients and their supporters any proposed procedure and other concerns.

Box 2.1 Standards required by all doctors

1 Good clinical care
2 Maintaining good medical practice
3 Relationships with patients
4 Working with colleagues
5 Teaching and training
6 Health
7 Probity

The Royal College of Surgeons of England (2014). Royal College of Surgeons of England, "Good Surgical Practice". N.p., 2014. Web. 23 Feb. 2016. https://www.rcseng.ac.uk/surgeons/surgical-standards/professionalism-surgery/gsp/gsp

Box 2.2 Sample of standard operative notes

Patient name: Hospital ID: DOB:
Date and time:

NAME OF OPERATION PERFORMED

- *Type of procedure*: elective/emergency.
- *Name of*: supervising surgeon/operating surgeon/assistant(s)/scrub nurse/anaesthetist.
- *Type of anaesthesia, antibiotics, etc.*: GA/LA/spinal.
- *Incision*: midline, subcostal, 4 key holes, etc.
- *Findings/diagnosis*: perforated appendix, liver metastasis, etc.
  - Any problems/complications.
  - Procedure: in concise details.
  - Extra procedures performed with reasons.
  - Details of tissue removed, added, or altered.
  - Identification of any prostheses used, including serial numbers of prostheses and other implanted materials.
  - Anticipated blood loss
- *Closure*: sutures, layers, etc.
- *Post-operative care instructions*:
  - Monitoring: specific signs and schedule.
  - Level of allowed activity: bed rest for 4h, etc.
  - Diet and fluid: NBM for 24h, allow D&F, etc.
  - Physiotherapy.
  - Prophylactic: antibiotics, DVT, PPIs, etc.
  - Suture removal.
  - Follow-up.
- Signature.

Clinical assessment

- *Adequately assess your patient's condition*—ensure good history taking (including symptoms, psychological, and social factors) and physical examination where appropriate.
- Standard history taking and physical examination. See ➲ OHCM 10e Ch. 2.
- *Providing information*—patients, including children, should be given information about treatment options and any alternatives, main risks, side-effects, and possible complications.
- *Prioritization*—ensure that patients are prioritized and treated according to their clinical need.
- *Informed decision*—patients need the opportunity to make a fully informed and unharassed decision. Patients must agree to treatment suggested before proceeding. Where appropriate, they should indicate by signature their willingness to proceed (see ➲ Chapter 6, pp 51–54).
- Intimate examinations can be embarrassing or distressing for patients. You should be sensitive to what they may think of as intimate, including (occasionally) any examination where it is necessary to touch or even be close to the patient. Before conducting intimate examination, you should explain to patient the need and what will it involve, get the patient's permission, and offer a chaperone. Stop the examination if the patient asks you to.

Record keeping

- *Ensure accurate records*—all records should be timed and dated, legible, complete, signed, and contemporaneous. Any changes in treatment plans should be recorded.
- *Ensure labelled records*—always use patient's identification details on relevant records. The name of the most senior surgeon should be used to label the visit and ward round.

Performing procedures

Know your limits

- Always carry out surgical procedures within the limits of your competence and in a timely and safe manner.
- Ensure that unfamiliar operative procedures are performed only if there is no clinical alternative, if there is no more experienced colleague available, or if transfer to a specialist unit is considered a greater risk.

Know your results

- You should always be aware of your immediate results, results obtained by peer groups, and where possible, personal and published audits of long-term outcomes.
- Ensure that patients receive satisfactory post-operative care and that relevant information is promptly recorded and shared with the caring team, the patient, and their supporter(s).

Write legible operative notes—typed if possible

See Box 2.2

- Notes should accompany the patient into recovery and then to the ward, and should be in sufficient detail to enable effective continuity of care by the team.

Discharge patients and handover practice

- *Safe discharge*—provide appropriate information to the patient and/or their carer(s) on discharge. Follow-up notes should be sufficiently detailed to allow another doctor to continue the care of the patient at any time.
- *Safe handover*—ensure a proper formal handover of patient's condition to the appropriate colleagues following your period on duty.

Dealing with emergencies

- *Emergency has priority*—patients should be treated according to the priority of their clinical need.
- *Accessibility*—you should be able to respond promptly to a call to attend an emergency patient. Surgeon in charge should be available, either within the hospital or within a reasonable distance of the hospital, to give advice throughout the duty period.

Working with colleagues

- *Know your limits*—utilize the knowledge and skills of other clinicians and transfer the patient, when appropriate, to another colleague or unit where the required resources and skills are available.
- Avoid denigrating others.
- *Multidisciplinary team meetings*—should be regularly attended.
- Training other colleagues
  - Surgeons have responsibilities for creating a learning environment suitable for teaching, training, and supervising students, trainees, and other team members. Individuals with whom trainees can legitimately share concerns should be identified.
  - Consultant surgeons have the overall responsibility for any duties delegated to a trainee or other member of the staff. Duties and responsibilities can only be delegated to those competent in the relevant area of practice.
  - Be mindful that your behaviour serves as a role model to junior doctors and set an example to other colleagues in your team by behaving professionally and respectfully towards all team members.

Maintaining professional performance

- Surgeons are responsible for maintaining their competence in all areas of their practice, including competence in teaching, management, and research.
- The surgical royal colleges and surgical specialty associations recommend a minimum of 50 hours of CPD activity per year to maintain appropriate level of up-to-date knowledge and competency.
- Introduction of new clinical interventions and surgical techniques (including equipment) that deviate significantly from established practice and are not part of an NHS local ethics committee research programme must be underpinned by rigorous clinical governance processes, having the patient's interests as the paramount consideration.

Safety and quality

- Surgeons have a duty to contribute to and comply with systems and processes that aim to reduce risk of harm to patients by measuring and monitoring performance and quality of care.
- The use of outcome measures should be a regular part of day-to-day clinical practice.
- Surgeons should be fully versed in the principles and practice of the WHO Surgical Safety Checklist and its adaptation through the Five Steps to Safer Surgery and apply those as an essential part of your operating work wherever this takes place.
- Surgeons should submit all their activity data to national audits and databases relevant to their practice and present the results at appraisal for review against the national benchmark.
- Surgeons should play an active role in ensuring that audit returns and outcome results accurately reflect your practice.
- Surgeons should take part regularly in morbidity and mortality meetings and be familiar with local processes and agreed thresholds for recording adverse incidents.
- Surgeons should support a culture of openness, honesty, and objectivity where concerns can be raised safely by all staff members.
- Surgeons should act promptly to rectify, or notify those responsible for rectifying, any incidents of poor quality of care or shortfalls in resources that might compromise safe care.

Other relevant good practice guidelines

- *Writing a reference*—you must be honest and fair when providing references. Keep your comments objective and unambiguous. State the basis upon which you are making your assessment. Information provided should be relevant, i.e. will not mislead the employer about a specific issue or the overall suitability of a candidate. You should draw attention to any issues that could put patients at risk. You should not generally include personal information about the candidate.
- *Seeking advice on assistance to die*—be prepared to listen and discuss reasons for the patient's request. Provide full empathy and respect. It is a criminal offence to encourage or assist a person to commit or attempt suicide. Doctors are not required, however, to provide treatments that they consider will not be of overall benefit to patients, or which will harm the patient. Always respect competent patient's right to make decisions about their care, including the right to refuse treatment providing no illegal actions are taken.
- *Using visual and audio recordings of patients*—you must respect patients' privacy and dignity. Give patients the information they want, or need, about the purpose of the recording, and make recordings only where you have appropriate consent or other valid authority for doing so. Ensure that patients are under no pressure to give consent, and stop recordings if the patient requested that. Anonymize or code recordings before using or disclosing them for a secondary purpose. Store recordings securely, and follow local guidance and procedures for this. You must not disclose or use recordings for purposes outside the scope of the original consent without obtaining further consent. You must get consent before making recordings for teaching, training, and assessment of healthcare professionals and students. It is good practice to get the patient's written consent, but if this is not practicable, the patient's oral consent should be obtained. Certain anonymized recordings can be used for patient's care or secondary purposes, including public domains, without seeking additional consent: X-rays, pathology slides, and endoscopic slides.
- *Personal beliefs and medical practice*—you must treat patients fairly and with respect, whatever their life choices and beliefs. Doctors may practise medicine in accordance with their beliefs, provided that they act in accordance with relevant legislation and they do not treat patients unfairly, do not deny patients access to appropriate treatment, and do not cause patients distress. Doctors may choose to opt out of providing a particular procedure because of their personal beliefs and values, as long as this does not result in direct or indirect discrimination against, or harassment of, individual patients or groups of patients. You should usually provide procedures that patients request and that you assess to be of overall benefit to them. If the patient is a child, you should usually provide a procedure or treatment (such as circumcision for a male) that you assess to be in their best interests.
- Maintaining boundaries
  - To maintain the trust of patients and the public, you must never make a sexual advance towards a patient, display sexual behaviour,

or make an improper emotional relationship with a patient or someone close to them.

- If a patient pursues a sexual or improper emotional relationship with you, you should treat them politely and considerately and try to re-establish a professional boundary. If you find it necessary to end the professional relationship, you must follow the guidance in ending your professional relationship with a patient.
- You must consider the potential risks involved in using social media and the impact that inappropriate use could have on your patients' trust in you and society's trust in the medical profession.
- You must comply with the GMC guidance on protecting children and young people, raising and acting on concerns, treatment for end of life patients, acting as a witness, consenting to research, reporting to official bodies such as DVLA, reporting serious communicable diseases, and reporting gunshots and knife wounds.

Beyond the guidelines and the future

The authors are to be congratulated on emphasizing, at the beginning of the guide, the importance of a surgeon's professional responsibilities. Being a member of the profession of surgery creates expectations in the eyes of the public. The key characteristics of professionals *are persons who seek a broad understanding of their practice, paying attention not only to their developing competence, but also to the fundamental purposes and values that underpin their work*.[1]

A profession is an occupation exercising 'good' in the service of another; is specialized work in that it cannot entirely be understood by the layman; is not measured by financial reward alone; is ethically and morally based; has an esoteric and complex knowledge base; exercises discretion; and depends upon professional judgement. It requires the capacity of the professional to retain a fiduciary (trusting) relationship with a client or, in the case of the surgeon, a patient and a manager.[2] Patient safety relies on surgeons making wise professional judgements, involving complex deliberation.[3,4]

Self-regulation is a key part of a profession's responsibility. Recognizing this, and in order to clearly set out how it expects members and fellows to conduct themselves, the Royal College of Surgeons of England has recently revised 'Good Surgical Practice'.[5] These standards will be an important reference point for the process of recertification of surgeons. *Ms Linda De Cossart, Vice President of the Royal College of Surgeons of England.*

1 Golby M. Educational research in educational research: trick or treat? Exeter Society for Curriculum Studies 1993; 15 (3): 5–8.
2 de Cossart, L. A question of professionalism: leading forward the surgical team. Ann R Coll Surg Engl 2005; 87: 238–41.
3 de Cossart L, Fish D. *Cultivating a Thinking Surgeon*. TfM Press, 2005.
4 Fish, D, de Cossart, L. *Developing the Wise Doctor*. RSM Press, 2007.
5 The Royal College of Surgeons of England. Good Surgical Practice. London. 2008.

Further reading

The Royal College of Surgeons of England (2014). Royal College of Surgeons of England,. "Good Surgical Practice". N.p., 2014. Web. 23 Feb. 2016. https://www.rcseng.ac.uk/surgeons/surgical-standards/professionalism-surgery/gsp/gsp

General Medical Council (2013). Good medical practice, http://www.gmc-uk.org/guidance/good_medical_practice.asp

The Royal College of Surgeons of England (2007). Safe handover: guidance from the Working Time Directive working party.

General Medical Council (2006). Good medical practice. Fitness to practice cases. Case number 215.

Implementation Manual WHO Surgical Safety Checklist 2009 Safe Surgery Saves Lives. 1st ed. World Health Organization, 2009. Web. 23 Feb. 2016.

http://www.nrls.npsa.nhs.uk/resources/collections/10-for-2010/five-steps-to-safer-surgery 2016. Web. 16 Jan. 2018.

Medico-legal aspects of surgical practice*

The British legal system 28
Appearing in court 30
Writing a statement 31
Mental Health Act 32
Brain stem death 33
Confidentiality 34
Clinical governance 36
Clinical negligence 37
Disciplinary bodies and procedures 38
Consent 40
Further reading 40

Key guidelines
- The Royal College of Surgeons of England (2014). Good surgical practice.
- GMC (2013). Good medical practice.
- GMC (2010). Treatment and care towards the end of life.
- GMC (2017). Confidentiality: good practice in handling patient information.
- Mental Health Act 2007.
- Data Protection Act 1998.

---

* The guidelines in this chapter have been sourced and summarized from different UK, European, and international government sources, professional organizations, and medical specialty societies. Leading guidelines have been listed in the further reading section at the end of this chapter.

The British legal system

- *Medical law*—is a branch of law concerns the responsibilities of healthcare professionals and the rights of patients. *Criminal law* involves the public interest and it usually relates to a crime that directly and seriously threatens the well-being of the general population. *Civil law*, in contrast, is the law related to private matters where the injured party (the claimant) usually initiates the proceedings. This include four branches: family law (e.g. child welfare), property law (e.g. patents), contract law (e.g. partnerships, insurance), and law of torts (e.g. actionable wrongs such as medical negligence). *Other branches of law* include admiralty law (governs maritime questions and offences), service law (law applied to all serving members of army, etc.), industrial law (e.g. condition of employment), and ecclesiastical law (church affairs).
- *Sources of law*—are the common law (known as case or judge-made law) that is derives from judgments made in decided case, and the statute law that is enacted by the parliament and supersedes common law. In England and Wales, the court system and judiciary system follows specific hierarchy (Fig. 3.1). Most cases are dealt with at the magistrates', county, crown, and coroner's courts. The legal system in Scotland and Northern Ireland is slightly different.
- *Solicitors* and *barristers* are legally qualified personnel through either a law degree (LLB) or a postgraduate qualification (CPE). Each follow a different postgraduate training route. Solicitors work mostly in private practice and deal with different aspects of law, while barristers become self-employed and can only be engaged by solicitors or similar professionals, not the public. They represent clients in court. Judges and sheriffs preside over court proceedings, either alone or as a part of a panel of judges. A *judge* hears witnesses, reviews evidence presented by

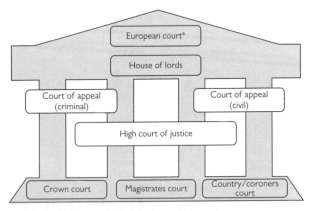

Fig. 3.1 Structure of the legal system in England and Wales
*subject to Brexit's final arrangements

parties of the case, assesses credibility and arguments, and then issues a ruling on the matter at hand. A *coroner* is a government official with a degree in a medical or legal field, who confirms and certifies the death of an individual within a jurisdiction. *Legal executives* work for solicitors doing the routine work.

- *Civil cases (litigation)*—are heard in the County and High Court in England and Wales, and Sheriff Court and Court of Session in Scotland.
  - Action usually begins with the injured party (the claimant) contacting a solicitor, who reviews the case and if convinced, sends a Letter of Claim, warning the defendant of litigation if settlement is not reached. Civil cases are usually heard before a single judge (with the right to be heard before a jury).
  - The outcome includes the claimant discontinuing the actions, parties reaching an agreement, or the court issuing a judgment. Over 95% settle before going to court.
  - If a trial takes place, then the claimant has to provide enough evidences, and judgment would be based on the *balance of probabilities*. Both parties can appeal the judgment.
  - Adjudication processes can also take place outside the court as Arbitration, where an impartial person makes a decision on a dispute that is binding on both parties.
- *Criminal cases (proceedings)*—are dealt with by the Crown Prosecution Service (CPS) in most cases. CPS engages barristers to conduct the prosecution in the higher court. The case is brought as R (Regina) or HMA (Her Majesty's Advocate) vs N (name of defendant).
  - The burden of proof is placed on the prosecution. They must call supporting evidence to prove that the defendant is guilty. The defendant then needs to prove that the evidence is unreliable and that the evidence does not prove guilt to the required standards, i.e. *beyond reasonable doubt.*
  - If the defendant (or the accused) pleads guilty, then no evidence is called and no trial takes place before sentencing. Otherwise, the judge may decide to run a hearing to decide sentencing, also known as a Newton hearing.
  - Arrest and prosecution can take place under the Police and Criminal Evidence Act (PACE) 1984, where a police officer may arrest anyone that he or she on reasonable grounds suspects is about to, or is in the act of, or has committed an arrestable offence. The detainee has certain rights and entitlements, including the right to remain silent and to have someone informed of his arrest.
- **Evidence** can be one of three types. *Direct*, which requires no mental processing by the judge or jury (such as eye witness); *circumstantial*, which requires the judge or jury to draw inferences (such as motives); and *hearsay*, which is a reported speech (e.g. a witness statement). **Witnesses** can be professional (providing professional evidence and opinion), witness of fact (providing facts only, i.e. what they saw, heard or read; opinions are not allowed), or expert witness (providing both facts and opinions).

Appearing in court

- Healthcare professionals are likely to be asked to appear in courts as witnesses at some stage in their professional life. Few become the subject of civil litigation for alleged negligence. Others might follow the route as expert witnesses.
- *Court preparation*—should be practised well in advance. Dress smartly and arrive in time. Provide your name and trial details to the Witness Service. Enquire how to address the judge or magistrate appropriately (Sir, Madam, Your Honour, etc.). Bring any contemporary notes and any relevant imaging or letters with you. Read your statement and bring a copy with you to the court (you are not allowed to read it in the court). Expert witnesses, however, are generally allowed to read from their expert reports.
- *In the court*—professional witnesses are only allowed to enter the courtroom once required to provide their evidence. You will be guided to the witness box, where you will be asked for your wish to swear on a holy book or to give the oath of affirmation.
  - Your main aim is to convince the jury or magistrates that you are a healthcare professional with adequate qualifications and enough experience to give valid, reliable, and important evidence. You must address your evidence to the magistrate or jury. Your evidence should be given orally (unless agreed otherwise). Do not use abbreviations without clarification. Do not use complex and technical language. Speak clearly and loudly enough so the judge or jury can hear you properly. You must ask if you can refer to your notes (this is almost always allowed after requesting permission).
  - You will then be cross-examined by the opposing party. Do not volunteer information, and do not hesitate to keep repeating your answer if necessary. Do not hesitate to request clarification or rephrasing of the question if need be. Never speak or argue with the barrister.
- *After giving evidence*—remain in witness box until you are given leave by the judge. Do not leave the court until you are released, as you might be required to hear subsequent evidences or recalled to give further evidence. Make sure you have been given a claim form and travel expenses form.

Writing a statement

- A statement is a written summary explaining your involvement in the treatment of a patient. Apply the same principles of writing valid clinical notes to writing a statement: legible, accurate, complete, factual, impartial, and easily understandable. Specific forms (MG11 in England and Wales for example) are supplied by the police for this purpose. Your statement should ONLY be issued upon receiving written confirmation that the patient agrees to disclose their confidential clinical information.
- Statements should include specific details about you (employment, qualifications, etc.) and the patient (name, age, etc.), as well as a declaration of authorship (for example: 'I believe that the facts stated in response to the above questions are true.') among other things.
- Legal obligations to write a statement only apply (as a contractual obligation) for forensic medical examiners or similar healthcare professionals.

Mental Health Act

- The Mental Health Act 1983 (substantially amended in 2007) is the law in England and Wales that allows people with a 'mental disorder' to be admitted to hospital, detained, and treated without their consent—either for their own health and safety, or for the protection of other people. Different sections of the Act are used depending on circumstances. For example, Section 2 is used to admit someone for assessment, Section 3 for treatment, and Section 4 in an emergency. The Act also allows people to be put on Community Treatment Orders (CTOs), following a period of compulsory treatment in hospital.
- Decision in applying the Act should be taken by an approved mental health professional (AMHP), approved clinician, and/or Section 12 approved doctor. All are professionals who have been trained and 'approved' to carry out particular duties under the Act. Responsible clinician refers to clinicians under whose care the patient is treated for the specific disease. AMPH is responsible to identify the person's 'nearest relative', who will be given certain power by the Act.
- Specific guiding principles apply within the Act. The person who is detained and treated against their will, for example, must be as fully involved in planning treatment as possible, and their wishes should be taken into account. The treatment should be provided in the least restrictive way possible.
- In emergency situations, Section 4 allows people to be admitted and detained for up to 72h after one responsible doctor has said that urgent admission is needed. AMHP is responsible for applying and approving this. A second doctor should review the patient within the 72h period and move the decision into section 2 or 3.
- Section 35-49 gives a Crown and Magistrates' Court the power to send someone who is accused of a crime or convicted to hospital either for treatment, or for a report to be made about their mental health. Section 136 allows the police to take someone from a public place to a place of safety, if they think he or she needs immediate care or control. Section 7 allows for people who have a 'mental disorder' to be given a guardian in the interests of their own welfare or to protect other people.
- The Care Quality Commission (CQC) is responsible for protecting the interests of people detained and treated under the Mental Health Act in England, and for ensuring the Act is used correctly.

Brain stem death

- There is no statutory definition of death in the UK; the diagnosis remains a matter of clinical judgment. The irreversible loss of capacity for consciousness, combined with irreversible loss of capacity to breathe can be reliably considered as equating the death of a human being.
- Brain stem death refers to the irreversible damage to the centres that control breathing and circulation where mechanical life support is not believed to enable the patient to regain life. Retrieval of organs for transplantation should be considered in this state. Chapter 16 provides further details on the criteria for brain stem death diagnosis and confirmation.
- Information and guidance on the statutory requirements for completing death and cremation certificates is available from a number of sources including Home Office Guidance (2010) for doctors completing Medical Certificates of Cause of Death in England and Wales.

Confidentiality

- By definition, confidentiality is a set of rules or a promise that limits access or places restrictions on certain types of information. Patients have a right to expect that information about them will be held in confidence by their doctors. The GMC guidance (2017) on Confidentiality sets out the principles of confidentiality and respect for patients' privacy that all doctors are expected to understand and follow. The United Kingdom Central Council (UKCC) Code of Professional Conduct for registered nurses sets out confidentiality principles for nursing staff.
- As a general rule, doctors should seek a patient's express consent before disclosing any identifiable information for purposes other than the provision of their care or local clinical audit.
- Confidentiality principle applies to all patients' identifiable health data, including medical notes, photographs, video tapes, among others. Healthcare providers have a duty to inform patients that their personal information may be disclosed for the sake of their own care and for local clinical audit. This might include any party who might require this access to support the provision of care, as well as for service planning and medical research.
- *Exceptions*—confidentiality is an important duty, but is not absolute. Exceptions include:
  - *Disclosure required by law*—information should be disclosed to satisfy a specific statutory requirement, and various regulatory bodies have statutory powers to request that.
  - *Disclosure with the patient's consent*—you can disclose sensitive information (e.g. to a friend) if the patient gives consent to do so. Doctors should ensure that the patient is aware of the type and depth of information to be disclosed.
  - *Disclosure in the patient's interests*—you can share relevant confidential information with appropriate healthcare professionals whenever assistance in the management of patients is required. Unless the patient specifies otherwise, information can be shared with the assigned next-of-kin. Information necessary to allow emergency treatment can also be disclosed unless patient expressed otherwise.
  - *Disclosure in the public interest*—personal information may be disclosed in the public interest, without patients' consent, and in exceptional cases where patients have withheld consent, if the benefits to an individual or to society of the disclosure outweigh both the public and the patient's interest in keeping the information confidential. This includes where information is used to protect individuals or society from risks of serious harm, such as serious communicable diseases or serious crime; or to enable medical research, education, or other secondary uses of information.
  - *Disclosure to Driver and Vehicle Licensing Authority (DVLA)*—when patients' condition affect their safety to drive, a doctors should explain to them: a) that the condition may affect their ability to drive and b) that they have a legal duty to inform the DVLA about the condition. If a patient refuses to accept the diagnosis, or the effect of

the condition on their ability to drive, you can suggest that they seek a second opinion, and help arrange for them to do so. If a patient continues to drive when they may not be fit to do so, you should make every reasonable effort to persuade them to stop.

- If you do not manage to persuade the patient to stop driving, or you discover that they are continuing to drive against your advice, you should inform them of your duty to disclosed confiential information, and you should contact the DVLA immediately and disclose any relevant medical information, in confidence, to the medical adviser.

- *Disclosure under Data Protection Act 1998 (DPA)*—this Act creates rights for those who have their data stored, and responsibilities for those who store, process, or transmit such data. Personal data refers to information in relation to a living individual who can be identified from those data. Sensitive data include race, religion, criminal history, and sexual orientation. Personal data shall be obtained only for one or more specified and lawful purposes, and shall not be further processed in any manner incompatible with that purpose or those purposes. Personal data shall be adequate, relevant and not excessive in relation to the purpose. A person who has their data processed has the right to: a) view the data an organization holds on them, b) request that incorrect information be corrected, c) require that data is not used in any way that may potentially cause damage or distress, and d) require that their data is not used for direct marketing.

- When disclosing information about a patient, you must: a) use anonymized or coded information where practical, b) be sure the patient has not objected and has ready access to their information, c) have obtained the patient's expressed consent for identifiable information, d) keep disclosure to the minimum, and e) observe all relevant legal requirements.

- The Care Quality Commission has powers of inspection, entry, and to require documents and information under the Health and Social Care Act 2008. Sections 76 to 79 govern the Commission's use and disclosure of confidential personal information.

Clinical governance

- Clinical governance is a systematic approach to maintaining and improving the quality of patient care within a health system. In 1997, in the White paper 'The New NHS: Modern, Dependable', the government made it a statutory duty for all healthcare professionals to become involved in a quality agenda. Clinical governance has therefore been introduced as a framework through which NHS organizations are accountable for continually improving the quality of their services and safeguarding high standards of care by creating an environment in which excellence in clinical care will flourish.
- Clinical governance has seven components that should be ensured in any clinical practice: *Education and training* (including continuing professional development (CPD)), clinical audit (measurement of performance against agreed standards and refining of clinical practice accordingly), *clinical effectiveness* (refining clinical practice in light of emerging evidence of effectiveness—a measure of the extent to which a particular intervention works), research and development (implementing tools for research practice such as critical appraisal of literature, project management, and development of guidelines and protocols), *openness* (performance and practice should be appropriately open to public scrutiny, while respecting individual patient and practitioner confidentiality), *risk management* (risks to patients, practitioners, and organization should be identified and minimized and continuously reviewed), and *information management* (including the management and use of information within the healthcare systems).

Clinical negligence

- By definition, negligence is a failure to exercise the care that a reasonably prudent person would exercise in like circumstances. The area of tort law known as negligence involves harm caused by carelessness, not intentional harm. Intentional harm is dealt with by the Criminal Law (Harold Shipman's case for example).

- Allegation of negligence by a healthcare professional would only succeed if it proves that all of the following components are met: a) the defendant had a duty of care to the claimant, b) that there was a breach of that duty of care, c) that the claimant suffered actionable harm or damage, and d) that the damage was caused by the breach.

- A duty of care takes place whenever a named healthcare professional interacts with a patient to provide professional advice and treatment. A duty is breached when the healthcare professional fails to reach the level of proficiency of his or her peers (the Bolam Test), and applies equally to the duty to diagnose, give advice, and/or treat. An actionable harm or damage occurs when there is a quantifiable injury suffered by the claimant, and this injury is caused by the actions of the defendant on a balance of probabilities. The burden of proof is on the claimant who should prove that the defendant has been negligent. Under the Limitation Act 1980, actions of negligence should be brought within 3y of the date of knowledge.

Disciplinary bodies and procedures

- General Medical Council (GMC) is an independent statutory body, established by the Medical Act 1858, and made responsible for medical registration, regulation, education, and discipline in the UK. It gains its current power from the Medical Act 1983. The GMC helps to protect patients and improve medical education and practice in the UK by setting standards for students and doctors. The GMC support them in achieving and exceeding those standards, and take action when they are not met.

- The Council for Professions Supplementary to Medicine (CPSM) was replaced by the Health Professions Council on 1 April 2002, which became the Health and Care Professions Council (HCPC) on 1 August 2012. HCPC is a regulator, and was set up to protect the public. To do this, HCPC keeps a Register of health and care professionals who meet their standards for their training, professional skills, behaviour, and health. HCPC regulates the following professions: arts therapists, biomedical scientists, chiropodists/podiatrists, clinical scientists, dietitians, hearing aid dispensers, occupational therapists, operating department practitioners, orthoptists, paramedics, physiotherapists, practitioner psychologists, prosthetists/orthotists, radiographers, social workers in England, and speech and language therapists. Anyone using the titles 'physiotherapist', for example, must be registered with HCPC. It is a criminal offence for someone to claim that they are registered with HCPC when they are not, or to use a protected title that they are not entitled to use. HCPC will prosecute people who commit these crimes.

- The National Clinical Assessment Service (NCAS) has been an operating division of the NHS Litigation Authority (NHS LA) since 2013. NCAS contributes to patient safety by helping to resolve concerns about the professional practice of doctors, dentists, and pharmacists. NCAS provides expert advice and support, clinical assessment and training to the NHS and other healthcare partners.

- Healthcare professionals operating within an NHS hospital setting who are under allegation of misconduct follow locally agreed internal disciplinary procedures, which usually, but not always, follow a common pathway:
  - A person conducting repeated minor problems or more serious performance or discipline problems is issued with a First Written Warning by their supervisor/line manager (with right to appeal within 28 days of receipt of warning). Failure to correct behaviour attracts a Second Written Warning by the supervisor/line manager (appeal within 28 days). Further failure to correct behaviour attracts a Final Written Warning by the line manager plus human resources (HR) (appeal within 28 days).
  - Performance or behaviour that is not improved despite previous warnings results in Dismissal with Notice, issued by the Director plus one other appropriate Senior Manager plus HR (appeal within 28 days).

- A Gross Misconduct results in Summary Dismissal issued by the Director plus one other appropriate Senior Manager plus HR (appeal within 28 days). Personal Misconduct applies to behaviour unrelated to clinical skills (e.g. sexual harassment or fraud). Professional Misconduct applies when the behaviour arises during the exercise of clinical skills (e.g. illegal drug prescribing). Professional incompetence applies to inadequate or poor performance of clinical skills or judgment.
- Actions requiring suspension from duty results in suspension from duty on full pay pending further investigation and action. This is issued after authority from Chief Executive has been sought or from designated authority.

Consent

Consent, from the legal point of view, is the legislation of a process to allow someone to make invasive act against someone else's body integrity (or against their confidential information). Touching a patient without valid consent may therefore constitute a civil or criminal offence.

Chapter 6 deals with the consent process in detail.

Further reading

The Royal College of Surgeons of England (2014). Good surgical practice.
GMC (2013). Good medical practice.
GMC (2010) Treatment and Care towards the end of life GMC (2017) Confidentiality Mental Health
    Act 2007
Data Protection Act 1998
Jackson, E.Medical Law: Text, Cases, and Materials. OUP Oxford. 2013. SN - 9780199693603
Morris, Jones, M.A.Blackstone's Statutes on Medical Law. 8e. 2009. Oxford University Press.

Principles of admission management

Background 42
Admission process—good practice 42
Discharging patients from hospital 43
Further reading 44

Key guidelines
- Healthcare Commission. Guide to admissions management (UK).
- British Association of Day Surgery. Guidelines about the discharge process and the assessment of fitness for discharge.
- The Royal Pharmaceutical Society of Great Britain. Guidance on discharge and transfer planning.

Background

- The management of hospital elective and emergency admissions is one of the key responsibilities of both hospital doctors and NHS managers. It has a major impact on all aspects of the patient's experience, including the speed of access to diagnostic and treatment procedures, patient's choice, comfort, and safety.
- *Patient pathway*—the route that individual patients usually follow from their first contact with the NHS service (e.g. GP, A&E), through referral to the appropriate specialty, up to the completion of the treatment.

Admission process—good practice

Each patient should, on admission, be assessed according to the hospital policy. The following good practice points are recommended to ensure a safe and effective admission process:

- *Concise admission summary*—should be documented clearly by the admitting physician. Instructions for completing a full clinical history and physical examination as soon as appropriate should also be clearly documented and communicated.
- *Nursing assessment*—including social assessment, nutritional screening (where appropriate), and functional status screening should be performed by the appropriate healthcare staffing at the point of admission to ensure that the needs of the individual patient are fully met during their stay in the hospital, including appropriate provisions for their discharge.
- *Admission instructions*—documented and communicated to the junior doctors, on call team, and nurses in charge (Box 4.1).

Box 4.1 Admission instructions

1. Level of admission unit
2. Clinician in charge with his/her bleep/contact number
3. Admission diagnosis
4. Level of allowed activity
5. Diet, nursing assessments, monitoring schedule
6. IV fluid requirements, medications
7. Laboratory tests and imaging required

Discharging patients from hospital

- *Principles*—assessment of fitness for discharge is a multidisciplinary process and should be done with the highest attention to detail to ensure the patient is ready for discharge.
- *Discharge criteria*—patients can be discharged from hospital if their medical, physical, psychological, and social conditions permit (Boxes 4.2 and 4.3).
- *Scoring systems*—have been developed to support the discharge process and ensure a reproducible quality practice throughout the units.

Box 4.2 Discharging criteria

- *Stable medical condition*—stable vital signs (for at least 1h in the case of day surgery), full orientation to persons, place, and time, good pain control (including enough supply of oral analgesics), minimum complaint of nausea, vomiting or dizziness, minimum bleeding from the operative site, and ability to take oral fluid in case of day surgery.
- *Appropriate social condition*—availability of appropriate carer at home, full understanding and written instructions of post-operative care and contact numbers, and clear scheduled plan for follow-up.

Box 4.3 Information on discharge

- *Discharge medications*—clear instructions on prescribed analgesia, antiemetics, or antibiotics.
- *Care of wound*—e.g. change of dressing and suture removal.
- *Suitable timing*—for bath or shower.
- *Appropriate time*—to resume normal activities and work.
- *Expected symptoms after discharge*—and how to manage or call for help. All contact telephone numbers for any further enquiries or emergency situations must be written out for the patient and/or carers.

Further reading

Healthcare Commission. Guide to admissions management. (2006) (UK) URL: https://www.cqc.org.uk/sites/default/files/rv9_coreservice_acute_admission_wards_humber_nhs_foundation_trust_scheduled_20141003.pdf Accessed Feb 2016.

Joint Commission Mission. Hospital Accreditation. (US) Jointcommission.org. 'Joint Commission'. N.p., 2016. Web. 23 Feb. 2016.

British Association of Day Surgery. 'NURSE LED DISCHARGE'. N.p., 2016. Web. 23 Feb. 2016.

Chapter 5

Day case surgery

Background 46
Selection criteria 47
Discharging patients 48
How good your day surgery practice is—audit areas 49
Further reading 50

Key guidelines
- British Association of Day Surgery (2011). Day case and short stay surgery.
- Department of Health (2002). Day surgery: operational guide.

Background

- *Definition*—the admission of selected patients to hospital for a planned surgical procedure, returning home on the same day. Procedures not requiring full operating theatre facilities and/or general anaesthesia (like endoscopy or outpatient procedures) are not classified as a 'true' day surgery.
- *Benefits*—include patients, clinicians, staff, and trusts.
  - *Patients*—reduced disruption to normal daily life, avoidance of prolonged waiting lists and hospital stay, decreased hospital acquired infection rate, and avoidance of unexpected cancellation due to emergency cases. This mode of treatment is the preferred choice for most patients.
  - *Clinicians*—better organized and relaxing working environment, and ability to release inpatient beds for major cases.
  - *Staff*—better quality of work facilities and rewarding working environment.
  - *Trusts*—improved Integrated Care Pathway (ICP) setting, reduced waiting times, and facilitated 'choose and book' process.

Selection criteria

- Which procedure—any operation of relatively short duration, low incidence of post-operative complications, and minimum or no requirement for major perioperative interventions (blood transfusion, major analgesia, catheters, etc.). These include all intermediate and selected major operations where no specific contraindications exist.
  - Selection criteria should be collaboratively agreed by surgeons, anaesthetists, and nurses involved.
- Which patient—selection requires a balance between the extent of procedure, the fitness of patient, the use of general, regional, or local anaesthesia, the experience and particular skills of the clinicians, and the home conditions (Box 5.1).
- Full term infants >1mo are usually appropriate for considering as day surgery.

Box 5.1 Patient selection for day case surgery

Social circumstances

- Accompanying responsible carer—to stay with patient for 24–48 hours post-discharge.
- Suitable transport method—to be available on going home.
- Private telephone—to be accessible for emergency and unexpected situations.
- Distance to home—not to exceed 1–1.5h.

Age limits

- Arbitrary limits for age are increasingly considered inappropriate. Associated medical conditions (hypertension, obesity, smoking, asthma, and gastro-oesophageal reflux) are the most important factors, not the age per se.

Body mass index (BMI) limits

- Upper BMI ceiling limits for safe and effective day surgery differs between units. A BMI of 30–40 was later challenged with super obese patients' series up to 62.7kg/m^2 with no weight-related complications. Obesity is not an absolute contraindication to day care in expert hands and with appropriate resources and agreements. Associated medical conditions
- Type 1 diabetes mellitus, depending on its control and the extent of the procedure, can be managed as a day case if they are fit to eat and drink post-operatively. Asthma should be well controlled.

Other factors

- Times of operating, e.g. easier to get patients home if their operation is on a morning list. Where possible, configure morning lists with the more complex surgical and/or anaesthetic problems.

Discharging patients

Medical care
- Patients must have good analgesic control—local anaesthetic (LA) infiltration or block; oral or suppository medication (e.g. NSAID/paracetamol/codeine); and sufficient medications to maintain this state with clear instructions.
- Post-operative nausea and vomiting must be avoided where possible and controlled adequately before discharge. Anaesthetists will advise if they think prophylactic antiemetics should be prescribed (e.g. after a laparoscopic cholecystectomy).
- Constipation should be anticipated and aperients supplied if thought necessary.

Instructions
- Verbal and written instructions must be given. The patient should be advised not to drink alcohol, operate machinery, or cook until the following day. Advice should be given on the levels of activity and when to commence driving depending on the surgical procedure. Clear information must be given about dressings, suture removal, and district nurse or general practice attendance as well as appointments back at the hospital if necessary.
- Discharge summaries to be available when the patient leaves the unit. See ➋ Chapter 2, pp. 11–16.
- Sick note provided if necessary.

Follow-up
- Generally post-operative support and follow-up of patients occurs by telephone and is provided by day surgery nurses. Patients are given emergency contact numbers for expert nursing advice.
- Generic discharge criteria are difficult to draw, and common sense with sensible judgment should be used at all times.

How good your day surgery practice is—audit areas

- Is information given to patients before planned day surgery sufficient, comprehensible, and on time to reduce patients' anxiety and increase their satisfaction?
  - Standard—quality and quantity of information and their effect on patients.
  - Indicators—% of procedures and information leaflets meeting the criteria; % of satisfied patients.
- Is the pre-admission assessment effective enough in choosing appropriate patients for day surgery to improve their experience and reduce cancellation rate?
  - Standard—agreed selection criteria by the unit.
  - Indicators–% of patients been assessed using protocols; % been refused day surgery; % cancelled within 2d of operation.

Other audit suggestions

- Effectiveness of the pain management plan in controlling post-operative pain and increasing patient satisfaction.
- Is theatre utilization efficient enough to meet the government targets of doing 75% of elective surgery as a day case?
- Effectiveness of the discharge protocols in achieving safe and effective discharge process.

Expert opinion

Clinicians who recognize the quality benefits of day surgery are surprised and exasperated by the failure of so many to exploit the advantages it brings to patients and their health communities. The NHS Modernisation Agency final report on the ten changes in the NHS that would have the greatest impact listed treating day surgery as the norm at the top of the list. Day surgery will increase, but as is so often the case, predicting the catalyst and speed of change is difficult. Day surgery enthusiasts, surgeons, anaesthetists, and nurses working together will continue to broaden the scope of procedures suitable for the day surgery environment. The British Association of Day Surgery (BADS) Directory of Procedures gives an idea of what is achievable in dedicated facilities with appropriate equipment and trained staff. To many, day surgery is the simple and less fulfilling end of the surgical spectrum of procedures. This Directory shows that is not the case.

Surgery will continue to become less and less invasive with the help of new technology and surgical skills. In parallel, day surgery anaesthetic practice will exploit the value of regional and local anaesthetics to avoid systemic upset caused by strong analgesia, reduced surgical trauma aiding this change of practice. Mortality is an easily recognized measure of failure. Although obviously important, it is infrequent and not a good measure of the surgical experience. Quality of recovery affects all and is the standard by which the surgical experience should be judged. The ultimate is minimal upset by either drugs or trauma of an ever increasing range and complexity of surgical procedures such that patients need only leave home for their time in the operating theatre. In the years to come, this will be the norm. The likely catalyst will be the expansion of dedicated day surgical units led by clinicians and managers who have day surgery as their priority. *Mr Roddy Nash, Council Member, British Association of Day Surgery (BADS) 2008.*

Further reading

British Association of Day Surgery. Integrated Care Pathways for Day Surgery Patients. (UK) 2011

Department of Health. Day Surgery: Operational Guide. (UK) 2002. URL: http://www.dh.gov.uk/en/Publicationsandstatistics/Publications/PublicationsPolicyAndGuidance/DH_4005487. Accessed May 2009.

Royal College of Nursing. Selection Criteria and suitable procedures. Royal College of Nursing Publications. www.spitalmures.ro/_files/protocoale_terapeutice/chirurgie/chirurgie_de_zi.pdf. Accessed Jan 2018.

Osborne GA, Rudkin GE (1993). Outcome after day-care surgery in a major teaching hospital. Anaesth Intensive Care 21, 822–7.

Watkins BM, Montgomery KF, Ahroni JH, Erlitz MD, Abrams RE, Scurlock JE (2005). Adjustable gastric banding in an ambulatory surgery centre. Obes Surg 15, 1045–9.

British Association of Day Surgery: Discharge Criteria. https://www.aagbi.org/sites/default/files/Day%20Case%20for%20web.pdf. Accessed Jan 2018.

The Royal College of Anaesthetists. Raising the standard: a compendium of audit recipes. Available from: https://www.rcoa.ac.uk/ARB2012

Chapter 6

Good consent practice

Background *52*
Providing sufficient information *52*
Who should obtain consent? *52*
Good consent practice *53*
Withholding information *54*
Patients lacking capacity *54*
Further reading *54*

Key guidelines
- General Medical Council (2008). Consent: patients and doctors making decisions together.
- The Royal College of Surgeons of England (2014). Good surgical practice.

Background

- By definition, a person can give consent when he/she can appreciate and understand the facts and implications of an action. Consent principles apply to any interaction with patients.
- Recognize that seeking consent for surgical intervention is a process of providing information to enable the patient to make a decision and undergo a specific treatment. Consent requires time, patience, and clarity of explanation.
- 'You must' is an imperative in much of the advice rather than 'you should'. This must be borne in mind when gaining consent. Good documentation is advisable at all times.

Providing sufficient information

- *How sufficient*—information should be understandable enough to enable weighing risks and benefits of any procedure and for making appropriate informed decisions about care. Sufficient information is a right for patients and is protected by law.
- *How much information*—varies between individual patients. Factors affecting this include the type and complexity of treatment, possible side-effects and risks, patients' beliefs, culture, occupation, level of education, and patients' wishes. Decision should be based on an individual basis and the patients' views respected. Patients must be told if there is a potential serious outcome, even if the likelihood is very small (Chester vs Afshar).
- *Consent scope and limits*—if treatment has to be delivered in stages, for example, or has to involve more than one specialty, then information about whether or when to move from one form of treatment to another should be fully discussed with patient and documented. The need to seek further consent at a later stage should be clarified.

Who should obtain consent?

- *Best person*—the clinician doing the investigation and providing the treatment.
- *Delegation*—is only acceptable for appropriately trained and qualified staff with sufficient knowledge of delivery method of the procedure/investigation, main techniques, benefits, and risks. They do not have to be able to do the procedure themselves.
- If the patient agrees, you should involve the patient's supporter in the consent discussion. In case you have to act in your patient's best interests without the patient's consent, where possible seek affirmation from a consultant colleague.

Good consent practice

- *Work always in partnership with your patient*—no one else can make a decision on behalf of an adult who has capacity.
- *Review*—all available information before interviewing the patient.
- *Find appropriate time and setting*—where patients are able to understand and retain information.
- *Present information*—using up-to-date written and visual material, arrange for language and communication requirements as well as the presence of relatives or friends if requested by patient (offer the option), and give distressing information in a considerate way.
- *Discuss expected diagnosis*—what is the most likely diagnosis (if available) and possible outcome if disease left untreated. If the diagnosis is still uncertain, what further investigations prior to treatment are required?
- *Discuss options*—all available options for treating the condition, including the 'not to treat' option.
- *Discuss benefits and risks*
  - Main purpose and likely benefits of different options (diagnostic, curative, palliative, approved trial, etc.).
  - The common and serious possible side-effects.
- *Discuss main details*
  - Technical details (that can be understood by patient).
  - Perioperative experience.
- *Overall responsible doctor for the treatment*—and extent of doctor in training or medical students' involvement.
- *Reflection*—allow patients enough time to reflect on the appropriate decision, and involve nurses and other health care members in discussions.
- *Final reminder*—that patients can change their minds about their decision at any time and can seek a second opinion.
- *Questions*—should be answered fully, accurately, and honestly. Some questions might be difficult to answer. Seeking further advice from others is helpful.

Withholding information

* *Sharing information*—all relevant information necessary for decision making should be shared with the patient.
* *Exceptional circumstances*—include those where disclosing information may cause serious harm to the patient (serious harm does not just mean that the patient would become upset and refuse treatment); in special circumstances, withholding the selected information can be considered appropriate. Seeking help and advice in such cases is recommended. Keeping good records is essential.

Patients lacking capacity

* To facilitate decision making, the views of the patient's legal representative and the people close to the patient should be sought. Help should be requested when necessary. The care of the patient is the primary concern.

Know your results

Good consent practice—audit areas
Is consenting practice of acceptable quality?
* Quantity and quality of information, documentation, level of experience of consenting physician, etc.
  * Standard—quality and quantity of information.
  * Indicators—% of specific documented procedure, % of forms holding identifiable patient information, % of forms with documented site/side of operation, % of documented general/specific possible side effects, level of consenting physicians, etc.)

Other audit suggestions
* Patients' satisfaction/views on the consenting practice for specific operations/procedures.

Further reading

General Medical Council (2008). Consent: patients and doctors making decisions together. Available from: http://www.gmc-uk.org/guidance/ethical_guidance/consent_guidance/Consent_guidance.pdf.
The Royal College of Surgeons of England (2014). Good surgical practice. Available from: https://www.rcseng.ac.uk/standards-and-research/gsp (with kind permission).
Wikipedia. Informed consent. Available from: http://en.wikipedia.org/wiki/Informed_consent.

Chapter 7

Preoperative assessment

Background 56
General evaluation 58
Preoperative investigations 62
Further reading 66
Assessment of cardiovascular system 68
Further reading 72
Assessment of respiratory system 74
Further reading 78

Key guidelines
- NICE. The use of preoperative tests in elective surgery. (UK) 2016.
- NHS Scotland. Care before, during and after anaesthesia. (UK) 2003.
- CSI. Preoperative evaluation. (US) 2008.
- ACC/AHA Guideline. Perioperative guidelines. (US) 2014.
- ESC/ESA Guideline. Perioperative guidelines 2014.
- AAGBI and British Association of Day Surgery Guideline 2011.
- AAGBI. Pre-operative assessment and patient preparation. The role of the anaesthetist. (UK) 2010.
- National good practice guidance on preoperative assessment for day surgery. Modernisation Agency NHS 2005.

Background

- Patients undergoing operations should, wherever possible, have a preoperative assessment (face-to-face, telephone, or questionnaire) by a suitably trained individual.
- Objectives—to improve the surgical outcome by identifying any coexisting medical disorder, confirming its presence and severity with appropriate tests, treating conditions that may adversely influence the outcome, avoiding late cancellations, and/or deferring surgery if deemed necessary. Preoperative assessment can also be used to ensure that the patient has fully understood the proposed operation and is ready to proceed.

General evaluation

Apply the same principles of taking (or receiving) history and performing physical examination with special attention to risk factors.

- Clinical history
  - Proposed procedure—indications and any unexpected changes since being booked, urgency of surgery, previous anaesthetic records, and grade of surgery.
  - Systems review—as applied to the specific surgery. Grading patient's risk in clinic allows for better rationalization of investigations (Table 7.1). An interactive risk calculator, developed by the authors, is available as a tool on iOS devices: https://itunes.apple.com/gb/app/vascore/id1088581560?mt=8
  - Be familiar with the documentation being used in your own hospital.
  - Drug history—complete list of medications including over-the-counter and herbal products, and drug allergies, including previous reactions and if the patient was formally tested in an allergy clinic.
  - Social history—smoking, alcohol, drugs, other personal behaviour of importance.
- Physical examination—thorough and guided by clinical history.
- General impression—regardless of age, patients who live independently, do their shopping and gardening, or manage two flights of stairs or run a short distance are unlikely to have major serious medical disorders that would affect significantly the operative outcome in moderate surgical procedures.
- ASA grade—the American Society for Anaesthesiologists (ASA) grading system is commonly used to describe the patient's physical status. This grading is useful for record keeping, statistical analysis, and communication to colleagues. It is not intended as a measure of operative risk (Table 7.2).

Table 7.1 A traffic light system for preoperative assessment in major surgery, based on the Vascular Society of Great Britain and Ireland's Quality Improvement Programme.

GROUP I Questions—RED FLAG		
1. Recent (<3 mo) myocardial infarct or unstable angina/angina at rest?	Y	N
2. Recent (<3 mo) new onset of angina?		
3. History of poorly controlled heart failure? (nocturnal dyspnoea, inability to climb one flight of stairs due to shortness of breath)		
4. Severe/symptomatic cardiac valve disease? (e.g. aortic stenosis with gradient >60mmHg or requiring valve replacement, drop attacks)		
5. Poor respiratory function: i. FEV1<1.0L or <80% of predicted value; ii. PO_2<8.0kPa; iii. PCO_2>6.5kPa		

Patients with ANY positive finding from above are coded RED and should be reviewed by a specialist before proceeding to surgery. Specialist anaesthetists should also review the patient.

GROUP II Questions—AMBER FLAG		
1. Exertion breathlessness or on climbing one flight of stairs?	Y	N
2. Moderate renal impairment (creatinine >180mcmol/l); previous renal transplant?		
3. Recent (<6mo) treatment for cancer/life-threatening tumour?		
4. Poorly controlled diabetes mellitus? (HbAlc >7.5%, blood sugar >10mmol/l)		
5. Uncontrolled hypertension (sBP >190 and/or dBP >105)		
6. Recent (<6mo) transient ischaemic attack (TIA) or cardiovascular accident (CVA)?		

Patients with ANY positive finding from this group are coded AMBER and should be optimized before proceeding to surgery. Specialist anaesthetists should also review the patient.

LOW RISK PATIENTS—GREEN FLAG

Patients with NONE of the above are coded GREEN and are fit to proceed. Ensure that appropriate preoperative medications, core investigations (see Table 7.3), and special arrangements (ITU beds, duplex scanning, endoscopy, etc.) are made/requested.

http://www.vascularsociety.org.uk/doc-category/audit-qi/

Table 7.2 ASA grades*

ASA 1	normal healthy patient
ASA 2	mild systemic disease
ASA 3	severe systemic disease
ASA 4	severe systemic disease that is a constant threat to life
ASA 5	moribund patient who is not expected to survive without the operation
ASA 6	declared brain-dead patient whose organs are being removed for donor purposes

* (See also ➲ OHCM 10e Ch.13)

Preoperative investigations

- Rationale—tests should make an important contribution to the process of perioperative assessment and management without causing unnecessary disadvantage/harm.
- Possible disadvantages—unnecessary delay of surgery, false positive findings leading to costly and risky investigations, and diversion of hospital resources into unnecessary costly service.
- Choosing the appropriate preoperative tests in elective operations— have been recommended by NICE based on expert opinion using a consensus development process (level of recommendations: D). A derived practical algorithm is provided in Box 7.1 and Table 7.3, based on the three main factors recommended by NICE: patient age, surgery grade, and ASA grade.

Box 7.1 Recommendations relevant for all types of surgery.

NICE guidance is prepared for the National Health Service in England. All NICE guidance is subject to regular review and may be updated or withdrawn. NICE accepts no responsibility for the use of its content in this product/publication.

The recommendations in this NICE guideline were developed in relation to the following comorbidities: cardiovascular, diabetes, obesity, renal, and respiratory.

Communication
- When offering tests before surgery, give people information in line with recommendations (including those on consent and capacity) made in the NICE guideline on patient experience in adult NHS services.
- Ensure that the results of any preoperative tests undertaken in primary care are included when referring people for surgical consultation.

Considering existing medicines
- Take into account any medicines people are taking when considering whether to offer any preoperative test.

Pregnancy tests
- On the day of surgery, sensitively ask all women of childbearing potential whether there is any possibility they could be pregnant.
- Make sure women who could possibly be pregnant are aware of the risks of the anaesthetic and the procedure to the foetus.
- Document all discussions with women about whether or not to carry out a pregnancy test.
- Carry out a pregnancy test with the woman's consent if there is any doubt about whether she could be pregnant.
- Develop locally agreed protocols for checking pregnancy status before surgery.
- Make sure protocols are documented and audited and in line with statutory and professional guidance.

Sick cell disease or sickle cell trait test

(Continued)

Box 7.1 (contd.)

- Do not routinely offer testing for sickle cell disease or sickle cell trait before surgery.
- Ask the person having surgery if they or any member of their family have sickle cell disease.
- If the person is known to have sickle cell disease and has their disease managed by a specialist sickle cell service, liaise with this team before surgery.

HbA1c testing
- Do not routinely offer HbA1c testing before surgery to people without diagnosed diabetes.
- People with diabetes who are being referred for surgical consultation from primary care should have their most recent HbA1c test results included in their referral information.
- Offer HbA1c testing to people with diabetes having surgery if they have not been tested in the last 3 months.

Urine tests
- Do not routinely offer urine dipstick tests before surgery.
- Consider microscopy and culture of midstream urine sample before surgery if the presence of a urinary tract infection would influence the decision to operate.

Chest X-ray
- Do not routinely offer chest X-rays before surgery.

Echocardiography
- Do not routinely offer resting echocardiography before surgery.
- Consider resting echocardiography if the person has:
  - A heart murmur **and** any cardiac symptom (including breathlessness, pre-syncope, syncope, or chest pain) **or**
  - Signs or symptoms of heart failure.
- Before ordering the resting echocardiogram, carry out a resting electrocardiogram (ECG) and discuss the findings with an anaesthetist.

Table 7.3 Recommendations for specific surgery and ASA grades: colour traffic light tables.

Key	Meaning		
	Red light		
	Amber light		
	Green light		

Test	ASA 1	ASA 2	ASA 3 or ASA 4
Minor surgery (examples: excising skin lesion; draining breast abscess)			
Full blood count	Not routinely	Not routinely	Not routinely
Haemostasis	Not routinely	Not routinely	Not routinely
Kidney function	Not routinely	Not routinely	Consider in people at risk of AKI[1]
ECG	Not routinely	Not routinely	Consider if no ECG results available from past 12 months
Lung function/ arterial blood gas	Not routinely	Not routinely	Not routinely
Intermediate surgery (examples: primary repair of inguinal hernia; excising varicose veins in the leg; tonsillectomy or adenotonsillectomy; knee arthroscopy)			
Full blood count	Not routinely	Not routinely	Consider for people with cardiovascular or renal disease if any symptoms not recently investigated
Haemostasis	Not routinely	Not routinely	Consider in people with chronic liver disease • If people taking anticoagulants need modification of their treatment regimen, make an individualized plan in line with local guidance • If clotting status needs to be tested before surgery (depending on local guidance) use point-of-care testing[2]
Kidney function	Not routinely	Consider in people at risk of AKI[1]	Yes
ECG	Not routinely	Consider for people with cardiovascular, renal, or diabetes comorbidities	Yes

Table 7.3 (Contd.)

Test	ASA 1	ASA 2	ASA 3 or ASA 4
Lung function/ arterial blood gas	Not routinely	Not routinely	Consider seeking advice from a senior anaesthetist as soon as possible after assessment for people who are ASA grade 3 or 4 due to known or suspected respiratory disease

Major or complex surgery (examples: total abdominal hysterectomy; endoscopic resection of prostate; lumbar discectomy; thyroidectomy; total joint replacement; lung operations; colonic resection; radical neck dissection)

Test	ASA 1	ASA 2	ASA 3 or ASA 4
Full blood count	Yes	Yes	Yes
Haemostasis	Not routinely	Not routinely	Consider in people with chronic liver disease • If people taking anticoagulants need modification of their treatment regimen, make an individualized plan in line with local guidance • If clotting status needs to be tested before surgery (depending on local guidance) use point-of-care testing[2]
Kidney function	Consider in people at risk of AKI[1]	Yes	Yes
ECG	Consider for people aged over 65 if no ECG results available from past 12 months	Yes	Yes
Lung function/ arterial blood gas	Not routinely	Not routinely	Consider seeking advice from a senior anaesthetist as soon as possible after assessment for people who are ASA grade 3 or 4 due to known or suspected respiratory disease

Further reading

NICE (2003). The use of preoperative tests in elective surgery. (UK) available from: www.nice. org. uk/nicemedia/pdf/Preop-fullguideline.pdf. These guidelines are planned to be updated in April 2016 by NICE.

NHS Scotland (2003). Care before, during and after anaesthesia. (UK) available from: www. nhshealthquality.org/nhsqis/files/Anaesthesia National Overview - Sep2005.pdf

ICSI (2008). Preoperative evaluation. (US) available from: www.issi.org/preoperative_evaluation/ preoperative_evaluation_2328.html

ACC/AHA Guideline (2014). Guideline on Perioperative Cardiovascular Evaluation and Management of Patients undergoing Noncardiac surgery (US) available from: http://anesthesiology.med. miami.edu/documents.mm_articles/105.pdf

AAGBI (2010). Pre-operative Assessment and Patient Preparation. The role of the Anaesthetist. (UK) available from: www.aagbi.org/publications/guidelines/docs/preoperativeass01.pdf

Modernisation Agency NHS National Good Practice Guidance on Preoperative assessment for day surgery. available from: www.cancerimprovement.nhs.uk\documents\publications from NHS modernisation Agency/Pre-operative guidance for daycase surgery.pdf

Charles R, Smith R (1998). *Atlas of general surgery*, 3rd ed. Hodder Arnold, p. 124.

ESC/ESA Guideline (2014). Guidelines on non-cardiac surgery (Europe).

AAGBI and British Association of Day surgery (2011). Excellence in short stay surgery.

Assessment of cardiovascular system

Key guidelines
- ACC/AHA Guideline. Update on perioperative cardiovascular evaluation of the patient undergoing noncardiac surgery. (US) 2014.
- ESC/ESA Guideline. Guidelines on non-cardiac surgery: cardiovascular assessment and management. (Europe) 2014.
- NHS Scotland. Care before, during and after anaesthesia. (UK) 2003.
- ICSI. Preoperative evaluation. (US) 2008.

Background
Worldwide, non-cardiac surgery is associated with an average overall complication rate of 7–11% and a mortality rate of 0.8–1.5% depending on safety precautions.
- Up to 42% of these are caused by cardiac complications. Most occur within 72h of operation (peak at 48h). Perioperative infarction has a 50% risk of death. Detection and treatment of cardiac disorders in patients undergoing operative procedures can have significant impact on the surgical outcome.
- Major cardiac risk factors require further investigations and referral to a specialist. Intermediate risk factors require optimization.

Cardiac risk factors
Age
- In general, cardiac risk is higher in patients over the age of 70 (risk ratio (RR)×1.9). Age is a minor independent factor.

Ischaemic heart disease
- The risk is major with unstable coronary syndrome (acute or recent (<30d) myocardial infarction (MI) or unstable angina) and intermediate with stable coronary syndrome (stable angina, or previous MI by history or pathologic Q waves).

Congestive heart failure
- The risk is major with decompensated heart failure and intermediate with compensated or prior heart failure.

Arrhythmias
- Cardiac risk is major in patients with significant arrhythmias (high-grade AV block, symptomatic ventricular arrhythmias in the presence of underlying heart disease, or supraventricular arrhythmias with uncontrolled ventricular rate) and minor in patients with minimal ECG changes (left ventricular hypertrophy, left bundle branch block, ST–T abnormalities) or if the rhythm was not sinus (e.g. rate controlled atrial fibrillation).

Valvular heart disease
- In general, cardiac risk is higher when clinical findings suggest a significant valvular heart disease and major if valvular disease was severe.

Type of surgery
- High-risk surgery—include emergency major operations, aortic and other major vascular surgery, peripheral vascular surgery, and prolonged surgical procedures with associated large fluid shifts and/or blood loss. Estimated cardiac complication rate is >5%.
- Intermediate risk surgery—include carotid endarterectomy, head and neck surgery, intraperitoneal and intrathoracic surgery, orthopaedic surgery, and prostate surgery. Estimated cardiac complication rate is 1–5%.
- Low-risk surgery—include endoscopic procedures, superficial procedure, cataract surgery, and breast surgery. Estimated cardiac complication rate is <1%.

Other factors
- In general, cardiac risk is higher in the presence of cerebrovascular ischaemia (RR×2.9–4.7), insulin-dependent diabetes mellitus (IDDM) (RR×3.5), renal failure with serum creatinine above 2mg/dL (RR×5.2), and in poor general condition (RR×1.8).
- The risk is intermediate in diabetes mellitus and renal insufficiency, and minor in the history of stroke and in controlled systemic hypertension.

Cumulative cardiac risk index
- The Lee Index or 'Revised Cardiac Risk Index' was designed in 1999 to predict post-operative myocardial infarction, pulmonary oedema, ventricular fibrillation, and cardiac arrest by incorporating six variables (Box 7.2).

Box 7.2 Estimation of cardiac risk

Cardiac risk factors
1. Ischaemic heart disease—history of MI, current complaint of ischaemic chest pain or use of nitrate therapy, positive exercise test, or ECG with Q waves.
2. Heart failure—history of congestive heart failure, pulmonary oedema, paroxysmal nocturnal dyspnoea, presence of bilateral crepitations or S3 gallop, or the presence of pulmonary vascular redistribution.
3. High-risk surgery—see text.
4. Cerebrovascular ischaemia.
5. IDDM.
6. Serum creatinine >2mg/dL.

Risk estimation
1. No risk factors—0.4%.
2. One risk factor—1.0%.
3. Two risk factors—2.4%.
4. Three or more risk factors—5.4%.

• The more recent 2007 NSQUIP MICA Model with the primary endpoint being perioperative myocardial infarction or cardiac arrest up to 30d of surgery is considered by many clinicians and researchers as the best currently available cardiac risk prediction index in non-cardiac surgery. This model has five predictors, namely type of surgery, functional status, elevated creatinine, ASA score, and age. Interactive risk calculator, developed by the authors, is available as a tool on iOS devices: https://itunes.apple.com/gb/app/vascore/id1088581560?mt=8.

Action plan

• Major risk factors—require intensive investigations and management as appropriate, which may result in delay or cancellation of non-emergency surgery. Waiting 4–6wk after a myocardial infarction (MI) to perform elective surgery is recommended.
• Intermediate risk factors—are well-validated markers of enhanced risk of perioperative cardiac complications and justify careful assessment of the patient's current status.
• The use of plasma B-type natriuretic peptide (BNP) for prognostic purposes is not well established yet. Two meta-analyses showed a significant correlation between pre-operative BNP elevation and cardiovascular outcome (OR×20).

Further reading

NICE (2003). The use of preoperative tests in elective surgery. (UK) available from: www.nice.org.uk/nicemedial/pdf/Preop-fullguideline.pdf

NHS Scotland (2003). Care before, during and after anaesthesia. (UK) available from: www.nhshealthquality.org/nhsqis/files/Anaesthesia National Overview - Sep2005.pdf

ICSI (2008). Preoperative evaluation. (US) available from: www.issi.org/preoperative_evaluation/preoperative_evaluation_2328.html

ACC/AHA Guideline (2014). Update on Perioperative Cardiovascular Evaluation for Noncardiac Surgery. (US) available from: http://anesthesiology.med.miami.edu/documents/mm_articles/105.pdf

Mangano DT, Goldman L (1995). Preoperative assessment of patients with known or suspected coronary disease. *N Engl J Med*, 333, 1750–6.

Devereaux PJ, Goldman L, Cook DJ, Gilbert K, Leslie K, Guyatt GH (2005). Perioperative cardiac events in patients undergoing non-cardiac surgery: a review of the magnitude of the problem, the pathophysiology of the events, and methods to estimate and communicate risk. *CMAJ*, 173, 627–34.

Morris PJ, Wood WC (2001). *Oxford textbook of surgery*. Oxford University Press, Oxford.

ESC/ESA Guideline (2014). Guidelines on non-cardiac surgery: cardiovascular assessment and management. (Europe).

Assessment of respiratory system

Key guidelines
- NHS QIS Scotland. Care before, during and after anaesthesia. (UK) 2003.
- ICSI. Preoperative evaluation. (US) 2014.

Background
- Post-operative respiratory complications occur in 5–10% of major non-cardiac procedures and are more common than cardiac complications.
- Respiratory complications are significant if resulted in prolonged hospital stay or increased morbidity and mortality.
- Common significant respiratory complications—include bronchospasm, atelectasis, pneumonia, respiratory failure with prolonged mechanical ventilation, and exacerbation of underlying chronic lung disease.

Risk factors
- Advanced age—increases pulmonary risks significantly (RR×1.9–2.4). The correlation is mostly related to coexisting conditions, not to chronologic age.
- Obesity—slight non-significant increase in pulmonary complications (RR×1.3), contrary to common beliefs.
- Smoking—significant risk factor (RR×1.4–4.3). Stopping smoking >8wk preoperatively reduces the risk significantly (by 50%); stopping in <8wk may increase the risk.
- General health status—strong predictor, especially in patients with ASA grade above two (RR×1.5–3.2).
- Chronic obstructive pulmonary disease (COPD) patients—significantly at risk (RR×2.7–4.7).
- Controlled asthma—no effect on risk.
- Type of surgery
  - Site of surgery—risk of complications is higher in upper abdominal and thoracic surgery (10–40%) compared to lower abdominal surgery (0–15%). Risk is minimum in laparoscopic cholecystectomy (0.3–0.4%) as compared to open cholecystectomy (13–33%).
  - Duration of surgery—higher risk if surgery duration exceeds 3 hours (RR×1.6–5.2), and in surgery under general anaethetic (RR×1.2).

Predicting pulmonary risk
- Epstein and colleagues model—uses a sum of modified Goldman cardiac index plus main pulmonary risk factors. Factors include smoking, obesity, productive cough, diffuse wheezing, rhonchi, FEV1: FVC ratio <70%, and $PaCO_2$ >45mmHg. Most useful in lung resection operations. Some centres use percent of diffusing capacity to predict pulmonary complications in patients without COPD after lung resection.
- ARISCAT risk index predicts overall incidence of postoperative respiratory complications (Table 7.4) and can be used for quick clinic screening tool. Gupta scoring system for reparatory failure (http://goo.gl/9PpqyS) and pneumonia (http://goo.gl/fk5Sl9) are available online.

Table 7.4 ARISCAT (CANET) Risk Index

Factor	Risk score
Age	age >80: 16
	age 51–80: 3
Emergency surgery	8
Surgical incision	Thoracic: 24
	Upper abdominal: 15
Surgical duration	>3h: 23
	2–3h: 16
Respiratory infection <1mo	17
Hb <10g/dL	11
Preoperative PO_2	<90%: 24
	91–95%: 8
Total risk score	**Respiratory complication rate**
High: >45	~40%
Intermediate: 26–44	~15%
Low: <26	~2%

Reproduced with permission from Canet, Jaume; Gallart, Lluís, Prediction of Postoperative Pulmonary Complications in a Population-based Surgical Cohort, Anesthesiology, Volume 113, Issue 6, p.1338, Copyright © 2010 Wolters Kluwer Health, Inc.

Risk reduction strategies

Preoperatively

- Encourage cigarette cessation for >8wk before surgery.
- Treat COPD as appropriate.
- Use antibiotics and possibly delay surgery in respiratory infections.
- Educate patient on lung expansion manoeuvres (able to reduce respiratory complications from 60% to 19%).

Intraoperatively

- Use spinal or epidural anaesthesia.
- Use laparoscopic approach if possible.
- Aim at operative duration of <3h.

Post-operatively

- Use epidural analgesia.
- Use nerve block.
- Use deep breathing exercises.
- Use continuous positive airway pressure if necessary.

Other preoperative issues—specific advice and organization

- Fasting, the pill, and prophylactic prevention of deep vein thromboses (DVTs) are dealt with in later chapters (see ⊃ Chapter 7, pp. 45–48; ⊃ Chapter 12, pp. 87–90).
- Smoking—although in general, smoking cessation should be advised, there is no strong evidence to recommend smoking cessation in the immediate short term prior to surgery as a means to achieve improved outcomes and reduce post-operative complications.
- Patients advised to take their normal medications (excluding anticoagulants, see ⊃ Chapter 12, pp. 87–90), and particularly important to continue with B-blockers. Aspirin and statins for the prevention of MI or CVA should be continued unless instructed by local protocol.
- Procedure and anaesthetic leaflets provided to aid informed consent.
- The patient should have telephone contact if a day patient.
- A responsible adult and home support must be available.
- Home circumstances, e.g. stairs and transport, need to be enquired about.
- Advice given about getting back to normal activities and work.
- A contact point at the hospital if needed in the post-operative period at home.

Further reading

NHS QIS Scotland (2003). Care before, during and after anaesthesia. NHS Scotland.

ICSI (2014). Preoperative evaluation. ICSI, Bloomington, USA.

Hata TM, Moyers JR (2006). Preoperative evaluation and management. In: Barash PG, Cullen BF, Stoelting RK, eds. *Clinical anaesthesia*. 5th ed. Lippincott Williams & Wilkins, Philadelphia.

Smetana GW (1999). Preoperative pulmonary evaluation. *N Engl J Med*, 340, 937–44.

Epstein SK, Faling LJ, Daly BD, Celli BR (1993). Predicting complications after pulmonary resection. Preoperative exercise testing vs a multifactorial cardiopulmonary risk index. *Chest* 104, 694–700.

Ferguson MK, Gaissert HA, Grab JD, Sheng S (2009). Pulmonary complications after lung resection in the absence of chronic obstructive pulmonary disease: the predicting role of diffusing capacity. *J Thoracic Cardiovasc*, 138, 1297–302.

Canet J, Gallart L, Gomar C, et al. (2010). Prediction of postoperative pulmonary complications in a population-based surgical cohort. *Anesthesiology*, 113, 1338.

Perioperative fasting*

Background *80*
Healthy adults—'the 2 and 6 rule' *81*
Children undergoing elective surgery—'the 2, 4, and 6 rule' *82*
Higher risk adults and children *83*
Post-operative oral intake in elective surgery *83*
Exceptions from the guidelines *83*
Further reading *84*

Key guidelines

- European Society for Clinical Nutrition and Metabolism—ESPEN (2017). Guidelines on enteral nutrition: non-surgical oncology.
- Royal College of Anaesthetists (2012). Raising the standard: a compendium of audit recipes.
- The Royal College of Nursing (2013). Perioperative fasting in adults and children.

---

* The guidelines on this chapter have been sourced and summarized from different UK, Europe, and international government sources, professional organizations, and medical specialty societies. Leading guidelines have been listed in the further reading section at the end of this chapter.

Background

- *Rationale*—fasting policy ensures high patient comfort, adequate hydration, and safe anaesthesia. The common practice (or malpractice) of complete abstention from food and drink for 8–12h before anaesthesia should be discouraged.
- *Approach*—both patients and carers should be made aware of current recommendations, understand decision making in terms of risks and benefits, and have the opportunity to ask questions. Effective application of these guidelines should be achieved within a collaborative interdisciplinary approach.

Healthy adults—'the 2 and 6 rule'

- *Healthy adults*—are adults with ASA grade 1 or 2 and no significant gastrointestinal disorder or on drugs such as opioids that slow gastric emptying.
- *Diet and fluid*—see Table 8.1.
- *Oral medications*—safe to take any oral medication if there is no need to stop or convert into parenteral (Box 8.1). Water (up to 30mL) can be given orally to help in swallowing [D].
- *Oral premedications (benzodiazepines, etc.)*—safe to take as per the recommendation for water and clear fluid [A].
- *Delayed operation*—consider giving a drink of water (safe and beneficial practice) [D].

Box 8.1 Medication check preoperatively

Steroids, anticoagulant, oral contraceptives, antiplatelets etc.

See also individual chapters and Ch. 9 'Perioperative medical complications'

Table 8.1 Fasting recommendations in healthy adults

Diet type	Recommendations	Grade
Water	Safe and beneficial to drink with unlimited amounts up to 2h before induction	[A]
Clear fluids	Clear tea, black coffee, etc.—safe to drink with unlimited amounts up to 2h before induction	[A]
Free fluid	Milk, tea with milk, coffee with milk—safe to drink up to 6h before induction	[B]
Solid food and sweets	Safe to take up to 6h before induction	[D]
Chewing gum	Unsafe to use on the day of operation and should not be permitted	[B]

Children undergoing elective surgery—'the 2, 4, and 6 rule'

- *Diet and fluid*—see Table 8.2.
- *Oral medications*—safe to take any oral medication if there is no need to stop or convert them into parenteral (Box 8.1). Water up to 0.5mL/kg (30mL) can be given orally to help in swallowing [D].
- *Oral premedications (benzodiazepines, etc.)*—safe to take as per the recommendation for water and clear fluid [A].
- *Delayed operation*—consider giving a drink of water or other clear fluid as a safe and beneficial practice. Water or clear fluid should be given if the delay is expected to be >2h [D].

Table 8.2 Fasting recommendations in healthy children

Diet type	Recommendations	Level
Water	Safe and beneficial to drink with unlimited amounts up to 2h before induction	[A*]
Milk	Breast milk—safe up to 4h before induction Formula milk/cow's milk—safe up to 6h before induction	[D]
Solid food and sweets	Safe to take up to 6h before induction	[D]
Chewing gum	Unsafe to use on the day of operation and should not be permitted	[D]

Level of recommendation is A for ≥1y and D for <1y

Higher risk adults and children

- *Higher risk patients*—are those with a significant risk of regurgitation and aspiration. Patients with gastro-oesophageal reflux disease, obesity, and diabetes are examples.
- *Fasting guidelines*—follow the one for healthy adults or children, unless contraindicated [D].
- *Special manoeuvres*—may be considered in high-risk patients for safety issues [D]:
  - H2-receptor antagonists and proton pump inhibitors.
  - Sodium citrate and gastrokinetic agents.
  - Rapid sequence induction.
  - Tracheal intubation.
  - Nasogastric tube.
- *Emergency cases*—treat as full stomach and apply manoeuvres to reduce aspiration [D].

Post-operative oral intake in elective surgery

- *Adults*—encourage drinking when patients feel ready for it, providing there are no contraindications [A].
- *Children*—offer oral fluids when fully awake from anaesthesia, providing there are no contraindications [A]. Clear fluids or breast milk should be considered first [D].

Exceptions from the guidelines

Patients having a procedure under sedation should follow the unit protocols. Instructions on post-operative fasting in major abdominal surgery or gastro-intestinal tract should be planned individually with the surgeon in charge.

Further reading

The Royal College of Nursing (2013). Perioperative fasting in adults and children. Available from: http://www.rcn.org.uk/professional-development/publications/pub-002779

Royal College of Anaesthetists (2012) Raising the standard: a compendium of audit receipes. Third edition

Levy DM, Pre-operative fasting- 60 years on from Mendleson. Continuous Education Anaesthesia Critical Care and Pain (2006) 6(6):215–218

Perioperative medical complications*

Cardiovascular complications 86
Further reading 90
Respiratory complications 92
Further reading 96
Renal complications 98
Further reading 101
Neurological complications 102
Further reading 104

* The guidelines on this chapter have been sourced and summarized from different UK, Europe, and international government sources, professional organizations, and medical specialty societies. Leading guidelines have been listed in the further reading section at the end of this chapter.

Cardiovascular complications

Key guidelines
- Scottish Intercollegiate Guidelines Network (2004). Postoperative management in adults.
- Scottish Intercollegiate Guidelines Network (2007). Acute coronary syndromes.
- National Institute for Health and Clinical Excellence (2014). Atrial fibrillation.
- ESA/ESA (2014). Cardiovascular guidelines for non-cardiac surgery.
- ACC/AHA (2014). Guideline on perioperative cardiac evaluation
- National Institute for Health and Clinical Excellence (2009). Thoracoscopic epicardial radiofrequency ablation for atrial fibrillation.
- Advanced Life Support (ALS) (2011). Sixth edition.

Perioperative myocardial infarction (PMI)
- *Incidence*—affects about 2–3% of patients perioperatively after major non-cardiac surgery. Myocardial injury after noncardiac surgery (MINS) is defined as prognostically relevant myocardial injury due to ischaemia that occurs during or within 30 days after noncardiac surgery. Minimal risk in patients with no clinical atherosclerotic disease, and highest incidence (4–7%) in patients with known coronary disease. MINS are estimated to affect ~ 20% of patients of moderate to high-risk surgery (VISION study).
- *Presentation*—many (~65% in POISE trial) have no specific complaints. Few (~15%) complain of chest pain. Present occasionally with signs of congestive heart failure (e.g. short of breath).
- *Diagnosis*—maintain a high index of suspicion in high-risk patients, males, and elderly (See also ➔ OHCM 10e Ch. 5).
  - Review patients' risk factors.
  - *Seek specialist medical advice*—early on clinical suspicion [CS]*
  - *Obtain 12-lead electrocardiogram (ECG)*—immediately [D]. High-risk asymptomatic patients should always have ECG performed on admission (baseline), immediately after surgery, and daily for two days post-operatively [CS].
  - *Check troponin levels (I or T)*—raised levels can be detected in almost all patients within 6–9h after PMI onset (earlier using sensitive assays and low cut-off values). Sensitivity, specificity, positive and negative predictive values are remarkably high (>90%). High-risk asymptomatic patients can be considered for troponin levels measurement before surgery, and 48–72 h after surgery [B].
  - *Confirm diagnosis*—this can be established (within appropriate clinical and ECG findings) on finding raised (or fall from raised) troponin levels in 12h from onset of symptoms, with no other explanation (e.g. PE, AF) [B].
- *Treatment*—see Box 9.1 (See also ➔ lumbar puncture OHCM 10e Ch.18).

Box 9.1 Post-operative MI—treatment

- Level of care—admit to a specialist cardiology unit [C]. Use continuous ECG monitoring to detect the potentially lethal but treatable arrhythmias and manage according to ALS protocol [D].
- Level of care—admit to a specialist cardiology unit [C]. Use continuous ECG monitoring to detect the potentially lethal but treatable arrhythmias and manage according to ALS protocol [D].
- Secure IV access, draw blood samples.
- Aspirin—300mg immediately [A]. Aspirin reduces the rate of further vascular event (death, stroke, MI) by 30 and 50% in unstable angina and MI, respectively.
- Nitroglycerine, as sublingual glyceryltrinitrate (tablet or spray), unless the patient is hypotensive or extensive RV infarction is suspected.
- Morphine or diamorphine (5–10mg)(with metoclopramide). Pain relief is of paramount importance and drugs should be titrated to control symptoms, but avoiding sedation and respiratory depression.
- Other types of treatment—intensive blood glucose control in hyperglycaemic or diabetic patients is required for at least 24h [B]. Other types of treatment should be applied following specialist advice (B-blockers etc.).
- Thrombolytic agents—contraindicated and should not be used.

Atrial fibrillation (AF)

- *Incidence*—supraventricualr arrhythmias and AF are more common than ventricular arrhythmias in the perioperative period. The aetiology of these arrhythmias is multifactorial, but the sympathetic response to surgery is an important trigger for AF.
- *Aetiology*—multifactorial. Commonly associated with sepsis, electrolyte disturbances (especially potassium and magnesium), hypoxia, hypovolaemia, and drug toxicity (mainly theophylline, adenosine, and digitalis). Other risk factors include hypertension (RR ×1.42), recent or active MI (AF occurs in 6–10%), rheumatic valvular disease, heart failure (AF occurs in 10–30%), obesity (BMI >35kg/m^2), and in binge drinkers (AF occurs in 10–30%).
- *Presentation*—many episodes are asymptomatic. Patients may complain of dizziness, weakness, palpitations, and dyspnoea. More serious presentations include angina, hypotension, and heart failure.
- *Diagnosis*—ECG should be performed in all patients, and typically shows rapid and irregular atrial waves (350–600/min) with irregularly irregular ventricular response (90–170bpm). Look for evidence of left ventricular hypertrophy, bundle branch block, prior MI, and arrhythmias on earlier ECGs. Measure important intervals (P wave duration and morphology, RR, QRS, and QT). Other investigations include CXR, U&Es, ABGs, and echocardiogram.
- *Prevention*.
  - Correct electrolyte abnormalities, anaemia, and hypoxia [D]. Keep potassium levels above 4mmol/L (common practice). Correct magnesium levels as appropriate.
  - Perioperative pain should be effectively controlled (see ➔ Chapter 19).

- Routine ECG and troponin check should always be considered in high-risk asymptomatic patients (see above).
- Preoperative B-blockers and nitrates—never stop without alternatives [B].
- Prophylactic medications—recommended in cardiothoracic and other high-risk operations (e.g. vascular surgery). Consider using amiodarone [A], B-blocker [A], sotalol [A], or a rate-limiting calcium antagonist [B]. Digoxin should not be used as prophylaxis [B].
- *Treatment*—see Box 9.2 (see also ➲ OHCM 10e Ch. 3).
  - *Thoracoscopic epicardial radiofrequency ablation for atrial fibrillation*—small series and short-term follow-up showed evidence of efficacy. The procedure should only be performed within appropriate clinical governance setting and by well-trained physician. Patient selection should involve a multidisciplinary team.
  - *Indications*—when drug treatment is ineffective or not tolerated.
  - *Efficacy*—within limited patient numbers and follow-up period, 81–93% of patients were in sinus rhythm at 6–18mo.
  - *Safety*—few complications were reported, including atrial oesophageal fistula, pleural effusion, and pneumothorax.

Box 9.2 Post-operative AF—treatment

Principles—follow same recommendations as for AF in non-surgical patients [D]

Haemodynamically unstable patient.
- Features—ventricular rate >150bpm, ongoing chest pain, or shock.
- Start IV heparin (heparin 5,000–10,000U IV) if no or subtherapeutic anticoagulation exists.
- Life-threatening cases—use electrical cardioversion immediately [D].

Non-life-threatening unstable cases.
- First-time AF (or unknown history)—electrical cardioversion if readily available. Otherwise, use IV amiodarone (rhythm control) [D].
- Known AF (or known history of coronary symptoms, age >65, contraindications to anticoagulation or antiarrhythmias)—control ventricular rate (digoxin: loading dose 500µg/12h × 2, followed by maintenance dose 0.125–0.25mg/24h) [D].
  - Use β-blockers or rate-limiting calcium antagonists as alternative. Otherwise, use amiodarone.

Haemodynamically stable patient
- Refer to a medical specialist.
- Correct underlying abnormalities.
- Anticoagulation—start IV heparin as above for acute AF <48h (cardioversion for AF >48h is probably safe if no signs of cardiac thrombus exist). Consider warfarin in high-risk patients for recurrent AF, stroke (formal stroke risk assessment), or if AF persists >48h [D].
- Persistent AF—consider rhythm control or rate control.
  - Rhythm control for symptomatic, young, first-time patients.
  - Rate control for over 65, known coronary heart diseases, or contraindications to anticoagulation.

Further reading

Devereaux PJ, Goldman L, Yusuf S, Gilbert K, Leslie K, Guyatt GH (2005). Surveillance and prevention of major perioperative ischaemic cardiac events in patients undergoing non-cardiac surgery: a review. CMAJ 173, 779–88.

Bursi F, Babuin L, Barbieri A et al. (2005). Vascular surgery patients: perioperative and long- term risk according to the ACC/AHA guidelines, the additive role of post-operative troponin elevation. Eur Heart J 26, 2458–60.

Krahn AD, Manfreda J, Tate RB, Mathewson FA, Cuddy TE (1995). The natural history of atrial fibrillation: incidence, risk factors, and prognosis in the Manitoba Follow-up Study. Am J Med 98, 476–84.

Scottish Intercollegiate Guidelines Network (2004). Postoperative management in adults. Available from: http://www.sign.ac.uk/pdf/sign77.pdf.

Scottish Intercollegiate Guidelines Network (2007). Acute coronary syndromes. Available from: http://www.sign.ac.uk/pdf/sign93.pdf.

National Institute for Health and Clinical Excellence (2014). Atrial fibrillation. Available from: https://www.nice.org.uk/guidance/cg180

ACC/AHA/ESC (2006). Guidelines for the management of patients with atrial fibrillation—executive summary: a report of the American College of Cardiology/American Heart Associatin Task Force on Practice Guidelines. J Am Coll Cardiol 48, 854–906.

National Institute for Health and Clinical Excellence (2009). Thoracoscopic epicardial radiofrequency ablation for atrial fibrillation. Available from: http://www.nice.org.uk/ nicemedia/pdf/IPG286Guidance.pdf.

Wong CK, White HD, Wilcox RG et al. (2000). New atrial fibrillation after acute myocardial infarction independently predicts death: the GUSTO-III experience. Am Heart J 140, 878–85.

Dries DL, Exner DV, Gersh BJ, Domanski MJ, Waclawiw MA, Stevenson LW (1998). Atrial fibrillation is associated with an increased risk for mortality and heart failure progression in patients with asymptomatic and symptomatic left ventricular systolic dysfunction: a retrospective analysis of the SOLVD trials. Studies of Left Ventricular Dysfunction. J Am Coll Cardiol 32, 696–703.

Wang TJ, Parise H, Levy D et al. (2004). Obesity and the risk of new-onset atrial fibrillation. JAMA 292, 2471–7.

Ettinger PO, Wu CF, De La Cruz C Jr, Weisse AB, Ahmed SS, Regan TJ (1978). Arrhythmias and the 'Holiday Heart'. Alcohol-associated cardiac rhythm disorders. Am Heart J 95, 555–62.

2014 ACC/AHA Guideline on Perioperative Cardiovascular Evaluation and Management of Patients Undergoing Noncardiac Surgery

2014 ESC/ESA Guidelines on non-cardiac surgery:cardiovascular assessment and management. Advance Life Support Manual (ALS) Fourth Edition 2011

Botto, Fernando, et al. "Myocardial injury after noncardiac surgery: a large, international, prospective cohort study establishing diagnostic criteria, characteristics, predictors, and 30-day outcomes." Anesthesiology 120.3 (2014): 564–578.

Respiratory complications

Key guidelines
- Scottish Intercollegiate Guidelines Network (2004). Postoperative management in adults.
- American College of Physicians (2006). Risk assessment for and strategies to reduce perioperative pulmonary complications for patients undergoing non-cardiothoracic surgery.
- Scottish Intercollegiate Guidelines Network (2008). British guideline on the management of asthma.
- Resuscitation Council (UK) (2008). Emergency treatment of anaphylactic reactions.

Post-operative atelectasis
- *Incidence*—very common. Most likely cause of transient hypoxamia post-operatively, which complicates the recovery of 30–50% of patients following abdominal surgery. Endotracheal intubation and mechanical ventilation may be required in 8–10% of cases.
- *Pathophysiology*—atelectasis refers to collapse or loss of lung volume (clinically or radiologically) without evidence of respiratory infection. This results from altered compliance of lung tissue, impaired regional ventilation, and retained airway secretions in the perioperative period. Post-operative pain (especially in abdomino-thoracic surgery) contributes significantly to the reduction of functional residual capacity (FRC) and the development of atelectasis.
- *Presentation*—may remain asymptomatic, or progresses into respiratory infection or respiratory failure.
- *Diagnosis*—suspect in patients with abnormal respiratory rate (>25 or <10 breaths/min), tachycardia (>100bpm), or reduced conscious levels [CS]. Diagnosis is based on clinical examination, ABGs, sputum culture, and ECG. CXR should be reserved for patients with major lung collapse [CS].
- *Prevention*—most important (see Ch. 7). Consider continuous positive airway pressure (CPAP) in selected cases.
- *Treatment*.
  - In general, patients without significant secretions benefit from continuous positive airway pressure. For patients with significant secretions, chest physiotherapy and suctioning are most appropriate.
  - Early mobilization and breathing exercises are sufficient for most cases.
  - Extensive lobar or pulmonary collapse (unresponsive to respiratory therapy)—consider extraction of secretions using bronchoscopy (unproven efficiency).
  - Respiratory infection—maintain oxygenation, clear blocked airways, expand collapsed alveoli, and clear infection.
  - Oxygen therapy—can be delivered using nasal catheters (variable performance and low flow), Venturi masks (high flow; oxygen concentrations up to 60%), and reservoir masks (up to 70% oxygen delivery). Patients with type 2 respiratory failure due to COPD require special attention as they have chronic CO_2 retention, and therefore, are dependent on hypoxic drive. Oxygen is required to return SpO_2 to its normal (or subnormal, but acceptable) level.

Bronchospasm and asthma-like reaction

- *Incidence*—common in the post-operative period.
- *Pathophysiology*—abnormal constriction of bronchial smooth muscles, triggered by aspiration of gastric contents, medications (tubocurarine, morphine, atracurium), suctioning, endotracheal intubation, and/or exacerbation of underlying COPD or asthma.
- *Presentation*.
  - Acute severe cases—patient unable to complete a sentence in one breath, wheezy, tachycardic (>110bpm), tachypnoeic (>25rpm), and have low peak expiratory flow (PEF) if spirometry in use (33–50% of predicted).
  - Life-threatening cases—patient exhausted, confused, in coma, silent chest, cyanotic, bradycardic, hypotensive, and hypoxic (SpO2 <92%, PEF <33% of best or predicted).
- *Management*—see Box 9.3 (See also OHCM 10e Ch. 3).

Anaphylactic reaction

- *Definition*—severe, life-threatening, generalized or systemic hypersensitivity reaction that may cause death. Anaphylaxis is a much broader syndrome than 'anaphylactic shock'.
- *Pathophysiology*—sudden, systemic degranulation of mast cells or basophils with release of mediators (histamine, etc.) into the circulation.
  - Might be immunologic-mediated (IgE, IgG, immune complex) or non-immunologic-mediated (no immunoglobulin involved).
  - Organ dysfunction results from abnormal systemic vascular response (increases vascular permeability, coronary artery vasospasm, etc.), respiratory compromise (upper airway oedema, petechial

---

Box 9.3 Management of bronchospasm

Immediate management.
- Acute severe cases.
  - Oxygen 40–60%.
  - Salbutamol 5mg (or terbutaline 10mg) via nebulizer.
  - Ipratropium 0.5mg via nebulizer.
  - Consider for very ill patients—IV hydrocortisone 100mg or oral prednisolone 40–50mg or both; CXR if consolidation is expected.
  - Sedatives are contraindicated.
- Life-threatening/persistently severe cases.
  - Involve ITU team.
  - Increase nebulizers' frequency—salbutamol 5mg/15–30min or 10mg continuously hourly.
  - Magnesium sulphate 1.2–2g IV over 20min.
  - Consider (experienced staff)—IV B2 agonist, IV aminophylline, or mechanical ventilation.

Follow-up management.
- Keep the patient on:
  - Oxygen 40–60%.
  - Salbutamol and ipratropium nebulizers 4–6 hourly.
  - Prednisolone 40–50mg daily or IV hydrocortisone 100mg 6 hourly.
- Monitor for 24h, then give advice. Full instructions to GP to follow.

haemorrhages, bronchospasm, and mucus plugging), mucocutaneous vascular changes (generalized hives, flushing, pruritus, swollen lips-tongue-uvula), and increased consumption of oxygen in peripheral tissues despite decreased perfusion, leading to rapid onset of anaerobic metabolism.

- *Presentation*.
  - First impression—suspect in any patient who becomes suddenly ill (usually within minutes) upon exposure to a trigger (allergen).
  - Signs and symptoms.
    - —Skin—up to 90% of cases. Present with generalized itching, flushing, urticaria, periorbital oedema, and conjunctival swelling.
    - —Respiratory—up to 70%. Present with nasal congestion, voice changes, choking sensation, cough, wheezing, and short of breath.
    - —Gastrointestinal—up to 40%. Present with abdominal cramps, nausea, vomiting, and diarrhoea.
    - —Cardiovascular—up to 35%. Presents with dizzy feeling, tachycardia, hypotension, and peripheral collapse.
  - Criteria of diagnosis—the presence of the following three criteria makes the diagnosis of anaphylaxis most likely.
    - —Timing—sudden onset and rapid progression.
    - —ABC compromise—life-threatening disorder in airways, breathing, and/or circulation.
    - —Mucocutaneous—skin and/or mucosal changes.
    - —Supportive (but not essential) to diagnosis is the recent exposure to allergen. Notice that skin changes alone cannot be considered a confirmation criteria if unaccompanied by the other two.
  - Laboratory diagnosis—mast cell tryptase for recurrent idiopathic anaphylaxis. This is useful in follow-up, but should not delay initial assessment and management.
- *Treatment*—follow ABCDE protocol. See Box 9.4 (see also OHCM 10e Ch. 19).
  - Follow-up—keep patient for 6h in a clinical area where facilities are available for treating life-threatening conditions.
  - Early recurrence (biphasic reaction) occurs in 1–20% of cases. Patient might require 24h observation.
  - Consider antihistamine and steroids for 3d, especially in the presence of urticaria.

Box 9.4 Management of anaphylaxis

- Position the patient—supine, comfortable with elevated legs. Patient may prefer to sit up (easier for breathing), might require recovery position (unconscious) or left side position (pregnancy).
- Remove the trigger—if possible. Stop suspected drug, remove the bee sting, and do not attempt to induce vomiting in food anaphylaxis.
- ABCDE protocol—apply as appropriate (see ➜ Chapter 15, pp. 102–106).
  - Oxygen—high oxygen flow if necessary with Venturi system.
  - Crystalloid fluid bolus—500–1000mL IV. Repeat as needed.
  - Monitor—pulse oximetry, ECG, and blood pressure.
- Specific immediate management.
  - Adrenaline—give 300–500µg (0.3–0.5mL of 1:10000) IM. Repeat as required (every 3–5min). Consider IV for refractory cases (experienced staff).
- Consider also (second line).
  - Chlorpheniramine (H1 blocker)—IM or slow IV, 5–10mg (age >6y), especially for itching.
  - Hydrocortisone—IM or slow IV, 100–200mg (age >6y).
  - Bronchodilators—for wheezing (asthma-like) symptoms.

Further reading

Qaseem A, Snow V, Fitterman N et al. (2006). Risk assessment for and strategies to reduce peri-operative pulmonary complications for patients undergoing non-cardiothoracic surgery: a guide-line from the American College of Physicians. Ann Intern Med 144, 575–80.

Scottish Intercollegiate Guidelines Network (2008). British guideline on the management of asthma. Available from: http://www.sign.ac.uk/pdf/sign101.pdf.

Resuscitation Council (UK) (2008). Emergency treatment of anaphylactic reactions. Available from: http://www.resus.org.uk/pages/reaction.pdf.

Platell C, Hall JC (1997). Atelectasis after abdominal surgery. J Am Coll Surg 185, 584–92.

Squadrone V, Coha M, Cerutti E et al. (2005). Continuous positive airway pressure for treat- ment of post-operative hypoxaemia: a randomized controlled trial. JAMA 293, 589–95.

Scottish Intercollegiate Guidelines Network (2004). Postoperative management in adults. Available from: http://www.sign.ac.uk/pdf/sign77.pdf.

Sampson HA, Munoz-Furlong A, Campbell RL, et al (2006). Second symposium on the definition and management of anaphylaxis: summary report–Second National Institute of Allergy and Infectious Disease/Food Allergy and Anaphylaxis Network Symposium. J Allergy Clin Immunol 117:391.

Renal complications

Key guidelines
- NICE. Acute Kidney Injury (2013).
- The Renal Association (2002). Treatment of adults and children with renal failure.
- BMJ Clinical Evidence (2008). Acute renal failure.

Acute kidney injury (AKI)
- *Incidence*—accounts for 1% of all hospital admissions and complicates ~15% of inpatient episodes. Cases requiring dialysis have in-hospital mortality rate of 50% or more, especially when associated with sepsis in critically ill patients. Only 50% of patients with AKI receive 'good' care.
- *Definition and classification*—AKI is the abrupt and sustained decline (over hours or days) in renal excretory function, with resultant accumulation of urea and other chemicals in the blood. AKI occurs when there is a rise of creatinine >26mcmol/l in 48h, 50% rise in 7d, fall in eGFR >25% over 7d, or fall in urine output <0.5ml/kg/h over 6h (adults) or 8h (children). Based on the degree of change in serum creatinine concentration and severity of oliguria, RIFLE classification can reliably be used (Table 9.1).
- *Pathogenesis*—most in-hospital cases (>70%) are due to pre-renal (decreased renal perfusion) or acute tubular necrosis (ATN).
  - Pre-renal.
  - Fluid loss—gastrointestinal (diarrhoea, vomiting, bleeding), renal (diuretics, osmotic diuresis), skin or respiratory (sweat, burns),

Table 9.1 The RIFLE classification of ARF.

	GFR criteria*	Urine output criteria
Risk	• Increased serum creatinine ×1.5 • Decreased GFR >25%	<0.5mL/kg per h for 6h
Injury	• Increased serum creatinine x2 • Decreased GFR >50%	<0.5mL/kg per h for 12h
Failure	• Increased serum creatinine 3 • Decreased GFR >75% • Serum creatinine >4mg/dL	<0.5mL/kg per h for 24h, anuria for 12h
Loss	• Complete loss of kidney function for >4wk	
ESRD	• Complete loss of kidney function for >3mo	

GFR = actual (not estimated) glomerular filtration rate

Reproduced with permission from John Kellum, Nathan Levin, Catherine Bouman, et al. Developing a consensus classification system for acute renal failure, *Current Opinion in Critical Care*, 8 (6), 509–14, Copyright © 2002 Wolters Kluwer Health, Inc.

third space (crush injury). Hypotension—severely decreased blood pressure can result from shock (myocardial or septic) or treatment of severe hypertension.

- Decreased perfusion—severe hypotension and shock, congestive heart failure, nephrotic syndrome, and cirrhosis.
- Renal ischaemia—bilateral renal artery stenosis and hepatorenal syndrome.
- ATN—results from severe persistent pre-renal diseases or the presence of nephrotoxins (aminoglycosides, radiocontrast media, haemopigments, and others).
- Other causes—post-renal urinary tract obstruction (10%), acute glomerulonephritis, vasculitis, atheroemboli, etc.
- High risk patients include elderly (>65y) patients, chronic kidney disease (eGFR <60), heart failure, liver disease, diabetes, hypovolaemia, use of nephrotoxic drugs, symptoms of urologic obstruction, sepsis, neurologic impairment, and use of iodinated contrast agents within 1 wk.
- Risk of AKI can be quantified using online tools: http://ajlyon.co.uk/education

- Clinical presentation—asymptomatic, oliguria and dark urine, signs of renal failure (oedema, hypertension, weakness, fatigue, anorexia, mental changes), and/or signs of underlying causative disorder (shock, sepsis, etc.).
- Diagnosis.
  - Careful history and scrutiny of charts—best method to find the most likely underlying factor, and the timing and pattern of progression.
  - Urinalysis should be performed in all patients, testing for blood, protein, leucocyte, and nitrates. Do not routinely offer ultrasound of urinary tract if underlying cause is established.
  - Standard blood tests—U&Es, FBC, coagulation screen, and urine test. Consider testing for C-reactive protein (CRP), ABGs, immunologic tests, virology tests, and kidney-ureter-bladder (KUB) ultrasound scan.
  - Estimated GFR—this is only reliable in stable kidney disease and is not accurate enough in AKI. The change in values of estimated GFR is a useful marker for progression.
- Management.
  - Prevent AKI when using contrast agents by offering IV volume expansion (isotonic sodium bicarbonate or 0.9% sodium chloride) [Grade 1A], stopping ACE inhibitors temporarily, use low osmolality contrast medium, and discussing with a nephrologist beforehand.
  - Measure urine output, weight (twice daily), urea, creatinine, electrolytes, and consider measuring lactate, blood glucose, and blood gases.
  - Seek nephrology advice if stage 3 AKI, no clear cause of AKI, underlying cause requires specialist treatment, inadequate response to treatment, associating complication, renal transplant, or CKD stage 4 or 5.
  - Treat underlying factors (obstruction, hypovolaemia, etc.).
  - Using a single dose aminoglycoside is less nephrotoxic and appears to have similar benefits.
  - Data does not support using other agents (mannitol, theophylline, and calcium channel blockers) in AKI.

- Fluid management.

  IV sodium chloride (0.9%)—can reduce the incidence of AKI in high-risk patients when compared with unrestricted oral fluid regime.

  Loop diuretics plus fluids have adverse effect on renal function and can only be used for hypervolaemia or established oedema while renal function is recovering or patient awaiting/receiving renal replacement therapy.
- Treat/protect from complications—infection, hyperkalaemia, pulmonary oedema, bleeding.
- Consider dialysis in appropriate cases—refractory pulmonary oedema, severe metabolic acidosis (pH <7.2 or base excess <10), severe persistent hyperkalaemia (K+ >7mmol/L), or complicated uraemia (uraemic encephalopathy, pericarditis, etc.).

  There is no supportive evidence for prophylactic renal replacement therapy with haemofiltration in reducing the risk of contrast nephropathy.
- In haemofiltration, a patient's blood is passed through a set of tubing (a filtration circuit) via a machine to a semipermeable membrane (the filter) where waste products and water (collectively called ultrafiltrate) are removed by convection. Replacement fluid is added and the blood is returned to the patient. In dialysis, blood flows by one side of a semi-permeable membrane, and a dialysate, or special dialysis fluid, flows by the opposite side. Smaller solutes and fluid pass through the membrane, but not larger ones (red blood cells, large proteins, etc.). The counter-current flow of the blood and dialysate maximizes the concentration gradient of solutes between the blood and dialysate, which helps to remove more urea and creatinine from the blood.

Further reading

The Renal Association (2002). Treatment of adults and children with renal failure. Available from: http://www.renal.org/Standards/RenalStandards_2002b.pdf.

Kellum J, Leblanc M, Venkataraman R (2008). Acute renal failure. BMJ Clin Evid 9, 2001.

Bellomo R, Ronco C, Kellum JA, Mehta RL, Palevsky P (2004). Acute renal failure—definition, outcome measures, animal models, fluid therapy and information technology needs: the Second International Consensus Conference of the Acute Dialysis Quality Initiative (ADQI) Group. Crit Care 8, 204–12.

Bagshaw SM, Langenberg C, Wan L, May CN, Bellomo R (2007). A systematic review of urinary findings in experimental septic acute renal failure. Crit Care Med 35, 1592–8.

Pepin MN, Bouchard J, Legault L, Ethier J (2007). Diagnostic performance of fractional excre-tion of urea and fractional excretion of sodium in the evaluations of patients with acute kidney injury with or without diuretic treatment. Am J Kidney Dis 50, 566–73.

Hilton R (2006). Acute renal failure. Clinical review. BMJ 333, 786–90.

NICE (2013). Acute kidney injury: Prevention, detection and management of acute kidney injury up to the point of renal replacement therapy.

Neurological complications

Key guidelines
- Royal College of Physicians (2012) National clinical guidelines for stroke.
- Scottish Intercollegiate Guidelines Network (2010). Management of patients with stroke.
- BMJ Clinical Evidence (2008). Stroke management.

Transient ischaemic attack (TIA) and stroke
- *Incidence*—infrequent in surgical practice, but remains the third most common cause of death in most developed countries. About 0.3–3.5% of in-hospital general surgical patients develop a stroke, depending on the age and the presence of atherosclerotic risk factors. Most cases (85%) occur post-operatively, and few intraoperatively.
- *Pathogenesis*—mostly due to occlusive ischaemic injury to the brain following thromboemboli rather than haemorrhage. Possible sources of emboli are cardiac (AF) or carotid stenotic lesion (see ⊃ Chapter 47, pp. 457–460).
- *Clinical presentation*—rapid development of focal or generalized loss of cerebral function (lasting >24h in stroke) and/or leading to death.
- *Outcome*—about 10% die within 30d of onset. Nearly half of survivors experience some level of disability developing over 6mo period.
  - *Clinical disabilities*—may include arm, hand or leg weakness, sensory loss, aphasia, dysarthria, visual field defect, and cognitive impairment.
  - *Physical limitations*—walking, dressing, toileting, feeding, and bathing. Urinary and faecal incontinence are common.
  - *Common complications*—depression, anxiety, general pain, epileptic seizures, pressure sores, venous thromboembolism, and chest and urinary tract infection.
- *Diagnosis*—See also ⊃ Computed Tomography OHCM 10e. Ch 16.
  - Seek specialist advice [B].
  - *CT scan*—the first investigation of choice [B].
    —Indications—all patients.
    —Timing—as soon as possible. The maximum time between admission and brain scan is 12 hours [B], but the scan should be in the first hour if any of the following apply: patients with coagulation issues (anticoagulant treatment, bleeding tendency, possibility for thrombolysis), severe neurological defect (depressed level of consciousness, progressive or fluctuating symptoms, papilloedema or stiff neck, fever or severe headache on initial presentation.
  - *MRI scan*—reserve for patients with uncertain cause or equivocal results on CT scan.
  - *Other assessments*—risk of aspiration (50mL water swallow screening test), moving and handling requirements, and risk of pressure ulcers [B, C].
- *Treatment*—should be provided in specialized unit (Table 9.2) [A].

Table 9.2 Treatment of stroke

General management*		
Vital functions	• Maintain arterial oxygenation, blood glucose, hydration, and temperature within normal.	[B]
Blood pressure	• Only modest lowering of BP is indicated in the acute phase. Very high BP (mean BP >110 and diastolic BP >90) increases mortality (1.6). Rapid drop of BP may increase cerebral ischaemia.	[B]
Mobilization	• As soon as possible.	[B]
Special arrangements		
Antiplatelets	• Aspirin (300mg od)—for all patients, orally(NGT if dysphagic) or rectally, following exclusion of intracerebral haemorrhage by brain imaging • Clopidogrel (75mg od)—acceptable alternative for patients allergic to Aspirin.	[A]
Anticoagulation	• Start in every patient with AF (persistent or paroxysmal) if not contraindicated. Anticoagulation is otherwise not routinely used for ischaemic stroke	[A]
Statin		[A]
Surgical intervention		
Carotid endarterectomy	• Simvastatin 40mg. for every patient if not contraindicated. • Carotid artery territory stroke in patients with no severe disability should be considered for carotid endarterectomy. • Timing—Within 7d of onset of symptoms	[A]

* Other types of assessment, physiotherapy, interventions, and follow-up should be organized and provided by the specialist unit

Thrombolysis: Any patient, regardless of age or stroke severity, where treatment can be started within 3h of known symptom onset and who has been shown mot to have an intracerebral haemorrhage or other contraindications should be considered for treatment using Alteplase

Further reading

Royal College of Pysicians (2012) National Clinical Guidelinefor Stroke. Prepared by the Intercollegiate Stroke working Party. Fourth Edition.

Alawneh J, Clatworthy P, Morris R, Warburton E (2008). Stroke management. BMJ Clin Evid 9, 201.

Bell R, Merli G (1998). Perioperative assessment and management of the surgical patient with neurologic problems. In: Merli G, Weitz H, eds. Medical management of the surgical patient, pp. 283–311, WB Saunders, Philadelphia.

Principles of wound care*

Background *106*
Wound assessment *107*
Wound management *108*
Dressing selection *112*
Further reading *114*

Key guidelines
- NICE (2016) Chronic wounds advanced dressings.
- European Wound Management Association (2002–2008). Position documents.
- NICE (2014). Pressure ulcers.
- NHSSB (2005). Wound management manual.
- American Society of Plastic Surgeons (2007). Evidence-based clinical practice guideline: chronic wounds of the lower extremity.
- European Wound Management Association (2013). Debridement document.
- BMJ Clinical Evidence (2011). Diabetes: foot ulcers and amputations.

* The guidelines on this chapter have been sourced and summarized from different UK, Europe, and international government sources, professional organizations, and medical specialty societies. Leading guidelines have been listed in the further reading section at the end of this chapter.

Background

- *Definition of a wound*—disruption of normal skin structure and function due to internal or external injury. Chronic wounds are those unresponsive to initial therapy or persistent in spite of appropriate care.
- *Healing process*—very complex orchestral cascade of biochemical and cellular processes triggered by tissue injury.
  - *Wound scar strength*—achieves 30–50% of unwounded tissue strength in 4–6wk and 60% at 6mo. Never regains the same breaking strength as normal healthy skin. Ultimately acquires ~70–80% of the strength of uninjured skin.
  - *Healing phases*—vascular response, inflammatory response, proliferation, and maturation.
  - *Factors affecting healing (adversely)*—advanced age and smoking, underlying disorders (diabetes, cancer, malnutrition, dehydration), other treatment modalities (chemotherapy and radiotherapy), and poor wound care and surgical technique.

Wound assessment

- Accurate and thorough assessment—is essential in achieving effective treatment [C]. Baseline information helps to formulate a plan of care, evaluate healing process and efficacy of treatment regime, and ensure continuity and consistency during management period.
- Source of information—patient and family members on the extent of the problem (e.g. odour of wound and amount/type of exudate), nursing and medical notes, direct observation, and history and physical examination of other organ systems.
- Clinical history and physical examination—this should include a certain minimum set of information (Box 10.1) [B].

Box 10.1 Wound assessment

- *Duration*—current and previous wound complaints.
- *Wound site*—record and draw accurately.
- *Wound dimensions*—measure using appropriate method. The ruler-based assessment is simple and widely available. Measure the maximum width × breadth × depth. Other helpful methods include transparency tracings or grid camera.
  - Repeat measurement regularly while treating the wound; weekly recordings are usually sufficient.
- *Wound edges*—describe carefully: *rolled* (growing from centre), *everted* (growing from edges), *punched out* (vascular, neuropathic, or syphilitic—resulting from sloughing of the dead full thickness skin without concomitant repair), *flat sloping* (healing ulcer such as venous ulcers), or *undetermined* (pressure or tubercular ulcer—infected subcutaneous tissue).
- Wound bed base.
  - *Benefits of assessment*—indirect indicator of stage of healing and healthiness of the wound. Provides the basis for choosing a suitable dressing (see below).
  - *Colour classification of wounds*—black (necrotic), red (granulating), yellow (sloughy), pink (epithelialization), green (infected), or combination of them (e.g. 30% yellow/slough + 70% red/granulation). The colouring system (though not perfect) is used widely to provide a communication method and monitor progression.
- *Wound exudate*—look for the type, colour, and amount.
  - *Type and colour*—serous (clear fluid, no pus or blood or debris), sanguinous (almost entirely composed of blood), serosanguinous (clear fluid mixed with blood), or purulent (pus-like, viscous, and cloudy)
  - *Amount*—minimal or dry (no exudate), low (wound bed only is moist), moderate (wound bed and surrounding skin is moist), or high (surrounding skin is macerated).
- *Wound odour*—may have significant effect on quality of life.
  - *Described as*—absent (none), malodorous, very offensive odour only on taking off the dressing or filling the room.
  - *Effects of malodour*—can cause social isolation, nausea and vomiting, and even malnutrition.
  - *Cause of malodour*—should be established and treated appropriately (infection, dressing material, etc.).
- *Associated pain*—describe carefully: pain location (in or around the wound, in the leg/foot, intermittent claudication pain), frequency, and severity. Pain is a good indicator of current treatment efficacy.
- *Other organ systems*—should be checked as and where appropriate.
- Non-healing wounds may require biopsy to establish diagnosis [B].

Wound management

- *Principles*—four main principles: effective debridement, infection control, optimal dressing, and promotion of healing (Fig. 10.1) [B].
- *TIME*—the European Wound Management Association (EWMA) acronym 'TIME' refers to the same principles: Tissue management, Infection and inflammation control, Moisture balance, and Epithelial advancement.

Wound cleansing and pressure relief

- Universal precautions—should be followed at all times. These include washing and drying hands thoroughly, wearing plastic apron and gloves, and avoiding cross-contamination.
- Wound with no debris—does not require cleansing [C].
- Irrigate wound—with copious amount of physiologic saline 0.9% or ordinary tap water for leg ulcers [C]. Warm up the irrigating solution to room (or ideally body) temperature [B].
- Take swabs if necessary—best taken at this stage by using a zigzag motion with a vigorous rotation over the wound.
  - Take separate swabs for apparently separate infected areas (avoid cross-contamination). Place obtained swabs directly into the sample tube to avoid airborne contamination.

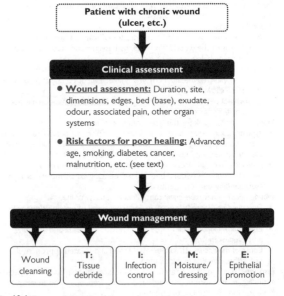

Fig. 10.1 Proposed algorithm for wound management.

- Pressure relief—this should be achieved by repositioning time schedule and using pressure-reducing devices (consider using pressure relieving devices such as mattresses, cushions, gutter, splints, etc. in limb oedema) [B].

Tissue management (debridement)

- *Indications*—all necrotic, poorly vascularized, and infected tissues must be adequately removed [B].
  - *Repeat as necessary*—serial sharp debridement helps to stimulate a healthy environment and promotes healing.
  - *Irrigate with saline*—under pressure. This reduces the bacterial surface contamination and is a recommended practice [B].
  - *Antiseptic solutions*—not recommended. They are toxic to human tissues and may delay healing [B].
- Dry hard eschar with normal looking surrounding skin—may be left alone [B], although some centres prefer to debride pressure ulcers so that the extent of the tissue damage can be assessed and aid quicker healing.
- Methods of debridement—include sharp (using a knife), autolytic (self-biologic process supported by appropriate dressing), enzymatic (using chemical enzymes), mechanical (using a wet-to-dry dressing), laser, larval therapy (using maggots to ingest dead tissues), water (using high pressure water jet), and low frequency ultrasound debridement.
  - Maggot therapy—proteolytic enzymes secreted by larvae liquefies necrotic tissue and allow for its digestion while leaving healthy tissue intact. Additional benefits include antimicrobial action and stimulation of wound healing. Maggot therapy increased slough percentage (67 vs 55% for traditional therapy|) and improved wound healing but not beyond one week of use.

Infection control

Definitions

- *Contamination*—wound acquires the pathogen transiently with no invasion or multiplication.
- *Colonization*—the microbial pathogen grows and multiplies, but does not invade the host or interferes with wound healing.
- *Wound infection*—the infecting organism interferes with the normal functioning of the host, utilizes the host's resources, and interrupts the normal healing process.

Diagnosis

- Criteria in Table 10.1 and Box 10.2 are adopted with modification from the international, multidisciplinary Delphi group consensus statement recruited by EWMA.
- Swabs for culture and sensitivity—must be obtained from relevant infected sites (separately) using aseptic technique.
- Topical antiseptics—iodine-based dressings reduce bacterial load and stimulate healing. Silver-based dressings have no proven advantages in improving wound healing in a Cochrane review. Honey provides high osmolarity and high concentration of hydrogen peroxide. There is good evidence of its benefits in burns but not enough evidence in venous ulcers.

Table 10.1 Diagnostic criteria for wound infection*

Diagnostic	Possible	Non-diagnostic
Acute wound		
• Pus/abscess • Cellulitis	• Delayed healing • Erythema ± induration • Exudate = haemopurulent, seropurulent, malodour • Wound breakdown/enlargement • Pocketing	• Increase in local skin temperature • Oedema • Pain/tenderness
Diabetic foot (adding to the above)		
• Purulent exudate • Lymphangitis • Phlegmon	• Joint crepitus • Swelling with increase in exudates • Localized pain in a normally asensate foot • Probes to bone	• Spreading dry necrosis • Exposed bone or tendon • Friable granulation tissue easily bleeds

*See original guidelines for full list

Box 10.2 Diagnostic criteria for superficial surgical site infection (SSI)

All suspected infections (localized pain or tenderness, localized swelling, redness, or heat) involving only the skin or subcutaneous tissue around the incision within 30d of procedure, with at least one of the following:
• Purulent discharge from the superficial incision.
• Pathogenic organisms isolated from an aseptically obtained culture of fluid or tissue from the superficial incision.
  The following are not reported as superficial SSI:
• Stitch abscess (minimal inflammation and discharge confined to the points of suture penetration).
• Infection of an episiotomy or neonate's circumcision site.
• Infected burn wound.
• Incisional SSI that extends into the facial and muscle layers (deep SSI).

Risk for osteomyelitis
• Suspect in the presence of exposed bone (or easily probed), open fracture, underlying internal fixation, gangrenous wound, persistent sinus tract, and non-healing wound [B]. Plain X-ray, bone scan, and/ or MRI scan should be considered to confirm and assess the extent of infection [B].
• MRI scan is the procedure of choice to establish the diagnosis in clinically high suspicious cases [B]. Bone culture and biopsy should be obtained [B].

Risk for endocarditis
See ➲ Chapter 22, pp.161–6.

Treatment
- Pain relief and patient reassurance.
- Surgical drainage and debridement—for abscesses and necrotic infected tissues [B]. Severe life-threatening infections may require extensive debridement and possible amputation [B]. Severe osteomyelitis requires aggressive resection and coverage with well-perfused tissue (e.g. muscles) [B].
- Systemic antibiotics—in all established wound infections as per approved unit protocols [A]. Prudent use is important to reduce the risk of antibiotic induced diarrhoea.
  - Common microbial pathogens:
        Aerobic—B-haemolytic *Streptococci*, *Staphylococcus aureus* and MRSA, *Escherichia coli*, and *Klebsiella*.
        Anaerobic—*Bacteroides*, *Clostridium tetani*, and *Clostridium welchii* (gas gangrene).
  - Type and route of antibiotics—depends on expected pathogen, unit protocols, and severity of infection. Commonly used regimes include cephalosporins, amoxicillin-clavulanic acid, macrolides, anti-staphylococcal penicillins, and fluoroquinolones [B].
  - Topical antibiotics—only use with caution in selected cases and under regular review [B]. Possible indications include wounds with poor blood supply (systemic antibiotics may not reach therapeutic levels), wounds with frequent contamination (e.g. faeces), unsuccessful long-term systemic antibiotics with bacterial resistance, antibiotic allergy, and planned delayed primary closure.
- Wound dressing—select the most appropriate (see below) and apply daily.

Dressing selection

- Ideal dressing—should protect, cleanse, optimize, and promote the wound healing process (Table 10.2) [B].
- Dressing types—differ in its source of origin and mechanism of action. They also have different capabilities to achieve one or more of the ideal dressing functions.
- Selection of dressing—depends on (Table 10.2):
  - Accurate assessment of wound—e.g. heavy or light exudative, odorous, sloughy, and/or infected.
  - Stage of healing process—one universally used approach is to use hydrogels (with other debriding agents) for debridement stage, foam and low-adherent dressing for granulation stage, and hydrocolloid and low adherent dressing for epithelisation stage.
  - Negative pressure wound therapy (VAC therapy) enhances healing process by reducing oedema, stimulating circulation, and promoting rate of granulation tissue formation. Data support the benefits of this therapy in significantly reducing the time to wound closure in diabetic patients, returning these patients to baseline more quickly and improving quality of life. Nevertheless, there is a need for better quality studies on this subject.
  - Skin graft—split and full thickness skin grafts should be considered to cover large wounds that are unlikely to heal appropriately with second intention.
  - Bioengineered skin substitutes—are composed of a live-cell construct that contains at least one layer of live allogenic cells, or from acellular scaffold. There is some evidence of their benefits in treating large wounds.
  - Hyperbaric oxygen therapy—has been used as an adjunct to wound care in the treatment of acute and chronic wounds. A Cochrane review indicates that most studies are limited by small sample size and are of low quality.
- All dressings are claimed to be effective, and current evidences cannot distinguish a clear benefit of one over the other, providing they are delivering one or more functions required for the particular wound type and stage.
- There is no evidence to support the routine use of antimicrobial (e.g. silver, iodine or honey) dressings ahead of non-medicated dressings.
- Experimental wound management—includes beta blocker cream (Timolol has limited evidence of promoting keratinocytes in unresponsive wounds), platelet-derived growth factor, epidermal growth factor, and granulocyte-macrophage colony stimulating factors.

Table 10.2 Dressing types

Alginate (e.g. Kaltostat®, Sorban®, Tegaderm®)	• Source—calcium and sodium salts of alginic acid polymer (seaweed). • Action—fibres absorb liquid and swell. Promote micro-environment. May be haemostatic. • Best in— heavily exudatitive wounds. • Protect - / cleanse +++ / optimize + / promote +.
Hydrogel (e.g. Nu-Gel®)	• Source— insoluble polymers. • Action—swell and increase in volume until saturated. • Best in—moderately exudative, not in heavily exudative or anaerobes. • Protect - / cleanse + / optimize ++ / promote +.
Hydrocolloids (e.g. DuoDerm®)	• Source—gel-forming polysaccharides and proteins that absorb water and swell. • Action—polymers absorb liquid and swell. Provides moist micro-environment. • Best in—moderately exudative and granulating wounds. • Protect + / cleanse ++ / optimize ++ / promote ±.
Surgical absorbent	• Source—cotton, gauze. • Action—absorbant, but allows leaking. Severely adherent to tissues. • Best as—second layer in heavily exudative wounds. • Protect ++++ / cleanse + / optimize -- / promote --.
Metronidazole gel	• Source—gel containing 0.8% w/v metronidazole. Provides moist environment. • Action—combats infection in malodorous wounds. • Best in—malodorous. • Protect - / cleanse ++ / optimize + / promote ±.
Low-adherent (e.g. NA Ultra®)	• Protect ++ / cleanse - / optimize + / promote ±.
Non-adherent foam (e.g. Mepilex®)	• Protect ++ / cleanse + / optimize + / promote ±.
Odour-absorbing (e.g. Carboflex®)	• Protect + / cleanse ++ / optimize - / promote ±.

Further reading

European Wound Management Association (2002–2008). Position documents (with kind permission). Available from: http://ewma.org/resources/for-professionals/ewma-documents-and-joint-publications/ewma-position-documents-2002-2008

NHSSB (2005). Wound Management Manual. Available from: https://openlibrary.org/books/OL16407175M/NHSSB_wound_management_manual

American Society of Plastic Surgeons (2007). Evidence-based clinical practice guideline: chronic wounds of the lower extremity. Available from http://www.plasticsurgery.org/Documents/medical-professionals/health-policy/evidence-practice/Evidence-based-Clinical-Practice-Guideline-Chronic-Wounds-of-the-Lower-Extremity.pdf

European Wound Management Association (2013). Document: Wound Debridement. Available from: http://lohmann-rauscher.co.uk/downloads/clinical-evidence/JWC_EWMA_Debridement.pdf

BMJ Clinical Evidence Wounds. (UK) Available from:: http://clinicalevidence.bmj.com/x/systematic-review/1902/overview.html

Department of Health (2007). Third prevalence survey of health care associated infections in acute hospitals in England 2006. Available from http://webarchive.nationalarchives.gov.uk/20081105143757/dh.gov.uk/en/Publicationsandstatistics/Publications/PublicationsPolicyAndGuidance/DH_078388

European Wound Management Association (2005). Identifying criteria from wound infection. Available from: http://www.cslr.cz/download/English_pos_doc_final.pdf

Lait ME, Smith LN (1998). Wound management: a literature review. J Clin Nurs 7, 11–7.

BNF. 56. Appendix 8. Avalable from: https://bnf.nice.org.uk/wound-management/

Opletalová K, Blaizot X, Mourgeon B, et al. Maggot therapy for wound debridement: a randomized multicenter trial. Arch Dermatol 2012; 148:432.

Lipsky BA, Hoey C. Topical antimicrobial therapy for treating chronic wounds. Clin Infect Dis 2009; 49:1541.

Vermeulen H, van Hattem JM, Storm-Versloot MN, Ubbink DT. Topical silver for treating infected wounds. Cochrane Database Syst Rev 2007;:CD005486.

Jull AB, Cullum N, Dumville JC, et al. Honey as a topical treatment for wounds. Cochrane Database Syst Rev 2015; 3:CD005083.

Tang JC, Dosal J, Kirsner RS. Topical timolol for a refractory wound. Dermatol Surg 2012; 38:135.

Ubbink DT, Westerbos SJ, Evans D, et al. Topical negative pressure for treating chronic wounds. Cochrane Database Syst Rev 2008;:CD001898.

Sanders, Lee, et al. "A prospective, multicenter, randomized, controlled clinical trial comparing a bioengineered skin substitute to a human skin allograft." Ostomy/wound management 60.9 (2014): 26-38.

Kranke P, Bennett MH, Martyn-St James M, et al. Hyperbaric oxygen therapy for chronic wounds. Cochrane Database Syst Rev 2012; 4:CD004123.

Preoperative assessment of bleeding risk*

Background *116*
Clinical assessment *116*
Laboratory assessment *117*
Management of bleeding tendency *118*
Further reading *119*

Key guidelines
- British Committee for Standards in Haematology (2008). Guidelines on the assessment of bleeding risk prior to surgery or invasive procedures.
- National Blood Authority Australia (2015). Preoperative bleeding assessment tool.

---

* The guidelines on this chapter have been sourced and summarized from different UK, Europe, and international government sources, professional organizations, and medical specialty societies. Leading guidelines have been listed in the further reading section at the end of this chapter.

Background

- Assessment of bleeding risk has been traditionally performed using unselected coagulation tests. Modern evidence-based practice should be based on focused clinical history, physical examination, and selected laboratory tests [B].

Clinical assessment

- *Screening clinical history*—all patients undergoing surgical interventions should be clinically screened for bleeding risk using three main questions [C]:
  - *Personal bleeding history*—any evidence of excessive post-surgical or post-traumatic bleeding.
  - *Family history*—any bleeding tendencies or excessive bleeding following surgery.
  - *Medications*—any current or previous use of anticoagulation or antithrombotic drugs.
- *Structured clinical history*—if screening questions were positive, in-depth clinical assessment should be performed. Negative screening clinical history in minor or moderate surgery (see below) requires no further in-depth history or coagulation tests [C].
  - *Accuracy*—in patients with normal screening bleeding history, the incidence of finding abnormal coagulation tests that require treatment is 0.3%. Positive abnormal screening history is associated with 15% chance of finding abnormal coagulation tests requiring treatment.
  - *General approach*—personal bleeding history depends on patients' perceptions of bleeding, which vary considerably. No uniform assessment exists, and effective dialogue between the patient and physician is essential for comprehensive assessment of the bleeding diathesis.
  - *Structured clinical history*—include:
    —Past bleeding complaints.
    —Current or previous history of iron deficiency anaemia.
    —Patient's usual response to physical trauma (surgical procedures, tooth extractions, accidents, etc.).
    —History of blood transfusion.
    —Character of menstrual cycle in females.
    —Dietary habits.
    —Certain complaints such as haematuria, melaena, and menorrhagia are often non-discriminatory and the underlying cause should be explored rather than accepting bleeding diathesis as the explanation.
- *Medications*—any prescribed, over-the-counter or herbal products, use of aspirin, warfarin, and/or Clopidogrel. Medication dose, frequency, and recent blood checks should be obtained. Recent use of antibiotics should also be documented.

Laboratory assessment

- *Indications*—for further coagulation screen include:
  - Positive screening (or detailed) clinical history [C].
  - Significant medical history (e.g. liver, renal, cardiac) [G].
  - Moderate or high-risk surgical interventions [G].
    - —Operating on vital organs—neurosurgery, vascular surgery, ophthalmic procedures.
    - —Extensive dissection—e.g. pelvic surgery, laparotomy, thoracotomy, mastectomy.
    - —Difficulty in securing direct haemostasis—closed liver or renal biopsies.
    - —Expected induced haemostatic defect—extensive malignancy, cardiopulmonary bypass surgery.
- *Coagulation screen tests*—include (as appropriate) haemogram (haemoglobin, blood smear, etc.), platelet studies (platelet count, morphology, function), prothrombin time (PT), activated prothromboplastin time (aPTT), fibrinogen, and bleeding time.
- *Local policies*—should be followed as appropriate.

Management of bleeding tendency

- Depends on the uncovered underlying abnormality. See Fig. 10.1.

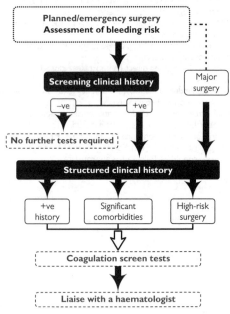

Fig. 10.1 Proposed algorithm for the assessment of bleeding risk in surgical patients.

Further reading

Chee YL, Crawford JC, Watson HG, Greaves M; British Committee for Standards in Haematology (2008). Guidelines on the assessment of bleeding risk prior to surgery or invasive procedures. Br J Haematol 140, 496–504.

Houry S, Georgeac C, Hay JM, Fingerhut A, Boudet MJ (1995). A prospective multicentre evaluation of preoperative haemostatic screening tests. The French Associations for Surgical Research. Am J Surg 170, 19–23.

National Blood Authority Australia (2015). Preoperative bleeding assessment tool.

Venous thromboembolism (VTE) prophylaxis

Basic facts *122*
Prophylaxis methods *123*
Current recommendations *124*
Further reading *126*

Key guidelines
- NICE (2017). Management of venous thromboembolic diseases and rule of thrombophilia testing.
- National Institute for Health and Clinical Excellence (2010). Venous thromboembolism. Reducing the risk of VTE in adults admitted to hospital.
- Scottish Intercollegiate Guidelines Network (2010). Prophylaxis of venous thromboembolism.
- BNF 2015: Section 2.8: Anticoagulants and protamine.

Basic facts

- Venous thromboembolism (VTE) (referring collectively to deep venous thrombosis (DVT) and pulmonary embolism (PE)) is the most common preventable cause of hospital death worldwide. VTE is responsible for about 25,000 deaths per year in the UK and 60,000 to 100,000 per year in the USA.
- Massive PE, the sudden killer, is estimated to occur in up to 5% of high-risk patients, not receiving prophylaxis, following high-risk surgery.
- Risk factors—see Table 12.1. Virchow's triad (factors causing stasis in blood flow, venous endothelial injury, and/or hypercoagulable state of blood) is a good concise summary of major processes leading to VTE. It is important to ensure an ultimate 100% compliance (target 90%) with the requirement for risk assessment of every individual patient admitted to the hospital. Risk assessment should be carried out on admission, again after 24h, and whenever the medical condition changes. A 'Risk Assessment for VTE' tool is available from the Department of Health.

Table 12.1 Major risk factors for VTE

Factor	Risk
Personal factors	
Age >60	×1.7 per each decade over 55
Obesity (BMI >30kg/m^2)	×2–3
Immobility (>3d bed rest, paralysis, plaster cast)	×10
Continuous traveler – trips >3h in the 4wk pre- or post-operatively	
Surgical factors	
Hospitalization (acute trauma, acute illness, surgery)	×10
Active cancer (or cancer treatment)	×7
CVP line in situ	
Severe infection	
Varicose veins with associated phlebitis	×1.5
Inflammatory bowel disease	
Medical factors	
Personal or family history of VTE	VTE recurrence rate 75% per y
Recent myocardial infarction or stroke	
Others: paraproteinaemia, paroxysmal nocturnal haemoglobinuria, Beçet's disease, antiphospholipid syndrome, inherited thrombophilia, myeloproliferative diseases, nephrotic syndrome	
Reproductive factors	
Use of oral contraceptives, hormonal replacement therapy, or tamoxifen/raloxifene	×3 (×6 for high-dose progesterone oils)
Pregnancy or puerperium	×10

Prophylaxis methods

- *General measures.*
  - Early mobility and leg exercises.
  - Adequate hydration—dehydration strongly correlates with VTE and should be avoided. Adequate hydration increases blood flow and reduces viscosity.
- *Mechanical measures.*
  - Graduated compression stockings (GCS)—effective in increasing deep venous blood flow velocity by 75% when correct pressures are applied (British Standard Class II and European Standard Class I stockings).
  - Intermittent pneumatic compression (IPC) devices—periodically apply moderate pressure on the calf/thigh muscles. Effective in reducing DVT risk by 56%.
  - Other mechanical methods—include mechanical foot pumps and electrical stimulation. Recommended for use when GCS inappropriate.
- *Pharmacological measures.*
  - Low-dose heparin—heparin is composed of heavy chains of polysaccharides that bind and accelerate the action of antithrombin and other coagulation factors/enzymes (X, IX, XI, and XII). Low-dose heparin reduces DVT risk by >50% (RR ×0.44), PE risk by 30% (RR ×0.70), and increases post-operative major bleeding risk by >46% (RR ×1.46). Prolonged use increases the risk of thrombocytopaenia and regular platelets count check should be performed. Low-dose heparin is recommended for patients with severe renal impairment or failure.
  - Low molecular weight heparin (LMWH)—short chains of heparin that bind less avidly to heparin binding proteins and allow for lower effective doses and more predictable levels. LMWH reduces DVT risk by >50% (RR ×0.49), PE risk by >60% (RR ×0.36), and increases post-operative major bleeding risk by >75% (RR ×1.77) when given preoperatively as compared to giving immediately before or early after surgery. The risk of thrombocytopaenia is less on using LMWH.
  - Fondaparinux and idraparinux—synthetic pentasaccharides that specifically and indirectly inhibit the activated factor Xa through its potentiation of antithrombin. Fondaparinux reduces DVT risk by 48% (RR ×0.52), PE risk by >60% (RR ×0.70), and increases the risk of major bleeding post-operatively compared to LMWH (RR ×1.49).
- Other measures—vena caval filters should be considered for surgical inpatients with recent (within 1mo) or existing VTE, and in whom anticoagulation is contraindicated.

Current recommendations

- General approach—depends on the type of operation (Table 12.2, Table 12.3).
- All medical patients—should, as part of a mandatory risk assessment, be considered for thromboprophylaxis measures. LMWH is the preferred prophylactic method. Aspirin is not recommended for thromboprophylaxis in medical patients.
- *Special precautions.*
  - Before admission—assess risk factors for each individual patient, advise on considering the cessation of combined oral contraceptives pills, HRT or tamoxifen/raloxifene for 4wk before elective surgery, and provide patients with verbal and written information on VTE.
  - On admission—offer all patients thigh-length GCS (or knee-length GCS if thigh-length not available or not tolerated) if not contraindicated. Wearing stockings requires active help by trained staff members. Best practice is to keep GCS on until normal mobility is resumed.
- Any tick for thrombosis risk should prompt thromboprophylaxis.
- Any tick for bleeding risk should prompt clinical staff to consider if bleeding risk is sufficient to preclude pharmacological intervention.

Table 12.2 Current recommendations for VTE prophylaxis

Type of operation	No extra risk factors*	>1 extra risk factors
General surgery	Mechanical	Mechanical + LMWH/fondaparinux**
Vascular	Mechanical	Mechanical + LMWH**

* See Table 12.1; ** If patient is not already on or requiring anticoagulation (therapeutic dose)

Table 12.3 Risk assessment for VTE prophylaxis

Thrombosis risk	Bleeding risk
Elderly and immobile patient	
• Age >60	
• Obesity (BMI > 30kg/m^2)	
• Significantly reduced mobility >3d	
Current significant disease	**Current significant disease**
• Dehydration	• Active bleeding
• Active cancer or cancer treatment	• Acquired bleeding disorders (such
• Hip fracture	as acute liver failure)
• Acute surgical admission with	• Acute stroke
inflammatory or intra-abdominal	• Uncontrolled systolic hypertension
condition	(230/120mmHg or higher)
• Critical care admission	
• Pregnancy or <6wk post partum	
Significant co-morbidities	
• Heart disease; metabolic, endocrine or	
respiratory pathologies; acute infectious	
diseases; inflammatory conditions	
Major surgery	**Special surgery/procedure**
• Total anaesthetic + surgical	• Neurosurgery, spinal surgery or
time >90min	eye surgery
• Surgery involving pelvis or lower limb	• Lumbar puncture/epidural/spinal
with a total anaesthetic + surgical	anaesthesia expected within the
time >60min	next 12h
• Surgery with significant reduction in	• Lumbar puncture/epidural/spinal
mobility	anaesthesia within the previous 4h
Thrombogenic status	**Bleeding disorder**
• Known thrombophilias	• Thrombocytopaenia (platelets
• Personal history or first-degree relative	<75×10^9/l)
with a history of VTE	• Untreated inherited bleeding
• Use of hormone replacement therapy,	disorders (such as haemophilia and
or oestrogen-containing contraceptive	von Willebrand's disease)
therapy	
• Varicose veins with phlebitis	

Data from National Institute for Health and Clinical Excellence (2010). Venous thromboembolism: reducing the risk of venous thromboembolism in patients admitted to hospital. Available from: URL: http://www.nice.org.uk/guidance/cg92

Further reading

National Institute for Health and Clinical Excellence (2017). Venous thromboembolism. https://pathways.nice.org.uk/pathways/venous-thromboembolism

Scottish Intercollegiate Guidelines Network (2010). Prevention and management of venous thromboembolism. Available from: http://www.sign.ac.uk/assets/qrg122.pdf

BNF 2015. Section 2.8: Anticoagulants and protamine. Available from: http://bnf.nice.org.uk/treatment-summary/oral-anticoagulants.html

Department of Health (2007). Report of the independent working group on the prevention of venous thromboembolism in hospitalized patients. Available from: http://www.venous-thromboembolism.org/reports/DH_073950.pdf

Centers for Disease control and prevention 2014. DVT & PE Data & Statistics. Available from: Centers for Disease control and prevention 2018. DVT & PE Data & Statistics. Available from: https://www.cdc.gov/ncbddd/dvt/data.html

Kikura M, Takada T, Sato S (2005). Preexisting morbidity as an independent risk factor for peri-operative acute thromboembolism syndrome. Arch Surg 140, 1210–7.

Tsai AW, Cushman M, Rosamond WD, Heckert SR, Polak JF, Folsom AR (2002). Cardiovascular risk factors and venous thromboembolism incidence: the longitudinal investigation of thrombo-embolism aetiology. Arch Intern Med 162, 1182–9.

National Collaborating Centre for Acute Care: Venous Thromboembolism: Reducing the risk in Surgical In-patients 2007. ISBN: 0-9549760_3_7

Prevention of infective endocarditis (IE)*

Basic facts *128*
Prophylaxis *129*
Further reading *130*

Key guidelines

- National Institute for Health and Clinical Excellence (2016). Antimicrobial prophylaxis against infective endocarditis.
- The Royal College of Physicians (2004). Prophylaxis and treatment of infective endocarditis in adults: concise guidelines.
- European Society of Cardiology (2009). Infective endocarditis: guidelines on prevention, diagnosis, and treatment.
- American Heart Association (2007). Prevention of infective endocarditis.

* The guidelines on this chapter have been sourced and summarized from different UK, Europe, and international government sources, professional organizations, and medical specialty societies. Leading guidelines have been listed in the further reading section at the end of this chapter.

Basic facts

- *Definition*—IE is an inflammation of the endocardium. The term can be used to refer only to infection in the endocardium or, more broadly, to include infections affecting native or prosthetic valves, atrial or ventricular endocardium, patent ductus arteriosus, arteriovenous shunts, pacemakers, and surgically created conduits.
- *Incidence*—about 2–6 annual cases per 100,000 population; male-to-female ratios range from 3:2 to 9:1. More than 50% of current cases occur in patients over 60.
- *Predisposing factors*—see Box 13.1.
- *Microbial pathogens*—staphylococci, oral streptococci, and enterococci account for 80% of cases.
- *Clinical presentation*—suspect in any patient with a well-recognized predisposing cardiac lesion who develops fever and heart murmur. Should also be suspected in patients with evidence of embolic events of unknown origin or patients with characteristic skin lesions (e.g. conjunctival or splinter haemorrhages).
- *Diagnosis*—depends on a thorough history, clinical findings, laboratory studies (especially blood cultures), and echocardiogram. Diagnosis can be confirmed using different criteria (e.g. Duke criteria).
- *Treatment*—appropriate antibiotics. Surgery is occasionally required.

Box 13.1 Predisposing factors to IE

- IV drug abusers.
- Acquired valvular heart diseases causing stenosis or regurgitation.*
- Prosthetic heart valve replacement*.
- History of previous IE* (recurrence occur in about 5%).
- History of hypertrophic cardiomyopathy.*
- Haemodialysis patients (risk increases by 30–100 times).
- Others—ventriculo-atrial shunts and patients undergoing liver, heart, and heart-lung transplantation.
- Structural congenital heart disease.* Patients with isolated atrial septal defect, fully repaired patent ductus arteriosus or ventricular septal defect (>6mo previously), and those with endothelialized closure devices are not at high risk.

* = high risk

Prophylaxis

General concepts
- Historically, IE, a serious condition that may result from bacteraemia, should be prevented in any exposure to invasive procedure, especially in high-risk patients.

Current understandings
- There is no consistent association between interventional procedures (dental or non-dental) and the development of IE.
- The risk is greater during regular tooth brushing than in patients undergoing a single dental procedure.
- Antibiotic prophylaxis has no solid proven effectiveness in protecting against IE.
- Fatal anaphylaxis resulting from antibiotic usage may cause more deaths than the theoretical death caused by the possible risk of sustaining IE and is not cost-effective.

Current recommendations
- Antibiotics should NOT be offered routinely to people undergoing dental or non-dental procedures to protect them from IE, even if they are from the high-risk group.
- Prophylactic antibiotics (that covers IE) should only be considered in patients at risk of IE if the operative site is suspected to be infected, and therefore, significant bacteraemia is to be induced [C]. This applies mainly to microorganisms that have the potential to cause bacterial endocarditis.
- European guidance echoes NICE but also recommends prophylactic antibiotics for high-risk patients having interventional dental work.

Further reading

National Institute for Health and Clinical Excellence (2016). Antimicrobial prophylaxis against infective endocarditis. Available from: http://www.nice.org.uk/guidance/CG64.

The Royal College of Physicians (2004). Prophylaxis and treatment of infective endocarditis in adults: concise guidelines. Available from: http://www.clinmed.rcpjournal.org/content/4/6/545.full.pdf+html

European Society of Cardiology. Endocarditis. (EU) Available from http://www.escardio.org/Guidelines-&-Education/Clinical-Practice-Guidelines/Infective-Endocarditis-Guidelines-on-Prevention-Diagnosis-and-Treatment-of: Acessed feb 2016

Wilson W, Taubert KA, Gewitz M et al. (2007). Prevention of infective endocarditis. Circulation 116, 1736–54.

Hill EE, Herijgers P, Claus P, Vanderschueren S, Herregods MC, Peetermans WE (2007). Infective endocarditis: changing epidemiology and predictors of 6-month mortality: a prospective cohort study. Eur Heart J 28, 196–203.

Tornos MP, Permanyer–Miralda G, Olona M, Gil M, Galve E, Almirante B, Soler–Soler J (1992). Long-term complications of native valve infective endocarditis in non-addicts. A 15-year follow-up study. Ann Intern Med 117, 567–72.

Ireland JH, McCarthy JT (2003). Infective endocarditis in patients with kidney failure: chronic dialysis and kidney transplant. Curr Infect Dis Rep 5, 293–9.

Chapter 14

Principles of blood transfusion*

Red cell blood transfusion 132
Fresh frozen plasma (FFP) transfusion 134
Platelets 134
Further reading 135

Key guidelines
- NICE. Blood Transfusion (2015).
- JPAC Advisory committee (2014). Handbook of transfusion medicine. UK Blood Services.
- The Association of Anaesthetists of Great Britain and Ireland (2008). Blood transfusion and the anaesthetist.
- National Comparative Audit Reports (2007–2012).

---

* The guidelines on this chapter have been sourced and summarized from different UK, Europe, and international government sources, professional organizations, and medical specialty societies. Leading guidelines have been listed in the further reading section at the end of this chapter.

Red cell blood transfusion

- *Benefits*—to increase the oxygen-carrying capacity of blood, with resultant more efficient delivery of oxygen to vital and non-vital organs.
- *Risks*—associated with blood transfusion, see Box 14.1.
- *Indications for transfusion*—always should weigh the expected benefits against possible risks. Clear valid justification for blood transfusion should always be available and documented in the patient's notes [D].
  - *Acute blood loss*
    —Acute blood volume loss of 30% can usually be replaced using crystalloids or synthetic colloids. Red cell transfusion to replace the oxygen-carrying capacity may be required only in later stages of shock.
    —Blood transfusion is indicated for class III shock (30–40% blood loss, i.e. 1,500–2,000mL) as initial modality. Less severe cases (classes I and II shock) do NOT require red cell transfusion for the only purpose of enhancing the blood oxygen-carrying capacity. Decision should be based on individual cases (e.g. patients over 65, those with pre-existing anaemia or reduced cardiorespiratory reserve may require red cell transfusion at an earlier stage).
  - *Low levels of haemoglobin*
    —Red cell transfusion is NOT required or justified if the level of current (or anticipated) Hb is >100g/L [D]. Transfusion should be considered if Hb level is <70g/L [D], aiming at reaching a target of 70–90g/L after transfusion. Patients with acute coronary syndrome with Hb of <80g/L should be considered for transfusion, aiming at reaching a target of 80–100g/L.
    —The same 'transfusion triggers' are applicable to patients with asymptomatic cardiovascular disease [C].
    —The number of units required depends on the clinical situation. Each unit of packed blood cells (300mL) in an adult would raise the Hb by 10g/L (within 15min of finishing the transfusion up to 12h) if no continued bleeding exists. Consider giving ONE unit of RBC at the time and assess the outcome clinically and with Hb level check before proceeding to the next unit.
    —Blood transfusion has no significant proven effect on cancer recurrence [B].
    —There is some evidence that limiting RBC transfusion is associated with decreased risk of health-care associated infections.
  - Preoperative blood transfusion.
    —Avoid transfusion if possible, especially if Hb is >100. Possible causes for anaemia should be investigated and treated preoperatively if possible [C].
  - *Erythropoietin*—offers new and alternative route for improving Hb concentrations, and should be used when appropriate (e.g. patients with objections to allogeneic transfusions) [D].
  - Pre-deposit autologous donation (PAD) does not significantly decrease the exposure of transfusion-related risks and should only be used in exceptional circumstances (e.g. patients with rare blood groups) [G].
  - RBC bags are kept at 4°C. Potassium leakage, pH drop, ATP depletion and loss of 2,3 DPG affect the RBC function, impairs cell flexibility, and may result in reperfusion injury.

Box 14.1 Risks of blood transfusion

Transfusion transmitted infections (TTI)

Definition—diagnosis made if no infection present prior to transfusion, the recipient has infection following the transfusion, and the blood component is contaminated or the donor of this component has evidence of the same infection.

Viral—HIV, HCV, HBV. Very low risk. Estimate risk for hepatitis C or HIV transmission: 1 in 1–2 million units transfused in UK and USA.

Bacterial—higher incidence. Estimated risk: 1 in 400,000 units of platelets transfused in UK and USA.

Others—prions (CJD—very rare), protozoa.

Transfusion reaction

Acute immune-mediated haemolysis—MEDICAL EMERGENCY.

Mechanism—results from complement-mediated intravascular haemolysis, where the recipient's plasma has existing antibodies (anti-A, anti-B, or rarely anti-Rh) to the donor's red blood cells (RBCs), causing rapid RBC destruction.

Risk—may lead to disseminated intravascular coagulation (DIC), circulatory shock, and acute tubular necrosis with acute renal failure.

Clinically—agitation, anxiety, fever, flushing, abdominal, back and chest pain, abnormal bleeding from puncture sites, tachycardia, hypotension, tachypnoea.

Treatment.

STEP 1—stop infusion, check identity, start ABCDE Management Plan (see Chapter 21).

STEP 2—send bloods for FBC, U&Es, clotting, and culture. Send urine sample.

STEP 3—inform the haematologist.

Delayed haemolytic reaction.

Mechanism—delayed antibody response after re-exposure to foreign red cell antigen. Occurs within 2–10d. Less severe.

Clinically—failing Hb, mild fever, slight increased bilirubin in serum.

Treatment—non-specific. Special care for future transfusions.

Febrile non-haemolytic reactions—most common reaction.

Mechanism—cytokines (interleukin (IL)-1, IL-6, IL-8, tumour necrosis factor-alpha (TNFα)) generated and accumulated during blood components' storage process.

Clinically—fever and chills within 1–6h of transfusion.

Treatment—stop infusion, exclude acute haemolysis, use paracetamol.

Anaphylactic reaction—LIFE-THREATENING CONDITION

Other reactions—urticarial reaction, post-transfusion purpura, transfusion-related acute lung injury, immunomodulation.

Procedural errors

Human errors can occur in one or more of the minimum 40 steps of transfusing blood to patients. The estimated incidence is 71:24,000 transfusions. Transfusion best practice should always be followed.

Fresh frozen plasma (FFP) transfusion

- *Preparation*—donors' whole blood using hard centrifugation or aphaeresis. Subject to strict quality monitoring, e.g. FFP should be rapidly frozen to −30°C to maintain the activity of labile coagulation factors. Level of electrolytes, platelet, and leukocyte depletion are monitored. Handling of the frozen, brittle plastic bags requires special care. Any discoloration or leak when subjecting the FFP pack to pressure should be investigated promptly.
- *Benefits*—FFP contain the same spectrum of haemostatic factors found in healthy blood. Level of each factor differs with time and method of preparation.
- *Risks*—hypersensitivity reaction (1–3%), leukocyte depletion, infection, and graft-versus-host defense.
- *Indications*—limited in surgical practice.
  - *Coagulation factor deficiencies and DIC.*
    - —Multi-factor deficiencies or DIC in association with severe bleeding (guided by coagulation tests). Not indicated where there is no evidence of bleeding.
  - *Reversal of warfarin effect—not indicated.*
    - —Vitamin K and/or activated prothrombin complex concentrate should be used dependent upon urgency of reversal.
  - *Liver disease with prolonged PT time.*
    - —FFP may be useful, but the response is unpredictable and repeated coagulation screening is essential to guide treatment.
  - *Surgical bleeding and massive transfusion.*
    - —FFP should be given in line with local Major Haemorrhage Protocol (e.g.: 4U FFP per 6U RBC).

Platelets

Consider platelet transfusions to patients with established thrombocytopenia who have clinically significant bleeding and a platelet count below $30 \times 10^9/l$.

Consider platelet transfusions to raise platelet count $> 50 \times 10^9/l$ in patients who are having invasive procedures or surgery. Consider transfusion at higher levels $(100 \times 10^9/l)$ in patients having surgery in critical sites (central nervous system, eye surgery, etc.).

Further reading

Handbook of Transfusion Medicine (2014). Joint UK Blood Transfusion and Tissue Transplantation Services Professional Advisory Committee. Available from: http://www.transfusionguidelines.org.uk/transfusion-handbook

The Association of Anaesthetists of Great Britain and Ireland (2016). The use of blood components and their alternatives. Available at : http://onlinelibrary.wiley.com/doi/10.1111/anae.13489/full

National Comparative Audit Reports (2009 – 2012). NHS Blood Transfusion Clinical Audit. Reports and tools. Available from: http://hospital.blood.co.uk/media/2315/ad578e8b-0ccc-45fd-ae73-4e0e4eb86d45.pdf

Serious Hazards of Transfusion (SHOT) UK 2013 report. Available from: http://www.shotuk.org/shot-reports/report-summary-supplement-2013/

Enright H, Davis K, Gernsheimer T, McCullough JJ, Woodson R, Slichter SJ (2003). Factors influencing moderate to severe reactions to PLT transfusions: experience of the TRAP multicentre clinical trial. Transfusion 43, 1545–52.

Wiesen AR, Hospenthal DR, Byrd JC, Glass KL, Howard RS, Diehl LF (1994). Equilibration of haemoglobin concentration after transfusion in medical inpatients not actively bleeding. Ann Intern Med 121, 278–80.

Guidelines for the use of fresh-frozen plasma, cryoprecipitate and cryosupernatant. British Committee for Standards in Haematology, Blood Transfusion Task force. 2004. British Journal of Haematology. 126;1. 11–28

Further reading

Perioperative anticoagulation management*

Background *138*
Warfarin *139*
Recommendations *140*
New oral anticoagulants *141*
Further reading *142*

Key guidelines
- British Committee for Standards in Haematology (2016). Perioperative management of anticoagulation and antiplatelet therapy.
- Scottish Intercollegiate Guidance Network (2009). Antithrombotics: indications and management.
- British Committee for Standards in Haematology (2008). Guidelines on the assessment of bleeding risk prior to surgery or invasive procedures.

---

* The guidelines on this chapter have been sourced and summarized from different UK, Europe, and international government sources, professional organizations, and medical specialty societies. Leading guidelines have been listed in the further reading section at the end of this chapter.

Background

- *General concept*—anticoagulant therapy is common among patients undergoing elective or emergency surgery. Perioperative effective management should be individualized and should balance the benefits of anticoagulation against the risk of causing significant bleeding.

Warfarin

- *Efficacy of warfarin*
  - Vitamin K antagonists reduce the risk of recurrent VTE by >80%.
  - In those with mechanical heart valves (MHV), warfarin decreases the incidence of thromboembolic (TE) resulting in death, stroke, or peripheral ischaemia requiring surgery from 4% to 1% per patient-year. When warfarin is stopped for 5d in patients with AF or a MHV, it is estimated that it will result in 0.5 TE events per 1,000 patients.
- *Anticoagulation dynamics*—on stopping warfarin, most patients will normalize in about 5d (warfarin half-life is 36h). Once warfarin is restarted, about 3d elapse before the international normalized ratio (INR) reaches the level of 2.0. Consequently, patients can be expected to have a sub-therapeutic INR for about 2d before surgery and 2d after. Partial protection against a TE event is still expected during this period but depending on the indication for warfarinization, bridging therapy may be required.
- *Heparin bridging therapy*
  - LMWH bridging therapy is effective in VTE prevention but there is less data for its use in AF and MHVs.
  - Bridging heparin will increase the risk of bleeding (13% vs 0.8%). However, the risk of bleeding being fatal is 3% vs the risk of TE stroke being fatal at 40%.
  - *Factors affecting perioperative bleeding*—include the type, extent, and duration of operation or procedure, the use of antiplatelet therapy, and the presence of other comorbidities that have a potential effect on haemostasis. (See ➲ Chapter 10, pp.75–80).

Recommendations

- *General approach*—individualized decisions must be made dependent upon the risks of bleeding vs the risks of TE.
- Patients with a target INR of 2.0 to 3.0 undergoing elective surgical procedure should stop oral anticoagulants for 5d before the procedure (4 clear days) [C]. The target INR should be <1.5 on the day of surgery. Ideally, INR should be determined 1d pre-op to allow for using PO Vitamin K if INR >1.5.
- *If INR is >2.5 on the day of surgery*—the risk of bleeding should be weighed against the urgency and required timing of the procedure by both the surgeon and anaesthetist.
- If rapid reversal of warfarin anticoagulation is required, warfarin should be stopped and 5–10mg of IV vitamin K should be used. Full reversal will be achieved in 4–24h.
- *Very high-risk patients*—i.e. those with an episode of VTE within the last 3mo, those who developed VTE whilst being on anticoagulation who have a target INR of 3.5, those with AF and a recent (<3mo) TIA or stroke, those with AF and CHADS2 score >4 (Congestive failure; Hypertension; Age ≥75 years; Diabetes mellitus; prior Stroke, TIA or thromboembolism), and those with MHVs, other than those with a bileaflet aortic valve, should be considered for a bridging therapy when INR drops below 2 [D] (see Box 15.1).
- *High risk patients*–i.e. patients with CHADS2 score <4, and those with a bileaflet aortic MHV with no other risk factors—do NOT require bridging therapy [A].

Box 15.1 An example of recommended management plan for anticoagulation warfarin bridging for prosthetic heart valves in the perioperative period

- Stop warfarin 5d preop [A].
- Commence treatment dose LMWH on d3, dose adjusted for abnormal renal function.
- Give last dose of LMWH 24h before surgery [B].
- Restart treatment dose LMWH 24h post-op for low bleeding-risk surgery and at 48–72h post-op for high bleeding-risk surgery.
- Increase treatment dose LMWH to 100U/kg twice daily the following morning, after reassessment and exclusion of post-op bleeding complications.
- Recommence warfarin at USUAL MAINTENANCE DOSE on the evening of or day after surgery depending upon haemostasis and bleeding risk.
- Continue therapeutic LMWH until warfarin is therapeutic. Teach injection technique if domiciliary self-medication required.
- Prior to discharge, ensure follow-up arrangements for repeat INR.
- Attention to hydration and mobilization as for routine thromboprophylaxis.
- The antigoagulation plan should be clearly documented in the patient notes.

- *Low-risk patients*—i.e low-risk AF or VTE >3mo earlier do NOT require bridging therapy but only need prophylactic LMWH [C].
- *High-risk surgery*—post-operative bridging should not be started until >48h postoperatively[C].
- *Vena caval filter*—should be considered if an absolute contraindication to therapeutic anticoagulation (or a failure of anticoagulation) exists associated with acute proximal venous thrombosis.

Direct oral anticoagulants (DOACs)

- The most common DOACs in use are dabigatran, rivaroxaban, and apixaban.
- Dagibatran etexilate (direct thrombin inhibitor) is recommended as an option for preventing and treating VTE. DOACs are also recommended for use in non-valvular AF with equivalent efficacy to warfarin and better safety.
- Due to their predictable pharmokinetics, routine coagulation monitoring is not required for patients on DOACs. Normal thrombin time (TT) should be considered as a marker of minimal concentration of circulating dabigatran. PT and aPTT are not useful as markers of DOACs activity (or lack of). [A]
- Optimal management depends upon the reason for anticoagulation, the type of DOAC and the type of surgery being undertaken.
- Bridging is not necessary with DOACs as the diminution of effect is predictable and short-term. However, patients with significant risk of thrombosis should be considered for a PROPHYLACTIC dose of an anticoagulation until starting the full dose of DOACs. [D]
- *High-risk surgery*—stop DOAC 48h before surgery (longer if CrCl <30ml/min, duration dependent upon type of DOAC). Restart after 48h at least. [B]
- *Low-risk surgery*—stop DOAC 24h before surgery (longer if CrCl <30ml/min, duration dependent upon type of DOAC). Restart in 6–12h if homeostasis is fully secured [B].
- *Procedures associated with immobilization*—LMWHs recommended 6–8h after procedure.
- Andexanet, when available, should be used to reverse rivaroxaban effect prior to emergency invasive procedures or surgery with a high bleeding risk [C].

Perioperative antiplatelet therapy

- Most invasive non-cardiac procedures (including neuroaxial anesthesia) do NOT require stopping of aspirin monotherapy when it is used as a secondary prevention [C]. If the bleeding risk is high, aspirin can be stopped 3d before and up to 7d after without any major risk.
- Dual antiplatelet therapy (for recent acute coronary syndrome or coronary artery stent) should continue perioperatively for low bleeding risk procedures [C].
- Dual antiplatelet therapy in high bleeding risk procedures—surgery should be postponed if possible till there is no need for a dual antiplatelet therapy. Otherwise, continue aspirin and stop clopidogrel 5d before the procedure.
- Patient on antiplatelet therapy who have excessive perioperative bleeding. Use IV tranexamic acid [C], and if this does not work (rare), then consider giving two pools of donor platelets [C].

Further reading

Keeling, D., Tait, R. C., Watson, H. and the British Committee of Standards for Haematology (2016), Peri-operative management of anticoagulation and antiplatelet therapy. Br J Haematol, 175: 602–613. doi:10.1111/bjh.14344

June U. SIGN 129 • Antithrombotics : indications and management. Key to evidence statements and grades of recommendations. 2013;(June).

De Jong PG, Coppens M, Middeldorp S. Duration of anticoagulant therapy for venous thromboembolism: balancing benefits and harms on the long term. Br J Haematol [Internet]. 2012 Aug [cited 2015 Jan 30];158(4):433–41. Available from: http://www.ncbi.nlm.nih.gov/pubmed/22734929

Cannegieter SC, Rosendaal FR, Briët E. Thromboembolic and bleeding complications in patients with mechanical heart valve prostheses. Circulation [Internet]. 1994 Mar [cited 2015 Jan 30]; 89(2):635–41. Available from: http://www.ncbi.nlm.nih.gov/pubmed/8313552

Keeling D, Baglin T, Tait C, Watson H, Perry D, Baglin C, et al. Guidelines on oral anticoagulation with warfarin - fourth edition. Br J Haematol [Internet]. 2011 Aug [cited 2014 Jul 21];154(3):311–24. Available from: http://www.ncbi.nlm.nih.gov/pubmed/21671894

Douketis JD, Spyropoulos AC, Spencer FA, Mayr M, Jaffer AK, Eckman MH, et al. Perioperative management of antithrombotic therapy: Antithrombotic Therapy and Prevention of Thrombosis, 9th ed: American College of Chest Physicians Evidence-Based Clinical Practice Guidelines. Chest [Internet]. 2012 Mar [cited 2015 Jan 30];141(2 Suppl):e326S – 50S. Available from: http://www.pubmedcentral.nih.gov/articlerender.fcgi?artid=3278059&tool=pmcentrez&rendertype=abstract

Garcia DA, Regan S, Henault LE, Upadhyay A, Baker J, Othman M, et al. Risk of thromboembolism with short-term interruption of warfarin therapy. Arch Intern Med [Internet]. 2008 Jan 14 [cited 2015 Jan 30];168(1):63–9. Available from: http://www.ncbi.nlm.nih.gov/pubmed/18195197

Evaluation HT. Dabigatran etexilate for the treatment and secondary prevention of deep vein thrombosis and / or pulmonary embolism. 2014;(September 2009).

Camm AJ, Lip GYH, De Caterina R, Savelieva I, Atar D, Hohnloser SH, et al. 2012 focused update of the ESC Guidelines for the management of atrial fibrillation: an update of the 2010 ESC Guidelines for the management of atrial fibrillation. Developed with the special contribution of the European Heart Rhythm Association. Eur Heart J [Internet]. 2012 Nov [cited 2015 Jan 22];33(21):2719–47. Available from: http://www.ncbi.nlm.nih.gov/pubmed/22922413

Lai A, Davidson N, Galloway SW, Thachil J. Perioperative management of patients on new oral anticoagulants. Br J Surg [Internet]. 2014 Jun [cited 2015 Jan 30];101(7):742–9. Available from: http://www.ncbi.nlm.nih.gov/pubmed/24777590

Chee YL, Crawford JC, Watson HG, Greaves M; British Committee for Standards in Haematology (2008). Guidelines on the assessment of bleeding risk prior to surgery or invasive procedures. Br J Haematol 140, 496–504.

Principles of care
of critically ill patients[*]

Key definitions 144
Recommended approach 148
Further reading 150

The authors would like to thank the Welsh Institute for Minimal Access Therapy (WIMAT) Medicare centre in Cardiff. Their dedication, enthusiasm and vision have contributed significantly to the concepts detailed in this chapter.

Key guidelines

- Intensive Care Society (2011). Guidelines for transport of critically ill adults.
- National Institute for Health and Clinical Excellence (2007). Acutely ill patients in hospital.
- Loftus I (2010). Care of the critically ill surgical patient (CCrISP) manual.
- American College of Surgeons (2008). Advanced trauma and life support (ATLS) program for doctors.

[*] The guidelines on this chapter have been sourced and summarized from different UK, Europe, and international government sources, professional organizations, and medical specialty societies. Leading guidelines have been listed in the further reading section at the end of this chapter.

'Key' definitions

- *Expectations*—surgeons should be competent in identifying and treating high risk patients in the perioperative period, including ability to identify, assess, and initiate treatment for organ dysfunction and circulatory shock, obtain and interpret blood gases, use blood products and fluid composites, support nutrition, treat sepsis, and identify and diagnose brain stem death (Box 16.4).
- *Critically ill patients*—are defined as:
  - Patients with no existing critical illness, but who are at higher risk to develop life-threatening condition (e.g. extreme age groups, significant comorbidities, high-risk operations).
  - Patients with existing but compensated critical illness (e.g. pre-shock patients with peripheral shutdown and tachycardia, but no end-organ failure, pre-respiratory failure patients with normal PaO_2 on high-flow oxygen).
  - Patients with existing critical illness (e.g. shock with end-organ failure, respiratory failure requiring ventilation).
- *Level of care*—the level of monitoring and intervention required for the individual patient critical case (Box 16.1).
- *Organ failure*—altered organ function (reversible or irreversible) requiring intensive intervention to achieve homeostasis (Box 16.2). Shock is the acute circulatory failure with inadequate tissue perfusion causing cellular hypoxia. Four different categories exist (Box 16.3).

Box 16.1 Levels of care for critically ill surgical patients

- Level 0—normal ward in acute hospital. Provides basic physiologic monitoring and a fairly low nurse-to-patient ratio.
- Level 1—acute ward with higher nurse-to-patient ratio and additional support from critical care (outreach) team, e.g. the Surgical Extended Care Unit (SECU).
- Level 2—more advanced physiologic monitoring and high nurse-to-patient ratio, with the ability to support a single failing organ system, e.g. the High Dependency Unit (HDU).
- Level 3—advanced physiologic monitoring and respiratory support with high nurse-to-patient ratio. Ability to support two failing organ systems or more, e.g. the Intensive Care Unit (ICU).

Box 16.2 Organ failure—diagnostic criteria

- Cardiovascular—inadequate organ perfusion with resultant hypoxia. Clinical criteria include:
  - Hypotension—BP <90mmHg or fall of >30–40mmHg.
  - Decreased renal perfusion—oliguria <20mL/h.
  - Decreased cerebral perfusion—confusion or restlessness.
  - Decreased limb perfusion—dry mucous membranes, cold peripheries.
- Respiratory—failure of gas exchange resulting from inadequate function of one or more components of the respiratory system. Clinical criteria include:
  - Hypoxaemia—PO_2 <8kPa2 (or <60mmHg) at sea level.
  - Hypercarbia—PCO_2 >7kPa2 (or >45mmHg).
  - PaO_2/FIO_2 <300 in acute lung injury (or <200 in ARDS).
  - Or (more frequently) a combination of more than one criteria.
  - Type I respiratory failure is defined as hypoxaemia with no hypercapnia, typically caused by ventilation/perfusion mismatch. Type II is defined as hypoxaemia with hypercapnia, commonly caused by inadequate alveolar ventilation.
- Renal—a significant decline in glomerular filtration rate (GFR) with retention of nitrogenous waste products, and disturbance of body fluid volume, electrolyte and acid–base balance. Clinical criteria include:
  - Oliguria—urine output <0.5mL/kg/h or <45mL every 2h despite adequate resuscitation.
  - Raised creatinine >0.5mg/dL or 44.2µmol/L.
  - Decreased GFR.
- Coagulopathy—INR >1.5 with the absence of anticoagulants or platelet count <100,000.
- Other parameters—lactate ≥4mmol/L.

Box 16.3 Types of shock

- Hypovolaemic—direct loss of effective circulatory blood volume, due to bleeding or fluid loss.
- Cardiogenic—a cardiac pump failure resulting from direct injury to cardiac muscle.
- Obstructive—venous return is prevented from returning to heart, e.g. pericardial effusion.
- Distributive—abnormal distribution of blood flow in small vessels, resulting in inadequate supply to end organs.
- Septic shock—early vasodilation and late pump failure due to infective process.
- Neurogenic shock—vasodilation due to disruption to autonomic pathways within the spinal cord.
- Anaphylactic shock—vasodilation and pump failure due to release of IgE antibodies, causing massive degranulation of mast cells in sensitised individuals.
- Endocrine shock—circulatory failure due to adrenal insufficiency.

Box 16.4 Definition of brain stem death

- Definition—a person is dead when consciousness and the ability to breathe are permanently lost, regardless of continuing life in the body and parts of the brain, and that death of the brain stem alone is sufficient to produce this state.
- Diagnosis—is made after pre-conditions are satisfied: a structured irreversible brain damage, excluding certain drugs or metabolic causes, with temp of 35°C. Testing by qualified personnel should confirm the absence of cranial nerve functions, absence of motor function, apnea test, and similar results on repeating the test after time interval. The test should be performed by at least two medical practitioners registered with the GMC >5yrs, with one at least being a consultant and both competent in the field.

A structured form with integrated guidance can be used to confirm brain stem death status. (http://www.gicu.sgul.ac.uk/resources-for-current-staff/organ-donation-including-brainstem-death-testing/BSTformStGeorges%20vJB.pdf/at_download/file)

Recommended approach

- *Immediate management*—see Fig. 16.1.
  - Always follow the ABCDE approach in the initial assessment of any sick patient (A: Airways, B: Breathing, C: Circulation, D: Disability, E: Exposure). (See also ➋ OHCM 10e Ch. 19.)
  - Remember to assess and manage simultaneously (e.g. identify tension pneumothorax and treat immediately; identify the shock state and commence fluid management).
  - This stage ends once the patient is physiologically stable enough and not in immediate danger. Airways should be secured, breathing and oxygenation should be effective (oxygen saturation >90–94%), and circulation should be fully assessed and fluid management established.
- *Full patient assessment*—follows the previous step and aims at gathering as much information as needed to establish a working diagnosis of the current problem and to formulate an effective management plan.
  - *History and systematic examination*—should be thorough and focused. Holistic approach is required, including significant comorbidities, patient's current quality of life, and family members' opinion. Repeated examination and revisiting the history (e.g. 10min later) maximizes the chance of picking up on missed information and is a recommended practice.
  - *Chart review*—be systematic in your approach (e.g. R: Respiratory, C: Circulation, S: Surgical). Look specifically on the absolute values and trends. Check drug charts for both prescribed and delivered medications (e.g. missed antihypertensives in uncontrolled hypertension crises).
  - *Notes and results review*—including routine bloods, recent investigations, and documented reviews. Maximize your chance of getting the blood results on time by maintaining a forward organization of your team. Waiting at the end of the bed to get the results from computers is more effective practice than promising to review later.
- *Decision and plan*—following the thorough review (and management of life-threatening conditions), the management strategy depends on the stability of the patient.
  - *Stable patient*—should be haemodynamically stable enough and progressing as expected. A full management plan should ensure clear instructions on the required monitoring schedule (and level of care necessary for the day, see Box 16.1), fluid balance, required and urgency of investigations, care of the surgical site (dressing, drains), medications, and other significant instructions for the day (e.g. physiotherapy, referrals, nutrition).
  - *Unstable patient*—include those with unstable vital signs, inappropriate progression, unexpected level of pain, and slow but established deterioration. Arrange appropriate (soon or immediate) investigations or procedure, request specialist opinion immediately, and decide on the level of care required.
- *Documentation*—essential final (or interval) step and should be done properly (see ➋ Chapter 2, pp.19–20).
- Further management of each organ failure is discussed further in ➋ Chapter 16, pp.144–150.

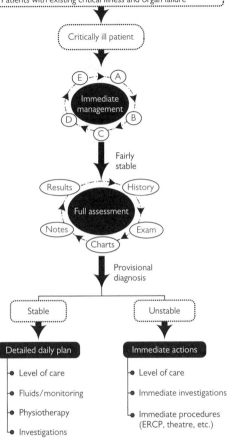

Fig. 16.1 Algorithm for approaching critically ill surgical patients.

Further reading

National Institute for Health and Clinical Excellence (2007). Acutely ill patients in hospital. Available from: http://www.nice.org.uk/Guidance/CG50.

Loftus I et al (2010). Care of Critically Ill Surgical Patient, 2nd edition.Hodder Arnold, London.

American College of Surgeons (2008). Advanced trauma and life support program for doctors, 7th ed. American College of Surgeons, Chicago.

Society of Critical Care Medicine. Learn ICU. Available from: http://www.learnicu.org/Pages/ default. aspx.

The Intensive Care Society. Available from: http://www.ics.ac.uk/.

European Society of Intensive Care Medicine. Guidelines. Available from: https://www.esicm.org/ resources/guidelines-consensus-statements/

Wikipedia. Intensive care medicine. Available from: http://en.wikipedia.org/wiki/Intensive_care_ medicine.

Webb AJ, Shapiro MJ, Singer M, Suter PM (1999). Oxford Textbook of Critical Care, Oxford University Press, Oxford.

Fauci AS, Braunwald E, Kasper DL et al. (2008). Harrison's Principles of Internal Medicine, 17th ed, McGraw–Hill Professional, Maidenhead.

Dellinger RP, Levy MM, Carlet JM et al. (2008). Surviving Sepsis Campaign: international guidelines for management of severe sepsis and septic shock. Crit Care Med 36, 296–327.

AoMRC (2008) A Code of Practice for the Diagnosis and Confirmation of Death.

Principles of trauma management[*]

Basic facts *152*
Principles of trauma management *154*
Specific organ trauma management *156*
Trauma management: special considerations *160*
Further reading *160*

Key guidelines

- NICE (2016). Major trauma.
- American College of Surgeons (2014). Resources for optimal care of the injured patient.
- American College of Surgeons (2008). Advanced trauma life support. 8th Edition.
- EAST Guidelines on trauma management (1998–2017).

[*] The guidelines on this chapter have been sourced and summarized from different UK, Europe, and international government sources, professional organizations, and medical specialty societies. Leading guidelines have been listed in the further reading section at the end of this chapter.

Basic facts

- *Major trauma* is defined as an injury or a combination of injuries that are life-threatening and could be life changing because they may result in long-term disability. Major trauma has a bimodal age distribution— under-20s and over-65s.
- *Impact of trauma*—is huge. Injuries from accidental trauma worldwide causes moderate to severe disability in >45 million people each year. Trauma is the biggest killer of people aged < 45 years. UK annual trauma cost is ~£0.35 billion in immediate treatment; subsequent financial costs are unknown. UK annual lost economic output due to major trauma is ~£3.5 billion.
- *Mechanism of trauma*—often determines resultant injury. Examples include head-on collision (injuries to face, lower limbs, and spine), rear-end collision (hyperextension of cervical spine, central cord syndrome), car rollover (crush injury, spinal compression fractures), steering wheel damage (sternal and rib fracture, cardiac contusion, and aortic injuries), low-speed pedestrian injury (tibia and fibula fracture, knee injuries), high-speed pedestrian injury (truncal injuries, tibia/fibula/femur injuries, craniofacial injuries), and high level fall (lower limbs fractures, pelvic fractures, cervical spine fracture, kidney injuries, visceral injuries).

Principles of trauma management

- Trauma management is challenging. Up to 40% of trauma patients have injuries that are initially missed, and up to 20% of these are clinically significant.
- *Regional trauma systems*—allow for transporting patients to appropriate centres in a timely and orchestrated manner. Resources for optimal care guidelines provide details of elements, integration, and coordination tactics of trauma systems and level of injury/care required. Effective trauma systems must have a lead hospital. Depending on resources and needs, this can be a level I or II facility, the difference in which is not in the initial definitive trauma care (which is provided in both levels regardless of the severity of injury), but in ability to lead in education and research, and to provide a highly specialized trauma care such as replantation. Level III trauma centre can provide prompt assessment, resuscitation, emergency operations, and stabilization and also arrange for transfer to a facility that can provide definitive trauma care.
- *Trauma team*—should be appropriately formed to achieve assigned level of care and prioritize management. This may include emergency physicians, trauma surgeons, emergency nurses, respiratory therapists, among others. Pitfall in trauma management arises from one or more of four domains: communication breakdown (plans not outlined clearly, key changes not effectively transferred), situational awareness failure (unrecognized developing shock, unrecognized blood transfusion needs), poor staffing (inadequately staff training or numbers), and unresolved conflicts (poor leadership style, perceived inadequacy of other team members).
- *Initial assessment and management*—primary survey should follow the ABCDE approach (see Chapter 16). Cervical spine immobilization should be assessed and managed as part of Airways. Primary survey simplifies priorities. Problems identified should be managed immediately, in the order they are detected, before moving on to next step.
- *Secondary survey*—should include a careful, head-to-toe assessment in all trauma patients determined to be stable upon completion of primary survey. This includes a detailed history, a thorough and efficient physical examination, and targeted diagnostic studies.
- *Emergency diagnostic studies*—include portable x-ray (lateral cervical spine, chest, and pelvis), possible CT scan (where appropriate), ultrasound FAST scan, electrocardiogram (ECG), and screening trauma laboratory tests (Hb, pregnancy test, coagulations studies, etc.).
- *Patient transfer*—should be immediately considered upon stabilizing the patient whenever sustained injuries are believed to be beyond the management capacity of the trauma centre.

- *Common presumptions to avoid pitfalls in trauma management*—include possible oesophageal intubation in ineffective airway management (0.5–6%), haemorrhagic shock in transient response to fluids, cardiac tamponade in unstable patient with normal jugular venous pressure (JVP), involvement of both thoracic and abdominal cavities in penetrating trauma to one of them (until proven otherwise), penetrating [subtle] bowel injury in any low velocity penetrating wounds (easily missed on FAST scan), open-book pelvic fracture (potentially life-threatening if manipulated) in any suspected fracture to pelvis, ocular injuries in all periorbital swelling and bruising, and a significant injury in elderly patients even if they appear well.
- *Pain management in trauma patients*—is essential. Short-acting agents (fentanyl or midazolam) are generally preferred.

Specific organ trauma management

- *Penetrating neck injuries*—are common. Gunshot wounds are associated with significant injuries in ~50% of victims (compared to ~15% in stab wounds). Zone I injuries, including the thoracic inlet, up to the level of the cricothyroid membrane, is treated as an upper thoracic injury. Zone III, above the angle of the mandible, is treated as a head injury. Zone II, between zones I and III, is an area of controversy.
  - Patients with hard signs of significant injury (active haemorrhage, expanding haematoma, subcutaneous emphysema, respiratory distress, etc.) require immediate operative exploration and management.
  - High resolution CT angiography, otherwise, offers appropriate diagnostic imaging with minimal risk, and is the initial diagnostic study of choice when available [Level II recommendation].
  - Selective operative management (vs mandatory exploration) of penetrating injuries to zone II have equivalent diagnostic accuracy. Selective management is therefore recommended to minimize unnecessary operations [Level I].
  - Either expedited contrast oesophagography or oesophagoscopy can be used to rule out an oesophageal perforation that requires operative repair. Morbidity increases significantly if repair is delayed >24h [Level II].
  - Carotid or vertebral artery injuries should be screened for whenever suspected [Level II] with a four vessel angiogram [Level II] or high resolution (eight slices or more) CTA (duplex scan is inaccurate). Grade I (intimal irregularity) or II (dissection or intramural haematoma) can be treated with antithrombotic agents such as aspirin or heparin only [Level II]; results for both are equivalent [Level III]. Grade III (pseudoaneurysm) should be considered for intervention as they rarely resolve [Level III], providing they remain asymptomatic. Grade IV (occlusion) should be treated with anticoagulation to prevent stroke (stroke rate ~45%). Grade V (transaction with extravasaion) has mortality rate of ~100%.
- *Blunt thoracic trauma*—should be assessed and treated using ATLS algorithm. Immediate life-threatening injuries include aortic injury, tension pneumothorax, haemothorax with severe, active bleeding, pericardial tamponade from myocardial injury, and tracheobronchial disruption.
  - Emergency department thoracotomy (EDT) rarely results in successful resuscitation. Patients most likely to survive an EDT neurologically intact are: a) pulseless patients with signs of life after penetrating thoracic injury, with no obvious non-survivable injury (e.g. massive head trauma, multiple severe injuries) [Strong recommendation], and b) patients with cardiac tamponade (diagnosed by ultrasound), with no obvious non-survivable injury [conditional recommendation].
  - Flail chest occurs when three or more adjacent ribs are each fractured in two places, creating one floating segment. Initial management consists of oxygen and close monitoring for early signs of

respiratory compromise. There is insufficient clinical evidence to recommend any type of surgical fixation of rib fractures [Level III]. Epidural catheter is the preferred mode of analgesia delivery [Level II]. A trial of mask CPAP should be considered in alert, compliant patients with marginal respiratory status, combined with optimal regional anaesthesia [Level III]. Patients with severe injuries, respiratory distress, or progressively worsening respiratory function require endotracheal intubation and mechanical ventilatory support [Level II].

- *Blunt aortic trauma*—occurs in 1–2% of blunt thoracic trauma and is a major cause of rapid death (20% survival rate). Main risk factor is rapid deceleration (high-speed motor vehicle collision or falls). CT angio is the mainstay of diagnosis [strong recommendation]. Type I injury (intimal tear) can be treated non-operatively (aggressive heart rate and blood pressure management). Type II (intramural haematoma), III (pseudoaneurysm), and IV (rupture) requires repair endovascularly [strong recommendation], preferably in a delayed manner when possible (haemodynamic stable patients, esp. with multiple injuries) [strong recommendation].
- *Haemothorax*—is common, and should be investigated with ultrasound scan or a CT chest [Level II]. Video-assisted thoracoscopic surgery (VATS) in stable penetrating thoracoabdominal wounds is safe and effective [Level II]. All haemothoraces, regardless of size, should be considered for drainage [Level III], using tube thoracostomy and/or VATS. Intrapleural thrombolytics can be considered to improve drainage of loculated collections in non-acute setting [Level III]. Massive haemothorax should be assessed based on patient stability rather than the volume or rate of output [Level III]. Nevertheless, an output of >1500 ml in 24h should prompt consideration for an operation [Level II].
- *Pneumothorax*—can be observed if occult, regardless of the use of positive pressure ventilation [Level III], and should be considered for VATS if persistent leaking air on day 3 post-injury [Level II].
- *Traumatic brain injury (TBI)*—is the acute alteration in brain function caused by a blunt external force, with Glasgow Coma Scale (GCS) score of 13 to 15, loss of consciousness for ≤ 30min, and duration of posttraumatic amnesia of ≤24h. CT scan is always required in this case [Level II] where possible (or criteria-based selective CT where resources are limited) [Level II]. Isolated TBI and –ve brain CT can be safely discharged if no other injuries exist [Level II]. Special care should be given to elderly patients and those on warfarin [Level III]. Measurable deficits in cognition and memory usually resolve at 1 month. Postconcussive symptoms may persist for >3mo in 20–40% of cases. Biomechanical markers (S-100, etc.) and advanced imaging (MRI, etc.) should not be routinely used [Level II].
- *Blunt abdominal trauma*—should undergo exploratory laparotomy in unstable patients with positive FAST scan [Level II] or positive diagnostic peritoneal lavage (DPL) (aspiration of gross blood, RBC >100k/mm³, WBC>500/mm³, bile or faeces) [Level I]. Negative FAST and DPL in unstable patient should prompt further resuscitation and searching for

other source of injury [Level III]. Stable patients with equivocal findings (abdominal tenderness, multiple rib fractures, associated neurologic injury, or multiple extra-abdominal injuries) should be investigated with a CT scan [Level I], or repeated USS [Level II], and admitted for observation if no significant injuries are found. Exploratory laparotomy is indicated where free fluid is identified on CT scan and no solid organ injury is identified [Level II].

- *Liver injuries*—are the most common in blunt abdominal trauma. Operative treatment is required in ~15% of cases. Laparotomy is indicated in haemodynamically unstable patients or in presence of diffuse peritonitis [Level I]. Otherwise, a trial of non-operative management should always be considered in suitable centres (average success rate 94%) [Level II]. Contrast CT scan is indicated in all stable patients [Level II]. Patients with higher grade injuries fail non-operative management more commonly; nevertheless, they should still be offered non-operative management as long as they remain hemodynamically stable. The severity of hepatic injury (Grade I to VI), neurologic status, elderly patients, or the presence of associated injuries are NOT absolute contraindication to conservative management [Level II]. Angiography with embolization should be considered in stable patients with evidence of extravasation.

- *Splenic injuries*—are common. Operative treatment is required in ~30% of cases. Laparotomy is indicated in haemodynamically unstable patients or in diffuse peritonitis [Level I]. Otherwise, a trial of non-operative management should always be considered in suitable centres [Level II]. Contrast CT scan is indicated in all stable patients [Level II]. Patients with active contrast extravasation or contrast blush on CT scan, or those with grade III injuries (Haematoma: subcapsular, >50% of surface area OR expanding, ruptured subcapsular or parenchymal haematoma OR intraparenchymal haematoma >5cm or expanding. Laceration: >3cm in depth or involving a trabecular vessel) or above should be considered for embolization [Level II]. Failure of embolization indicates the need for surgery.

- *Pancreatic injuries*—should be diagnosed as early as possible [Level III], but diagnosis can be challenging due to reduced sensitivity of CT scan and amylase/lipase levels [Level III]. Low grade injuries (I or II: minor or major contusion of laceration without duct injury or tissue loss) can be managed by drainage alone (gastrointestinal decompression and nutritional support) [Level III], with repeated imaging in 5–7d. Grade III injuries (distal transection or parenchymal/duct injury) and above should be managed with wide closed suction drainage, pancreatic duct repair, and/or resection [Level III]. Mortality following pancreatic and duodenal injury is ~15–20%.

- *Renal injuries*—should be treated conservatively in the absence of major renal lacerations associated with devascularized segments [Level II]. Shattered but perfused kidneys in haemodynamically stable patients with minimal transfusion requirements should be treated conservatively as well [Level I]. Operative exploration can be considered in patients with major blunt renal injuries with a devascularized segment (complication rate 40–80%) [Level II]. Angiographic embolization can be used as adjunct treatment modality [Level II].

- *Bladder injuries (including ruptured bladder)*—should be treated with a transurethral catheter (results are similar to primary suturing) [Level III].
- *Posterior urethral injuries*—may be treated either with delayed perineal reconstruction or primary endoscopic realignment (equivalent outcomes) [Level III].

- *Penetrating abdominal injuries*—should undergo emergency laparotomy in unstable, diffusely peritonitic patients, and those with evisceration of intra-abdominal organs, or with gastrointestinal haemorrhage [Level I]. Stable patients should be further investigated (using CT scan preferably) and monitored [Level II]. Serial physical examination is reliable in detecting significant injuries after penetrating trauma to the abdomen, if performed by experienced clinicians [Level II]. Stab wounds to the abdomen, flank, or back can often be locally explored and/or closed. Persistently stable and asymptomatic patients can be discharged (immediately or within 24h) [Level III]. Patients with penetrating injury isolated to the right upper quadrant of the abdomen may be managed without laparotomy in the presence of stable vital signs [Level III]. Diagnostic laparoscopy may be considered as a tool to evaluate diaphragmatic lacerations as well as peritoneal penetration [Level III]. Gunshot wounds should be thoroughly exposed and examined, followed by exploratory laparotomy in unstable and/or peritonitic patients. The absence of evidence of peritoneal penetration (on CT scan, DPL, endoscopy, and/or serial examination) justifies a more conservative approach. Colonic penetrating injuries can be primarily repaired in stable patients with non-destructive injuries (involvement of <50% of the bowel wall without devascularization) [Level I], or should undergo resection with primary anastomosis (in stable clean cases) or with colostomy formation (otherwise) in destructive injuries [Level II].

- *Penetrating lower limbs arterial injuries*—should undergo surgical exploration in the presence of hard signs (pulse deficit, pulsatile bleeding, bruit, thrill, expanding haematoma), further investigations using CT angiogram (where potential injury is suspected [Level I]), or be assessed and discharged (in the absence of hard signs, lowered ABPI, or other injuries requiring admission) [Level II]. Non-occlusive arterial injuries can be safely observed, and possibly treated at a later stage [Level III]. Endovascular interventions (apart from embolization of profunda or tibial arteries) are generally not indicated [Level III]. Four-compartment fasciotomy should be considered when needed [Level III].

Trauma management: special considerations

- *Trauma in pregnant patients*—all female patients of childbearing age with significant trauma should have β-HCG testing and be shielded for X-rays whenever possible [Level III]. Best initial treatment for the fetus is the optimum resuscitation of the mother and early assessment of the fetus [Level III]. Kleihauer–Betke analysis should be performed in all pregnant patients >12 week-gestation, and all pregnant women >20-week gestation with trauma should have cardiac monitoring for a minimum of 6h [Level II]. Caesarean section should be considered in any moribund pregnant woman of ≥24-week gestation, and should take place within 20min of maternal death (ideally within 4min of maternal arrest [Level III].

- *Prehospital fluid resuscitation*—can be problematic. Placement of vascular access at the scene of injury should not be performed (delays transport and has no evidence of any benefits) [Level II]. Attempts at peripheral intravenous access should be limited to two attempts during prehospital transport. If failed, alternative methods (intraosseous, central access) should be considered where appropriate [Level III]. Intravenous fluid resuscitation should be withheld until active bleeding/haemorrhage is addressed [Level III]. Small volume boluses (250mL) of 3% and 7.5% hypertonic saline (HTS), where needed, are sufficient [Level I]. Administration of blood in the prehospital setting is safe and feasible [Level III].

Further reading

NICE (2016) Major Trauma. https://www.nice.org.uk/guidance/ng39

American College of Surgeons (2014) Resources for optimal care of the injured patient. Available from: https://www.facs.org/quality-programs/trauma/vrc/resources

American College of Surgeons (2008) Advanced Trauma Life Support. 8th Edition. https://www.facs.org/quality%20programs/trauma/atls

EAST (2017). https://www.east.org/education/practice-management-guidelines/category/trauma

Chapter 18

Sepsis and septic shock*

Basic facts *162*
Recommended management plan *164*
Further reading *168*

Key guidelines
- Surviving Sepsis Campaign Guidelines (2016).
- Care of the critically ill surgical patient (CCrISP) 2010.

---

* The guidelines on this chapter have been sourced and summarized from different UK, Europe, and international government sources, professional organizations, and medical specialty societies. Leading guidelines have been listed in the further reading section at the end of this chapter.

Basic facts

- *Definitions*—sepsis is a syndrome of systematic inflammatory process caused by infection. The spectrum ranges in severity from mild sepsis to refractory septic shock (Box 18.1).
- *Incidence*—sepsis accounts for over 25% of potentially preventable in-hospital deaths. Septic shock is associated with >40–50% mortality rate.
- *Clinical features*—related to the severity of sepsis and organ dysfunction (Box 18.1; Box 16.2, ⊃ p.145).
- *Level of recommendations*—the 2016 Surviving Sepsis Campaign divide recommendations into: Strong (S): recommended practice; weak (W): suggested practice; and Best Practice Statement (BPS).

Box 18.1 Definitions in sepsis

Infection—inflammatory response to microorganism invasion.

Systemic inflammatory response syndrome (SIRS)—the presence of two or more of the following:

Temperature >38.3°C or <36.0°C; heart rate >90bpm (or >2SD of normal value for age); respiratory rate >20 breaths/min; positive fluid balance (>20mL/kg in 24h); change in mental state.

WBC count >12,000 cells/mL or <4,000 cells/mL or >10% immature (band) forms; CRP >2SD of normal values; hyperglycaemia (blood glucose >7.7mmol/L) in non-diabetic patients.

Sepsis—SIRS in the presence of documented infection (e.g. positive culture for blood, urine, sputum, or normally sterile body fluid; clear focus of apparent infection).

Severe sepsis—sepsis with signs of organ dysfunction of moderate severity (e.g. oliguria or change in mental status).

Septic shock—severe sepsis with inadequate tissue perfusion refractory to fluid management (e.g. mean BP <60mmHg after 40–60mL/kg normal saline solution, the need for norepinephrine or epinephrine of >0.25µg/kg/min to maintain mean BP >60mmHg).

Intensive Care Medicine, Levy, 2001 SCCM/ESICM/ACCP/ATS/SIS *International Sepsis Definitions Conference*, 29 (4), 530–38, Copyright © 2003. With permission of Springer.

Data from Dellinger et al. Surviving Sepsis Campaign: International Guidelines for Management of Severe Sepsis and Septic Shock: 2012, *Critical Care Medicine*, 41(2), 580–637, Copyright © 2013 Society of Critical Care Medicine

Recommended management plan

- Follow surviving sepsis campaign guidelines strictly and thoroughly to obtain best results (Table 18.1).
- Immediate resuscitation—should start promptly (first 3h) once sepsis has been recognized [S]. Resuscitation should follow agreed protocols and aims at achieving identifiable targets (goal-directed) [BPS] (Fig. 18.1). Sepsis-related mortality can be reduced significantly using this approach (reduction by >15%).
- Confirm the source, type, and site of infection—using appropriate cultures (e.g. blood, sputum, wound, and urine—Box 18.2) and imaging (aspiration of potential source of infection).
- *Infection source control.*
  - *Antimicrobial therapy*—should start promptly (Box 18.3) using a broad spectrum antibiotic [S] following appropriate cultures (within the first hour in septic shock [S]). Each hour of delay in starting antibiotics in the first 6h can reduce survival rate by 7–8%. Antibiotic spectrum should be based upon culture results [BPS].
  - *Source control*—should be achieved as soon as possible (e.g. operative management of peritonitis, endoscopic management of cholangitis) [BPS]. This is best done ASAP after identification in severe septic cases. Minimal invasive procedures are always preferable when appropriate. Any intravascular access devices should be removed and replaced if they are possible source of infection [BPS].

Table 18.1 Surviving sepsis bundle

To complete within first 3 hours*	To complete within first 6 hours
Measure lactate level	Apply vasopressors for hypotension that does not respond to initial fluid resuscitation to maintain MAP ≥65mmHg
Obtain blood cultures	In the event of persistent arterial hypotension despite volume resuscitation (septic shock) or initial lactate ≥4 mmol/L (36 mg/dL): • Measure central venous pressure (CVP)* • Measure central venous oxygen saturation (ScvO$_2$)*
Administer broad spectrum antibiotics	Re-measure lactate if initial lactate was raised
Administer 30ml/kg crystalloid for hypotension or lactate ≥4.0	

* Time zero, or time of presentation, is defined as the time of triage in the emergency department or, if presenting from another care venue, from the earliest chart annotation consistent with all elements of severe sepsis or septic shock ascertained through chart review.

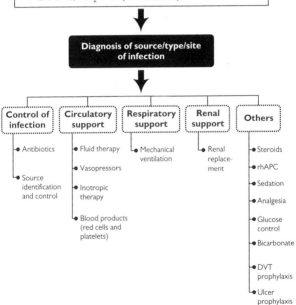

Fig. 18.1 Recommended approach to septic patients.

Box 18.2 Blood culture—good practice

Timing—before commencing antibiotics.

Number—two or more.

Site.

One percutaneously and one from each vascular access that has been inserted 48h or more.

Volume—10mL or more.

Data from Dellinger et al. Surviving Sepsis Campaign: International Guidelines for Management of Severe Sepsis and Septic Shock: 2012, *Critical Care Medicine*, 41(2), 580–637, Copyright © 2013 Society of Critical Care Medicine

Box 18.3 Antibiotic usage—good practice

Timing—soon (within 1h of identifying severe sepsis).

Type—start empirical antibiotics that have known broad-enough activity against most likely pathogen/s (and against MRSA where this is prevalent) [B]. Avoiding antibiotic resistance by reducing the spectrum is not recommended initially. Combination therapy should be considered in individual cases. Narrow the antibiotic spectrum once specific pathogen is identified.

Review—daily (more safe and cost-effective) [C].

Duration—7 to 10d, then stop (unless immunosuppressed or slow clinical response) [D].

Data from Dellinger et al Surviving Sepsis Campaign: International Guidelines for Management of Severe Sepsis and Septic Shock: 2012, Critical Care Medicine, 41(2), 580–637, 580–637, Copyright © 2013 Society of Critical Care Medicine

- *Circulatory support.*
  - *Fluid therapy*—using crystalloids [S]. Consider additional albumin if substantial amount of crystalloids are required [W]. Goal-targeted fluid therapy, fluid challenge technique up to 30ml/kg of rapid administration within 3h [S], and reduction of fluid administration upon reaching the target (normalized lactate) are recommended practices [W]. Consider vasopressors if initial mean arterial pressure (MAP) 65mmHg or below [S].
  - *Vasopressors*—norepinephrine is the 1st choice vasopressor to maintain the MAP at 65mmHg or above when fluid therapy fails to achieve this goal [S]. MAP of >65mmHg is associated with adequate blood flow and acceptable tissue perfusion (Box 16.4).
  - *Inotropes*—add vasopressin or epinephrine [W] to maintain MAP. Dopamine is only recommended in highly selected patients [W]. Dobutamine should be considered for patients resistant to fluid and vasopressors [W]. Increasing oxygen delivery to supranormal levels has no beneficial effect and is not recommended.
  - *Blood products*—indicated when Hb drops below 7g/dL [S]. The target Hb should be 7–9g/dL (see ➜ Chapter 13, pp. 91–96). Erythropoietin is not recommended [S]. Fresh frozen plasma is also not indicated to correct without bleeding [W]. Platelets should be transfused when <10k without bleeding, or <20k with bleeding [W].
- *Respiratory support.*
  - Mechanical ventilation, when indicated, should aim at achieving adequate tidal volume of 6mL/kg and plateau pressure of ≤30cmH$_2$O.

- *Renal support.*
  - Renal replacement, when indicated, can be applied intermittently or continuously (no significant difference) for acute renal failure. Continuous dialysis is recommended for accurate fluid management in unstable patients.
- *Other interventions in septic patients.*
  - *Steroid therapy*—indicated only in cases of refractory hypotension to fluid and vasopressor management [W] (Box 18.5).
  - *Recombinant human activated protein C (rhAPC)*—recommended for patients with severe sepsis and high risk of death (e.g. APACHE II score ≥25 or multi-organ failure), but not for low risk of death (e.g. APACHE II score <20 or one organ failure). The average total mortality reduction is 76%.
  - *Sedation, analgesia, and neuromuscular blockade*—sedation using agreed protocols (intermittent bolus or continuous with daily interruption) is recommended for ventilated patients (significant decrease of ventilation duration and tracheostomy rates). Neuromuscular blockade causes more harm (prolonged neuromuscular blockade) than benefits and should be avoided if possible.
  - *Glucose control*—using agreed protocols (sliding scale) to maintain serum glucose level at <150mg/dL is highly recommended (average mortality reduction of ~45% and absolute mortality reduction of 4–10%).
  - *Bicarbonate therapy*—not recommended for the sole purpose of improving the haemodynamic status in acidotic patients.
  - *Prophylaxis*—is recommended against DVT and stress ulcers (using H2 blockers or proton pump inhibitors).
  - Oral or enteral (if necessary) feedings, as tolerated, are better than complete fasting.
- See also ➲ Sepsis OCHM 10e Ch. 19.

Box 18.4 Vasopressors—good practice

Insertion of arterial catheter is recommended for accurate titration of vasopressors [D].

Noradrenaline and dopamine are recommended initially [C], with epinephrine used as alternative for refractory cases [C].

Renal—protection dose of dopamine is not recommended routinely [A].

Data from Dellinger et al Surviving Sepsis Campaign: International Guidelines for Management of Severe Sepsis and Septic Shock: 2012, Critical Care Medicine, 41(2), 580–637, pp. 580–637, Copyright © 2013 Society of Critical Care Medicine

Box 18.5 Steroids—good practice

No role for ACTH stimulation test—no clear clinical significance [B].

No role for dexamethasone if hydrocortisone exists [B].

No role for steroids once vasopressors have been discontinued [D].

No role of high doses (comparable to over 300mg hydrocortisone) as a treatment option for septic shock [A].

No role for treating sepsis without the presence of septic shock [D].

Data from Dellinger et al. Surviving Sepsis Campaign: International Guidelines for Management of Severe Sepsis and Septic Shock: 2012, Critical Care Medicine, 41(2), 580–637, pp.580–637, Copyright © 2013 Society of Critical Care Medicine

Further reading

Dellinger RP, Levy MM, Carlet JM et al. (2015). Surviving Sepsis Campaign: international guidelines for management of severe sepsis and septic shock.

Loftus I, et al. (2010). Care of the critically ill surgical patient, 3rd ed, Hodder Arnold, London.

Sasse KC, Nauenberg E, Long A, Anton B, Tucker HJ, Hu TW (1995). Long-term survival after intensive care unit admission with sepsis. Crit Care Med 23, 1040–7.

Rivers E, Nguyen B, Havstad S et al. (2001). Early goal-directed therapy in the treatment of severe sepsis and septic shock. N Engl J Med 345, 1368–77.

Kumar A, Roberts D, Wood KE et al. (2006). Duration of hypotension prior to initiation of effective antimicrobial therapy is the critical determinant of survival in human septic shock. Crit Care Med 34, 1589–96.

LeDoux D, Astiz ME, Carpati CM, Rackow EC (2000). Effects of perfusion pressure on tissue perfusion in septic shock. Crit Care Med 28, 2729–32.

Bernard GR, Vincent JL, Laterre PR et al. (2001). Efficacy and safety of recombinant human activated protein C for severe sepsis. N Engl J Med 344, 699–709.

van den Berghe G, Wouters P, Weekers F et al. (2001). Intensive insulin therapy in critically ill patients. N Engl J Med 345, 1359–67.

Antibiotic prophylaxis in surgery*

Background *170*
Risk factors for developing SSIs *171*
Risk of prophylactic antibiotics *172*
Current antibiotic prophylaxis recommendations *174*
Further reading *178*

Key guidelines
- Scottish Intercollegiate Guidelines Network (2014). Antibiotic prophylaxis in surgery.
- British National Formulary (2015). Summary of antibacterial prophylaxis.
- National Institute for Health and Clinical Excellence (2017). Surgical site infection: prevention and treatment of surgical site infection.

---

* The guidelines on this chapter have been sourced and summarized from different UK, Europe, and international government sources, professional organizations, and medical specialty societies. Leading guidelines have been listed in the further reading section at the end of this chapter.

Background

- *Main objectives*—to reduce the incidence of surgical site infection (SSI), a common and potentially avoidable problem in surgical practice. Emergency procedures with contaminated fields should be treated as established infection.
- *Definitions*—SSIs refer to infections affecting surgical wounds, body cavities, bones, joints, and other tissues within the surgical field, including infection of prosthetic implants. Prevalence of SSIs ranges from 2 to 20% depending on different factors (see below).
- *Impact of SSIs*—increased length of hospital stay (by 7–10d), increased rate of admission to intensive care, increased hospital readmission rate (×5), and increased mortality rate (×2). The costs of treating SSIs are substantial.
- *Efficiency*—properly used, prophylactic antibiotics can reduce the risk of SSIs by up to six times compared to controls.

Risk factors for developing SSIs

- *Operative field contamination*—operative procedures can be classified into four groups (Table 19.1) with incremental risk of SSI.
- *Comorbidities, patient's health, and ASA Grade*—ASA grade ≥2 has significant effect on SSI risk.
- *Surgical skills and technique*—e.g. operations taking longer than the 75th percentile for similar type of procedure have significantly higher SSI rate.
- *Risk index*—more reliable in estimating SSI risk than each factor alone (Table 19.2).

Table 19.1 Types of surgical wounds

Type	Description
Clean	No breach to a potentially contaminated organ (respiratory, alimentary, or genitourinary tracts). No inflammatory process or sepsis are found or entered, and no break to aseptic techniques.
Clean contaminated	Entering the respiratory, alimentary, or genitourinary tracts without significant spillage.
Contaminated	Operating on acute inflammatory process but no pus, or the presence of gross contamination of the wound (e.g. gross spillage from a hollow viscus).
Dirty	Operative field has gross pus, or operating on old (>4h) compound/open injuries.

Table 19.2 Risk index for developing SSIs*

Type of surgery	No extra factors**	One extra factor**	Two extra factors**
Clean	1%	2.5%	5.5%
Clean contaminated	2%	4%	10%
Contaminated	3.5%	7%	14%

* Numbers represent probability of wound infection rounded to the nearest 0.5. ** Extra factors include: 1. ASA grade ≥2, 2. duration of operation more than the 75th percentile.

Risk of prophylactic antibiotics

- *Antibiotic resistance*—rates increase significantly with increased total antibiotic exposure.
- *Antibiotic-associated colitis (C. difficile infection)*—risk increases with even a single dose of prophylactic antibiotics (especially third generation cephalosporins), and becomes significantly more common when antibiotics are given for >24h (see ➔ Chapter 18, p.186).
- *Increased cost of treatment.*
- *Adverse drug reactions*—e.g. allergy, toxicity.

Current antibiotic prophylaxis recommendations

- *Which procedure*—any clean operation involving the use of prosthesis or implant, clean contaminated, and contaminated operations. Otherwise, do NOT use prophylactic antibiotics.
- *Antibiotics choice* (Table 18.3)
  - Consider using for prophylaxis the same antibiotics used for active treatment of infections in this site.
  - The choice must reflect the local information on common pathogens and their antimicrobial sensitivity.
  - Infections occurring post-operatively usually are caused by the same bacteria that prophylactic antibiotics were given to protect against. Consider using different type of antibiotics if first prophylaxis did not achieve its targets.
- *Dose*—single dose should be the same as usual therapeutic dose [G].
- *Timing*—IV prophylactic antibiotics should be given within 60min before the incision is made or on starting the incision as practical [B].
- *Duration of effect*—the half-life of selected antibiotic should be sufficient to cover the operating time. Prolonged surgery or when significant blood loss has occurred would indicate a second dose.
- *Stopping the antibiotics*—post-operative doses of prophylaxis antibiotics (>24h) should not be given for any operation [A]. All doses should be administered immediately before or during the operation. Continuing antibiotics for prophylaxis reasons should be clearly justified (blood loss >1,500mL, haemodilution [B], or treatment of established infection).
- *Penicillin allergy history*—any anaphylactic reaction, urticaria, or rash occurring immediately after previous penicillin administration increases the likelihood that immediate hypersensitivity to penicillins exists. Beta-lactam antibiotics should be avoided in such cases [B].
- *MRSA*—a glycopeptide (e.g. vancomycin or teicoplanin) should be considered for prophylaxis in the carriers of MRSA undergoing high-risk surgery. Intranasal mupirocin may be used in MRSA carriers pre- and/or post-operatively to minimize carriage and the risk of subsequent infection (see ⊃ Chapter 18, p.184).
- *Inpatient requiring antibiotic prophylaxis*—the risk of *C. difficile* infection should be considered. If high risk for *C. diff*, then some antibiotics such as cephalosporins, carbapenems, and fluoroquinolones should be used with caution.
- See ⊃ OHCM 10e Ch. 13.
- Advise patients preoperatively on: take a shower or have a bath using soap, do NOT remove hair the night before, and use electric clippers same day of surgery if needed, use theatre wear.
- There is NO evidence of using: routine nasal decontamination with topical antibiotics, or routine mechanical bowel preparation.

Table 19.3 Types of surgical wounds

Operation	Common pathogens	R*	Type and dose	Grade
Gastric/ oesophageal surgery	Enteric gram –ve bacilli, gram +ve cocci	b	Single dose ** of: gentamicin (IV) or cefuroxime (IV) or Amoxiclav Δ	[A, D]
Colorectal surgery	Enteric gram –ve bacilli, enterococci, anaerobes	a	Single dose of gentamicin (IV) + metronidazole (IV) or cefuroxime (IV) + metronidazole (IV) or co-amoxiclav (IV) alone Δ	[A]
Appendicectomy	Ebteric gram –ve bacilli, enterococci, anaerobes	b	Single dose of gentamicin (IV) + metronidazole (IV) or cefuroxime (IV) + metronidazole (IV) or co-amoxiclav (IV) alone Δ	[A]
Biliary surgery (open)	Enteric gram –ve bacilli, enterococci, clostridia	b	Single dose of cefurozime (IV) or metronidazole (IV) or gentamicin (IV) + metronidazole (IV) or co-amoxiclav alone Δ	[A]
Laproscopic cholecystectomy		N***		[A]
ERCP	Enteric gram –ve bacilli, enterococci, clostridia	?	Single dose of gentamicin (IV) or ciprofloxacin (IV or PO)	[D]
Vascular surgery	S. aureus, S. epidermidis, anaerobes in diabetes, gangrene, or undergoing amputation	b	Single dose of cefurozime (IV) or ciprofloxacin (IV) + gentamicin (IV). Add metronidazole (IV) for suspected anaerobic infection or gangrene or co-amoxiclav (IV)	[A]
Lower limb amputation/ major trauma		b	Benzylpenicillin 300–600mg qds for 5d or (for penicillin allergic) metronidazole 400–500mg tds	[A]
Breast surgery		b	-	[C]

(Continued)

Table 19.3 (Contd.)

Operation	Common pathogens	R*	Type and dose	Grade
Inguinal/femoral hernia repair (open)		N	-	[A]
Inguinal/femoral hernia repair (laproscopic)		N	-	[B]
Surgery using mesh (e.g. gastric band)		N***	-	[B]
Clean contaminated procedures		b	-	[D]

*R = level of recommendation = highly recommended (unequivocal benefits)

b = recommended (highly likely to be beneficial); c = usually recommended but may be withdrawn as per local policy; N = not recommended (likely to cause harm more than benefit)

** Add extra dose for prolonged operations (>2-4h) *** Consider for high-risk patients Δ add teicoplanin if high risk of MRSA.

Beyond the guidelines and the future

Although some examples of appropriate agents have been shown in Table 19.3, many centres have extensively revised their antibiotic regimens in an attempt to reduce the incidence of *C. difficile*. In particular, the use of cephalosporins and quinolones for both treatment and prophylaxis has been markedly reduced.

Further reading

Scottish Intercollegiate Guidelines Network (2014). Antibiotic prophylaxis in surgery. A national clinical guideline. Available from: http://www.sign.ac.uk/assets/sign104.pdf

National Institute for Health and Clinical Excellence (2017). Surgical site infection: prevention and treatment of surgical site infection. Available from: http://guidance.nice.org.uk/CG74.

British National Formulary 75 (2015). Summary of antibacterial prophylaxis. Available from: http://www.bnf.org

Bratzler DW, Houck PM; Surgical Infection Prevention Guideline Writers Workgroup (2005). Antimicrobial prophylaxis for surgery: an advisory statement from the National Surgical Infection Prevention Project. Am J Surg 189, 395–404.

The Society for Hospital Epidemiology of America; the Association for Practitioners in Infection Control; the Centres for Disease Control; the Surgical Infection Society (1992). Consensus paper on the surveillance of surgical wound infections. Infect Control Hosp Epidemiol 13, 599–605.

Classen DC, Evans RS, Pestotnik SL, Horn SD, Menlove RL, Burke JP (1992). The timing of prophylactic administration of antibiotics and the risk of surgical wound infection. N Engl J Med 326, 281–6.

Culver DH, Horan TC, Gaynes RP et al. (1991). Surgical wound infection rates by wound class, operative procedure, and patient risk index. National Nosocomial Infections Surveillance System. Am J Med 91(3B), 152S–157S.

* Numbers represent probability of wound infection rounded to the nearest 0.5. ** Extra factors include: 1. ASA grade ≥2, 2. duration of operation more than the 75th percentile.

Chapter 20

Principles of infection control*

Background *180*
Personal protection equipment *182*
Safe use and disposal of sharps *183*
Methicillin-resistant *Staphylococcus aureus* (MRSA) *184*
Clostridium difficile-associated diarrhoea *186*
Management of short-term urinary catheters *188*
Further reading *189*

Key guidelines
- National Institute for Health and Clinical Excellence (2012). Infection control: prevention of health care-associated infection in primary and community care.
- Department of Health (2008). The Health Act 2006: code of practice for the prevention and control of health care associated infections.
- Department of Health (2008). Clean, safe care: reducing infections and saving lives.
- epic2: national evidence-based guidelines for preventing health care-associated infections in NHS hospitals in England (2007).
- World Health Organization (2004). Practical guidelines for infection control in health care facilities.
- Centres for Disease Control and Prevention (2007). Infection control guidelines.
- MRSA guidelines (Europe, UK).
- Updated guidance on the management and treatment of *Clostridium difficile* infection (2013)
- Healthcare Commission (2005). Management, prevention and surveillance of *Clostridium difficile*.
- National Institute of Clinical Excellence (2012), *Clostridium difficile* infection: Fidaxomicin

---

* The guidelines on this chapter have been sourced and summarized from different UK, Europe, and international government sources, professional organizations, and medical specialty societies. Leading guidelines have been listed in the further reading section at the end of this chapter.

Background

- *Definitions*—health care-associated infections (HCAIs—also known as nosocomial infections) are infections acquired in hospitals or as a result of health care interventions. Infection control is a strategy that applies epidemiologic and scientific principles to achieve effective prevention or reduction in HCAIs.
- *Prevalence*—the overall prevalence of HCAIs in England has remained relatively constant at about 8% over the last 25y. The particular challenge in management and cost from MRSA and *Clostridium (C.) difficile* infections has recently taken the infection control strategies to the top of the agenda. Infection with, e.g. *C. difficile*, can cost the hospital an extra £4,000–10,000 per patient, and cost the patients their lives!
- *Medico-legal issues*—prevention and control of infection is a legal obligation for the Department of Health, NHS Trusts, and their staff. Under the Health Act of October 2006, if a patient, visitor, or health care worker can prove that they acquired an infection in hospital that resulted in harm, they may be able to claim damages (e.g. for loss of earnings).
- *Common types of HCAIs*—include urinary tract infection, surgical site infection, chest infection, and skin and mucous membrane infection
- *The five main routes of transmission*—direct and indirect contact (dressing, contaminated gloves), droplets (coughing, sneezing), airborne (air conditioner, dust), common vehicle (food, water), and vector-borne (mosquitoes, flies).
- *People at high risk of HCAIs*—include extremes of age, immunodeficiency states, using invasive devices (Foley catheters, tracheostomies, etc.) as well as patients on antimicrobial therapy.

Hospital hygiene

- *General look*—hospitals must ensure a clean environment that is free from dust and spoilages and in acceptable condition to patients, visitors and staff [C].
- *Supplies*—good hygienic practice requires hospitals to provide their staff (and patients) with adequate supplies of clean water, liquid soap, handrub, towels, and sharps containers [D].
- *Staff responsibilities*—every individual working within the health care system should pay special attention to their responsibilities in maintaining a safe, clean, and appropriate care setting for patients and other staff [D].

Hand hygiene

- *Timing*—appropriate hand decontamination should be done before any direct contact/care with patients and after any potentially contaminating activity [C]. Hospital staff should be provided with appropriate training. Patients should be informed on their role in maintaining hygienic standards within healthcare facilities.

- *Agents*—liquid soap and water are the first-line decontaminating agents of choice for any visibly soiled or potentially grossly contaminated hands [A]. Alcohol-based handrub is preferred for use between caring for different patients if no visible hand contamination is present [A].
- *Technique*—effective hand washing techniques include preparation of hands by wetting them under running water, application of liquid soap, rubbing hands vigorously and thoroughly for 10–15s at least, rinsing hands, and drying them appropriately using paper towels [D].
- *Hand care*—hand cuts and abrasions should be covered with waterproof dressings, and fingernails should be kept short and clean with no nail polish. Wrist and hand jewelleries should be removed. Application of emollient hand cream should be considered on regular bases [D].
- *Efficiency.*
  - *Compliance*—historically low (<45%), even in controlled study conditions and ICUs. When hand washing is performed, proper techniques are usually not followed (e.g. less than 10s).
  - *Alcohol-based handrub*—resulted in significant improvement in compliance with hand hygiene standards, decreased in nosocomial infection rates (from 17% to 10%), and reduction in transmission of MRSA (from 2 to 1 episode per 10,000 patient days). Hands must be rubbed together thoroughly and vigorously until the solution is evaporated. Alcohol is not sufficient to destroy *C. difficile* spores, and liquid soup with water must be used.

Personal protection equipment

- *Gloves*.
  - *Usage*—for performing any invasive procedure, contacting sterile sites, mucous membranes, or non-intact skin [D, R*]. Gloves are single-use items. They should be put on immediately before use and removed on completing the task. Polythene gloves should not be used for clinical interventions. Gloves are clinical wastes and should be disposed of as appropriate [D, R].
  - *Efficiency*—wearing gloves does not replace proper hand hygiene. Studies showed that up to 15% of gloves have unrecognized perforations, mostly on the thumb and index finger. Selected pathogenic bacteria can also be recovered from hands after removing the gloves. Therefore, proper hand washing following removal of gloves is recommended [D, R].
- *Plastic aprons*.
  - *Usage*—to protect against contamination of staff clothing with blood, body fluid, and other biological materials [D, R]. Plastic aprons are single-use items for only one procedure or episode. They form part of clinical wastes and should be disposed of as appropriate [D, R].
  - *Eye protection and face masks*—should be used in procedures of high-risk of contaminations for the face or eyes with blood, body fluid, and other biological materials [D, R].

* R: Health and safety regulation]

Safe use and disposal of sharps

- *Handling*—all sharps must be handled carefully and should not be passed directly from hand to hand, bent, broken, or disassembled [D, R].
- *Sharps containers*—manufactured at certain standards, and should be used to discard used sharps at the point of use by the user. Sharps containers must not be filled above their mark [D, R].

Methicillin-resistant *Staphylococcus aureus* (MRSA)

- *Definition*—first described in 1961 upon introduction of methicillin antibiotics. Infection results from resistant strains of *Staphylococcus aureus* to methicillin and other beta-lactam antibiotics. Methicillin resistance is mediated by a special penicillin binding protein (PBP–2a) encoded by *mecA* gene. Five major MRSA clones emerged worldwide since 2002.
- *Impact on health care*
  - *Prevalence*—MRSA accounts for 1–40% of all *S. aureus* infections in Europe, being significantly higher in Southern Europe compared to Scandinavia. MRSA affects ~11–14 people per 100,000 population, about 5–10% of them are invasive infections.
  - *Impact*—MRSA infection causes significantly higher mortality (OR ×1.93), longer hospital stay (×1.29 fold for MRSA bacteraemia), and higher costs (×1.36 fold for MRSA bacteraemia) compared to methicillin-susceptible *S. aureus* infection.
- Detection.
  - High-risk patients.
    —Antibiotic use—independent risk factor. Risk is highest on using cephalosporin (up to 3 times for ≥5d usage), fluoroquinolone (OR ×3.4), and the use of more than one antimicrobial agent (OR rises from ~1.5 for one agent to ~6 for four agents).
    —Special hospital settings—frequent prolonged or readmission episodes to hospitals, proximity to others with MRSA colonization or infection, and residential care patients.
    —Medical condition—previous MRSA colonization, surgical site infection, HIV-positive patients, intensive care, and haemodialysis patients.
    —Transmission—occurs via transiently contaminated hands of hospital staff, contaminated environmental surfaces, and the direct contact with colonized or infected individuals.
  - *Screening*—should be performed on all high-risk patients admitted to general units and on all general patients admitted to high-risk units. Regular screening (weekly or monthly) should be performed on all patients in high-risk units.
    —Screening sites—anterior nares, groin and perineum, skin lesions and wounds, IV catheters sites, urine catheters, tracheostomy, and sputum from productive cough.
    —Staff screening—not recommended routinely. Screening is indicated if new MRSA carriers are found in the unit, and if transmission in the unit continued despite active control measures.
- *Management* (Box 20.1).
- *Prevention*.
  - Strict infection control measures—are essential.
  - Surveillance—must be performed regularly by infection control team.
  - Strict antibiotic policy.

Box 20.1 MRSA management

Decolonization.

Indications—recommended for certain patient groups under the advice of infection control team. This may include patients with documented recurrent MRSA infections, patients undergoing operative procedure, and carrier staff during outbreak time.

Techniques—nasal (mupirocin 2% in a paraffin base to the inner surface of each anterior nares three times a day for 5d), throat (systemic antibiotics), skin (4% chlorhexidine body wash/shampoo, 7.5% povidone iodine or 2% triclosan), and clean clothing, bedding, and towels after completion.

Strict infection control measures.

Physical setting—patient isolation is recommended depending on available facilities. Patient movement should be kept to the minimum. Patient equipment (stethoscopes, sphygmomanometers) should be single use or decontaminated before used for other patients. Topical and systemic prophylaxis (+/– prophylactic antibiotics) should be considered prior to performing any procedure (including placing patients at the end of theatre list). No special arrangements for prolonged eradication protocol on discharge from the unit are usually required.

Clostridium difficile-associated diarrhoea

- *Definition*—*C. difficile* is an anaerobic, Gram positive, spore-forming bacterium, capable of producing enterotoxins, and resulting in occasionally life-threatening antibiotic-associated colitis.
- *Prevalence*—*C. difficile* colonizes <5% of normal population (up to 20–50% of hospitalized elderly patients), and is usually kept under control by normal bacterial flora. About 20% of hospitalized patients become infected during their stay (cross infection), up to a third of them develop diarrhoea due to *C. difficile* toxins. Some types of *C. difficile* strains (type 027) can cause major outbreaks.
- Risk factors (Box 20.2).
- *Clinical presentation*—ranges from mild diarrhoea to severe pseudomembranous colitis, severe sepsis, and bowel perforation.
- *Diagnosis and treatment approach*—see Fig. 20.1.
- *Prevention*—six key measures can significantly reduce the burden of *C. difficile* within hospital setting: judicious antibiotic prescribing policy, early isolation of infected (or suspected) cases, enhanced environmental cleaning, strict hand hygiene, appropriate use of personal protective equipment, and staff education and training.

Box 20.2 *C. difficile* risk factors

Antibiotics—main risk factor.

Most frequent—broad-spectrum penicillins and cephalosporins, clindamycin, and fluoroquinolones. Receiving multiple antibiotics and long duration treatment increases the risk significantly.

Occasional—trimethoprim and sulphonamides.

Rare—metronidazole and vancomycin (usual treatment for *C. difficile*), aminoglycosides, and chloramphenicol.

Hospital admission factors—hospitalization of elderly, ICU stay, long hospital stay.

Disease- and procedure-related factors—severe underlying disease, gastrointestinal procedures, use of NGT, and receiving anti-ulcer drugs.

Development of outbreak—depends on the ability of a high infectivity. *C. difficile* strain to cause more than one new case in patients surrounded by individuals with high risk factors (hospitalized elderly treated with antibiotics in the same ward) where standards of infection control are low (high cross- contamination).

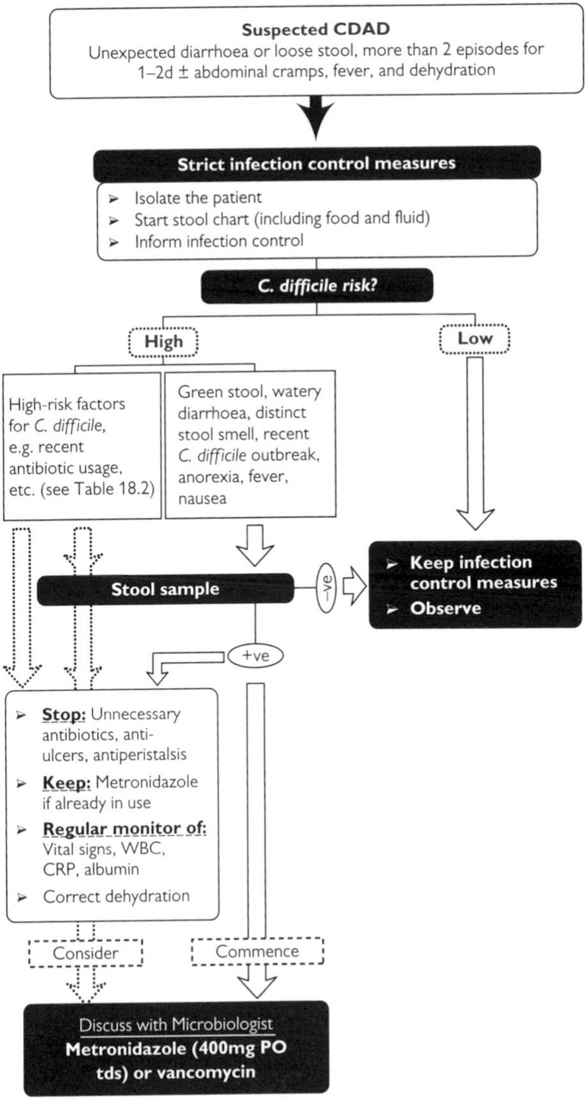

Suspected CDAD
Unexpected diarrhoea or loose stool, more than 2 episodes for
1–2d ± abdominal cramps, fever, and dehydration

Strict infection control measures
➤ Isolate the patient
➤ Start stool chart (including food and fluid)
➤ Inform infection control

C. difficile risk?

High

Low

High-risk factors
for *C. difficile*,
e.g. recent
antibiotic usage,
etc. (see Table 18.2)

Green stool, watery
diarrhoea, distinct
stool smell, recent
C. difficile outbreak,
anorexia, fever,
nausea

Stool sample –ve

➤ **Keep infection
control measures**
➤ **Observe**

+ve

➤ **Stop:** Unnecessary
antibiotics, anti-
ulcers, antiperistalsis
➤ **Keep:** Metronidazole
if already in use
➤ **Regular monitor of:**
Vital signs, WBC,
CRP, albumin
➤ Correct dehydration

Consider

Commence

Discuss with Microbiologist
**Metronidazole (400mg PO
tds) or vancomycin**

Fig. 20.1 Management algorithm for suspected *C. difficile*-associated diarrhoea
C18.F1 (CDAD).

Management of short-term urinary catheters

- Only to be used if absolutely necessary, always with full asepsis, and with the smallest gauge and 10mL balloon. Remove catheter as soon as possible [D].
- A single-use sterile lubricant should be used and a sterile closed drainage system which should be at a lower level than the bladder, but not in contact with the floor [D].
- When possible, self-catheterization should be encouraged. Relatives and carers must be educated on best practice and routine personal hygiene encouraged [D].
- Urinary drainage bags should be emptied frequently to maintain urine flow and prevent reflux
- Further guidelines on enteral feeding devices and vascular access instruments can be found in NICE (2012). Infection control: prevention of health care-associated infection in primary and community care.

Fidaxomicin has been evidenced in clinical trials to be non-inferior to vancomycin and may reduce recurrence rates. However, it has not currently been fully appraised by NICE. Refer to local guidelines/consult microbiologist.

Further reading

Department of Health (2008). The Health Act 2006: code of practice for the prevention and control of health care associated infections. Available from: http://www.rdehospital.nhs.uk/docs/patients/services/housekeeping_services/Health%20Act%202006.pdf

Department of Health (2008). Clean, safe care: reducing infections and saving lives. Available from: http://antibiotic-action.com/wp-content/uploads/2011/07/DH-Clean-safe-care-v2007.pdf

Pratt RJ, Pellowe CM, Wilson JA et al. (2007). epic2: national evidence-based guidelines for preventing health care-associated infections in NHS hospitals in England. J Hosp Infect 65 Suppl1, S1–64.

National Institute for Health and Clinical Excellence (2012). Infection control: prevention of health care-associated infection in primary and community care.

World Health Organization (2004). Practical guidelines for infection control in health care facilities. Available from: http://www.wpro.who.int/publications/docs/practical_guidelines_infection_control.pdf

Centres for Disease Control and Prevention (2007). Infection control guidelines. Available from: http://www.cdc.gov/ncidod/dhqp/guidelines.html.

The Groupement pour le Depistage, l'Etude et la Prevention des Infections Hospitalieres (1993). Guidelines for control and prevention of methicillin-resistant Staphylococcus aureus transmission in Belgian hospitals. Available from: https://www.health.belgium.be/sites/default/files/uploads/fields/fpshealth_theme_file/4448393/Guidelines%20for%20the%20control%20and%20prevention%20of%20methicillin-resistant%20Staphylococcus%20Aureus%20transmission%20in%20Belgian%20hospitals%20%28June%202005%29%20%28SHC%207725%29.pdf

Coia JE, Duckworth GJ, Edwards DI et al. (2006) Guidelines for the control and prevention of meticillin-resistance *Staphylococcus aureus* (MRSA) in health care facilities. J Hosp Infect 63 Suppl1, S1–44.

Bassetti, M. et al. European perspective and update on the management of complicated skin and soft tissue infections due to methicillin-resistant Staphylococcus aureus after more than 10 years of experience with linezolid. Clinical Microbiology and Infection, Volume 20, 3–18; Link: http://www.clinicalmicrobiologyandinfection.com/article/S1198-743X(14)60009-4/abstract

Updated guidance on the management and treatment of Clostridium difficile infection (2013) available at: https://www.gov.uk/government/uploads/system/uploads/attachment_data/file/321891/Clostridium_difficile_management_and_treatment.pdf

Haley RW, Culver DH, White JW et al. (1985). The efficacy of infection surveillance and control programs in preventing nosocomial infections in the US hospitals. Am J Epidemiol 121, 182–205.

Pittet D, Mourouga P, Perneger TV (1999). Compliance with handwashing in a teaching hospital. Infection Control Program. Ann Intern Med 130, 126–30.

Voss A, Widmer AF (1997). No time for handwashing!? Handwashing versus alcoholic rub: can we afford 100% compliance? Infect Control Hosp Epidemiol 18, 205–8.

Quraishi ZA, McGuckin M, Blais FX (1984). Duration of handwashing in intensive care units: a descriptive study. Am J Infect Control 12, 83–7.

Pittet D, Hugonnet S, Harbarth S et al. (2000). Effectiveness of a hospital-wide programme to improve compliance with hand hygiene. Infection Control Programme. Lancet 356, 1307–12.

Alrawi S, Houshan L, Satheesan R, Raju R, Cunningham J, Acinapura A (2001). Glove reinforcement: an alternative to double gloving. Infect Control Hosp Epidemiol 22, 526–7.

Voss A, Milatovic D, Wallrauch-Schwarz C, Rosdahl VT, Braveny I (1994). Methicillin-resistant Staphylococcus aureus in Europe. Eur J Clin Microbiol Infect Dis 13, 50–5.

Cosgrove SE, Sakoulas G, Perencevich EN, Schwaber MJ, Karchmer AW, Carmeli Y (2003). Comparison of mortality associated with methicillin-resistant and methicillin-susceptible Staphylococcus aureus bacteraemia: a meta-analysis. Clin Infect Dis 36, 53–9.

Cosgrove SE, Qi Y, Kaye KS, Harbarth S, Karchmer AW, Carmeli Y (2005). The impact of methicillin resistance in Staphylococcus aureus bacteraemia on patient outcomes: mortality, length of stay, and hospital charges. Infect Control Hosp Epidemiol 26, 166–74.

Schneider–Lindner V, Delaney JA, Dial S, Dascal A, Suissa S (2007). Antimicrobial drugs and community-acquired methicillin-resistant Staphylococcus aureus, United Kingdom. Emerg Infect Dis 13, 994–1000.

Starr J (2005). Clostridium difficile associated diarrhoea: diagnosis and treatment. BMJ 331, 498–501.

Riggs MM, Sethi AK, Zabarsky TF, Eckstein EC, Jump RL, Donskey CJ (2007). Asymptomatic carriers are a potential source for transmission of epidemic and non-epidemic Clostridium dif-ficile strains among long-term care facility residents. Clin Infect Dis 45, 992–8.

Health Protection Agency. Clostridium difficile guidelines. Available from: http://www.hpa.org.uk/webw/HPAweb&Page&HPAwebAutoListName/Page/1179745281238?p=1179745281238.

Surrey Primary Care Trust (2008). Guidance for the management of Clostridium difficile. Available from: http://www.transition.surreypct.nhs.uk/policies-and-procedures/clinical-policies/infection-control-guidelines/Management_of_Clostridium_Difficile._August_08.pdf.

National Institute of Clinical Excellence (2012). Clostridium Difficile infection:Fidaxomicin

Chapter 21

Principles of pain management*

Basic facts *192*
Recommended approach *194*
Further reading *198*

Key guidelines

- British Pain Society (2013). Guidelines for pain management program for adults.
- European Society of Regional Anaesthesia and Pain Therapy. Post-operative pain management—good clinical practice.
- Clinical Knowledge Summaries. Palliative cancer care—pain management.
- NHS Quality Improvement Scotland (2009). Best practice statement: post-operative pain management.
- American Society of Anaesthesiologists Task Force on Acute Pain Management (2004). Practice guidelines for acute pain management in the perioperative setting.
- European Federation of Neurological Societies (2006). Guidelines on pharmacological treatment of neuropathic pain.
- The Pain Society (2004). Recommendations for the appropriate use of opioids for persistent non-cancer pain.
- National Institute of Health and Care Excellence (2017): Neuropathic pain – pharmacological management.

---

* The guidelines on this chapter have been sourced and summarized from different UK, Europe, and international government sources, professional organizations, and medical specialty societies. Leading guidelines have been listed in the further reading section at the end of this chapter.

Basic facts

- *Definition of pain*—unpleasant sensory and emotional experience associated with potential or actual tissue damage. Pain is a subjective conscious experience: 'Pain is whatever the experiencing person says it is, and exists whenever he says it does.'
- *Pain types and transmission*—see Boxes 21.1 and 21.2.

Box 21.1 Types and transmission of pain

Nociceptive pain—any pain associated with tissue damage. Pain correlates well with the extent and location of damage.

- Nociceptive somatic—stimulus is transmitted by somatic nerves. Pain is often described as well-localized, sharp, aching, throbbing, and/or pressure-like.
- Nociceptive visceral—stimulus is transmitted by visceral nerves. Pain is usually poorly localized, cramping, or gnawing if tissue damage was in a hollow viscus, and aching or sharp if the damage was in a capsule or mesentery tissue.

Non-nociceptive pain—(also known as neuropathic pain) results from direct effect of a lesion on the somatosensory system, causing abnormal function (without tissue damage) in the central or peripheral nerves. Usually presents with burning, stabbing, or lancinating pain; initiated spontaneously or by thermal, chemical, or mechanical stimulants. Common conditions causing this pain include diabetes, stroke, post-incision chronic pain, vascular diseases, and amputation.

Idiopathic pain—this pain cannot usually be explained by any obvious organic abnormality.

Box 21.2 Pain transmission—therapeutic implications

Steps of pain perception.

- Transduction—of signals from damaged tissue.
- Transmission—of electrical impulses through spinal cord, to brain stem and thalamocortical regions.
- Modulation—of initial nociceptive stimulus (amplification).
- Perception—of nociceptive impulse stimulus (emotional and physical experience).

Management therapy— should aim at attacking all four stages of nociception: NSAIDs for reducing inflammatory process at the damaged tissue, local anaesthesia and neural blockage for blocking transmission of stimulus, opiates to activate the inhibition process at the modulation level, and proper education to reduce anxiety at the perception level.

Recommended approach

Post-operative pain

- *General approach*—should be multimodal. Management of post-operative pain requires a thorough preoperative assessment (with pre-emptive measures), post-operative assessment of vital organs and pain pattern, appropriate use (and adjustment) of analgesia, management of side-effects, and proper discharge plan.
- *Preoperatively.*
  - *Directed pain history*—is essential (Boxes 21.3 and 21.4).
  - *Pre-emptive measures*—should be instituted appropriately to achieve effective post-operative pain control.
    - —Options—include written and verbal information regarding the post-operative pain management procedures and routes (e.g. IV, PO, PCA), methods of non-pharmacologic interventions available (distraction including music and videos, relaxation including abdominal breathing and jaw relaxation, physical agents including cold and heat massage, and hypnosis including focused attention states), and full explanation of patient concerns with appropriate patient education [B].
    - —Efficiency—although literature is insufficient to evaluate the exact impact of such measures, individualized preoperative education can favourably alter the pain experience and is a recommended practice.
- *Post-operatively.*
  - *Immediate action*—should follow the ABCDE approach (see ➲ Chapter 16, p. 148).
  - *Assess the pain and recognize its pattern.*
    - —In general—the sudden increase in pain intensity or unexpected high degree of pain may indicate that a new condition or complication has developed which may require further investigation.
    - —Pain assessment—should be thorough and holistic (Box 21.4). Charting pain pattern should be undertaken with the same regularity as charting observations of other vital signs (the fifth vital sign) [B].
  - Review, initiate, and modify the pain management plan.
    - —Educate the patient/carers—on the importance of pain as a signal, the effectiveness of management options, and reinforce the basic pain management principles [B].
    - —Effective non-pharmacologic procedures—should be rechecked and applied as appropriate (e.g. distraction with films, raising a cellulitic limb, physiotherapy).
    - —Pharmaceutical interventions (painkillers)—checked for type, dose, route, frequency, interval, combination, and side-effects. ALWAYS GO MULTIMODAL AND STEPWISE (Box 21.5).
  - The following clinical scenarios should benefit from certain approaches:
    - —Minor outpatient surgery—use long-acting local anaesthesia when possible. Use short-acting opioid (e.g. fentanyl) boluses in recovery. prescribe paracetamol/opiod combination prior to discharge.

Box 21.3 Preoperative pain assessment

- Pain history—history of chronic pain, successful or unsuccessful pain control methods in the past, and previous side-effects of pain management.
- PC—expected post-operative pain in the planned procedure, type of procedure (e.g. elective or emergency, minor or major), current preoperative severity of pain (if any).
- PMH—associated significant medical problems (e.g. arthritis), history of neurologic disorders, prior trauma, infection or respiratory difficulties, history of spinal surgery, history of alcohol abuse or addiction.
- DH—anticoagulants, use of opiates for chronic pain, monoamine oxidase inhibitors (MAOIs), allergies to opiates, local anaesthetics or NSAIDs.
- Others—infection on site of needle insertion, anatomical abnormalities.

Box 21.4 Pain assessment

- Location—e.g. operative site, deep, chest, joints, calf, forefoot.
- Intensity—mild, moderate, severe (or by using visual scale).
- Frequency—e.g. persistent, an hour or so before having the next analgesic injection, during the night.
- Nature—e.g. sharp, cramps, dull.
- Associated symptoms—e.g. nausea and vomiting.
- Impact of pain—depression, suicidal thoughts.
- Aggravating and alleviating factors—e.g. certain positions, physio, distraction.
- Presence of support—for daily activities.

Box 21.5 Other therapeutic modalities for cancer pain

- Neuropathic pain—see below.
- High-dose dexamethasone—consider for severe bone pain, spinal cord compression, soft tissue swelling, etc. [C].
- Anticancer systemic therapy—consider aromatase inhibitors for metastatic breast cancer [A] and androgen blockade for prostate cancer [C].
- Radiotherapy—for painful bone metastasis [C].
- Bisphosphate—for multiple myeloma patients [A].
- Coeliac plexus block—for upper GI infiltrating cancer [A].

—Surgery on the limbs—perform regional block where possible, or insert perineural catheter for 2–3 days of pain relief with continuous local anaesthesia.

—Minimally invasive abdominal surgery/abdominal wall surgery—provide transverse abdominis plane block; use fentanyl when and as required; and consider prescribing paracetamol (regular), diclofenac (regular), oxycodone, and hydromorphone as needed.

—Major open abdominal or thoracic surgery—use continuous epidural analgesia, paracetamol, fentanyl, and have a low threshold for PCA.

- Treat side-effects.

—Nausea and vomiting—can be effectively treated (following exclusion of serious underlying abnormality) by changing the dose, route or type of analgesia, and adding appropriate antiemetics.

—Sedation and lethargy—can be effectively treated (following exclusion of serious underlying abnormality) by reducing the dose of analgesic agent and using reversal agent if necessary.

—Other side-effects—include itching, numbness, hallucinations, dysphoria, and urinary retention.

- Re-evaluate management plan—at regular intervals.

Cancer pain

- *General approach*—should be based on a risk/benefit balance and tailored to each individual case. A multimodal and stepwise (WHO analgesic ladder) approach is recommended [B]. The same principles of approaching pain should be followed, i.e. ABCDE approach, proper pain assessment, appropriate use (and adjustment) of analgesia, management of side-effects, and proper long-term plan.
- *Origin of cancer pain*—may be directly related to cancer (most common), cancer complications (bedsore, muscles spasms), therapeutic modalities (radiotherapy, surgical scar), or resulting from associated disorders (arthritis).
- *Patient education*—essential step to ensure appropriate compliance [A].
- *Pain assessment*—should be holistic (e.g. physical, functional, psychosocial) and performed by the patient him/herself [B].
- *Pain management plan*—should start at a level appropriate to the severity (and type) of pain (see also Table 21.1).
  - Mild pain—non-opioids adjuvants [A].
  - Mild to moderate pain—non-opioids + weak opioid ± adjuvants [B].
  - Moderate to severe pain—opioids as a first-line [B]. Oral route is always recommended if possible.
- *Appropriate use of morphine*—should ensure effective initiation and titration (5–10mg of morphine, 4-hourly, titrated to control the pain with minimum side-effects), effective management of breakthrough pain (one sixth of normal regular dose of oral morphine), active management of side effects (constipation, nausea, and vomiting, oversedation), proper management of toxicity effects, and switching to parenteral administration (subcutaneous diamorphine) when necessary.
- Other types of treatment—should also be considered (Box 21.5).
- Pain management programme based on cognitive behaviour principles are treatment choice for patients with chronic pain.

Table 21.1 Perioperative pain control options

	Mild*	Moderate**	Severe***
Non-opioids†	P + local infiltration + NSAIDs (if not CI)	+	+
Weak opioids††	±	+ Regional block ± PRN weak opioids	+
Strong opioids†††	±	±	+ Major peripheral nerve block/plexus block/epidural local anaesthesia ± IV PCA

P = paracetamol; CI = contraindicated; PRN = when necessary; PCA = patient-controlled analgesia; * = mild pain (inguinal hernia repair, varicose vein operations); ** = moderate pain (hysterectomy, hip replacement); *** = severe pain (aortic surgery, thoracotomy)

† = paracetamol, NSAIDs, gabapentin; †† = codeine, tramadol; ††† = morphine, pethidine, oxycodone

Neuropathic pain

- *Definition and aetiology*—see Box 21.1. Accurate diagnosis relies on a proper history and physical examination, supported by the use of validated assessment tools.
- *General approach*—should be multimodal using proper patient education, pharmacological, and non-pharmacological therapies.
- *Non-pharmacological therapies*—include avoiding bed rest if at all possible. Maintaining functional and active life is important.
- *Pharmacologic therapy*—options include:
  - Amitriptyline, duloxetine, gabapentin, or pregabalin as initial treatment
  - If not effective or tolerated, offer one of the remaining three drugs and consider switching again if still not effective or tolerated.
  - Tramadol only if acute rescue treatment required.
  - Consider capsaicin for those with localized neuropathic pain or for those who wish to avoid or cannot tolerate oral treatments
- *Spinal cord stimulation (SCS)*—14 SCS devices manufactured by three companies have received European approval to market. Patient selection should involve a multidisciplinary team, expert in managing chronic pain.
  - Indications—severe chronic pain (measuring at least 50 on visual analogue scale of 0–100) for over 6mo, which remains resistant to conventional medical management (CMM). SCS is not indicated for ischaemic pain unless within a robust clinical trial.
  - Efficacy—trials have shown ~50% reduction in pain (in over 50% of people in 6mo time) compared to ~10% in CMM patients, and ~35% in SCS vs 7% in CMM group at 12mo.
  - Safety—serious complications are rare.

Further reading

European Society of Regional Anaesthesia and Pain Therapy. Post-operative pain management—good clinical practice. Available from: http://www.postoppain.org.

Clinical Knowledge Summaries. Palliative cancer care—pain management. Available from: https://cks.nice.org.uk/palliative-cancer-care-pain.

NHS Quality Improvement Scotland (2004). Best practice statement: post-operative pain management. Available from: http://www.nhshealthquality.org/nhsqis/files/Post_Pain_COMPLETE.pdf.

American Society of Anaesthesiologists Task Force on Acute Pain Management (2004). Practice guidelines for acute pain management in the perioperative setting: an updated report by the American Society of Anaesthesiologists Task Force on Acute Pain Management. Anaesthesiology 100, 1573–81.

Attal N, Cruccu G, Haanpää M et al. (2006). EFNS guidelines on pharmacological treatment of neuropathic pain. Eur J Neurol 13, 1153–69.

The Pain Society (2013). Recommendations for the appropriate use of opioids for persistent non-cancer pain. Available from: https://www.britishpainsociety.org/static/uploads/resources/files/pmp2013_main_FINAL_v6.pdf

CREST (2008). Guidelines on the management of neuropathic pain. Available from: http://www.thblack.com/links/RSD/CRESTManagementNeuropathicPainGuidelines.pdf.

Scottish Intercollegiate Guidelines Network (2008). Control of pain in adults with cancer. Available from: http://www.sign.ac.uk/guidelines/fulltext/106/index.html.

NHS Quality Improvement Scotland (2006). Best practice statement—management of chronic pain in adults. Available from: http://www.healthcareimprovementscotland.org/previous_resources/best_practice_statement/chronic_pain_in_adults.aspx

NHS Quality Improvement Scotland (2009). Best practice statement—the management of pain in patients with cancer. Available from: http://www.healthcareimprovementscotland.org/previous_resources/best_practice_statement/cancer_pain_management.aspx

NHS Quality Improvement Scotland (2004). Best practice statement—post-operative pain management. Available from: http://www.nhshealthquality.org/nhsqis/files/20372%20NHSQIS%20Best%20Practice.pdf.

European Association of Urology (2012). Guidelines on pain management. Available from: https://uroweb.org/wp-content/uploads/EAU-Guidelines-Pain_Management-2012.pdf.

Wounds UK (2004). Best practice statement—minimizing trauma and pain in wound management. Available from: http://www.wounds-uk.com/pdf/content_8952.pdf.

Serpell M (2005). Anatomy, physiology and pharmacology of pain. Anaesth Intensive Care Med 6, 7–10.

McCaffery M (1972). Nursing management of the patient with pain, Lippincott, Philadelphia.

VHA/DoD Clinical Practice Guidelines for the management of postoperative pain (2006).

McCaffery M, Pasero C (1992). Assessment: underlying complexities, misconceptions, and practical tools. In: Pain: clinical manual, 2nd ed, Mosby.

British National Formulary 57. Available at: http://www.bnf.org/bnf/.

Hyllested M, Jones S, Pedersen JL, Kehlet H (2002). Comparative effect of paracetamol, NSAIDs or their combination in post-operative pain management: a qualitative review. Br J Anaesth 88, 199–214.

World Health Organization. WHO's pain ladder. Available from: http://www.who.int/cancer/palliative/painladder/en/.

World Health Organization (1990). Cancer pain relief and palliative care. Available from: http://www.who.int/bookorders/anglais/detart1.jsp?sesslan=1&codlan=1&codcol=10&codcch=804;

WHO (1996). Cancer pain relief, 2nd ed, WHO Geneva. Available from: http://books.google.co.uk/books?id=Fhall7PMHZcC&dq=WHO+Cancer+Pain+Relief&pg=PP1&ots=te8gl4CW6&sig=MMdO9v5E106I955jeJS1UWE0e8k&hl=en&sa=X&oi=book_result&resnum=4&ct=result#PPR1,M1.

Cancer Research UK (2008). Treating cancer pain. Available from: http://www.cancerhelp.org.uk/help/default.asp?page=5884.

National Institute for Health and Clinical Excellence (2017) Neuropathic pain – pharmacological management. Available from http://www.nice.org.uk/guidance/cg173/evidence/cg173-neuropathic-pain-pharmacological-management-full-guideline3

National Institute for Health and Clinical Excellence (2008). Spinal cord stimulation for chronic pain of neuropathic or ischaemic origin. Available from: http://www.nice.org.uk/nicemedia/pdf/TA159QuickRefGuide.pdf.

Chapter 22

Principles of nutritional support[*]

Basic facts *200*
Screening for malnutrition *202*
Nutritional support—requirements *203*
Nutritional support—oral *204*
Nutritional support—enteral *204*
Nutritional support—parenteral *205*
Further reading *206*

Key guidelines
- National Institute of Health and Clinical Excellence (2017). Nutrition support for adults: oral nutrition support, enteral tube feeding and parenteral nutrition.
- European Society for Clinical Nutrition and Metabolism – ESPEN (2017). Guidelines on enteral nutrition: non-surgical oncology.
- Council of Europe Resolution Food and Nutritional Care in Hospitals (2003). 10 key characteristics of good nutritional care in hospitals.

[*] The guidelines on this chapter have been sourced and summarized from different UK, Europe, and international government sources, professional organizations, and medical specialty societies. Leading guidelines have been listed in the further reading section at the end of this chapter.

Basic facts

- *Definition*—malnutrition is a state of poor nutrition resulting in measurable adverse effects on body composition, function, or clinical outcome.
- *Incidence*—some degree of significant malnutrition can be found in ~10–60% of in-hospital patients, compared to <5% of the general population at home.
- *Risk factors*—commonly found in hospitalized patients (Box 22.1).
- *Effect of malnutrition*—see Box 22.2.
- *Clinical assessment*—should be thorough and holistic (Box 22.3).
  - Clinical history—any existing or potential risk factors for malnutrition (Box 22.1).
  - Physical examination—includes clinical appearance, weight and height, and anthropometrics (e.g. mid-arm circumference, triceps skinfold thickness).
  - Laboratory evaluation—patients requiring nutritional support should be checked for FBC, urea and creatinine, glucose, LFTs, albumin, prealbumin, and CRP. Trace elements (Mg, PO4, Ca, zinc, copper, folate, and B12) are required for total parenteral nutrition (TPN) commencement.

Box 22.1 Malnutrition—risk factors

Original disease—effect varies depending on the severity and type of disease: elective operations (SF*×1.1), sepsis (SF×1.35), pancreatitis (SF×1.3–1.8), acute renal failure (SF×1.3), major surgery with compromised cardiopulmonary functions (SF×1.55).

Poor intake—depression, nausea, weakness, poor quality of food, inadequate food intake (patient unable to eat for >7d or has insufficient food intake (<60% of energy expenditure) for >10d).

Poor digestion/absorption—operations on GI tract.

Excess loss—fistulae, stomas, drains, etc.

*SF = stress factor reflecting the estimated increase in calorie needs.

Box 22.2 Effects of malnutrition

Impaired immune defence—e.g. the risk of bloodstream infection in critically ill patients increases (relative hazard ×1.27) when calorie intake is less than 25% of recommended.

Poor wound healing—with decreased rate of fibroblastic proliferation and neovascularization. This leads to slower rates of wound healing, but rarely leads to complete wound disruption.

Reduced muscle strength—skeletal, respiratory, etc.

Vitamin—deficiencies.

Fluid and electrolytes—disturbances.

Impaired psychosocial functions.

Box 22.3 Malnutrition—diagnostic criteria

At risk—poor eating for the last (or coming) 5d or more, existence of one or more risk factors:

- Clinical appearance—bi-temporal wasting, thin extremities, low mid-arm circumference, low triceps skinfold thickness, hair loss, xerosis, glossitis, bleeding or sore on the gums and oral mucosa.
- Laboratory findings—low albumin (<33g/L), low prealbumin (<150g/L), low transferrin (<1,500mg/L), absent cutaneous hypersensitivity, decreased total lymphocyte count (<1,500 cells/L).

Confirmed—BMI ≤18.5kg/m^2 (or ≤20kg/m^2 with associated weight loss of >5% over 3–6mo), unintentional weight loss of >10% over 3–6mo.

Screening for malnutrition

- *Patient selection*—nutritional screening should be offered to all
  patients upon their hospital or care home admission, first outpatient
  appointment, on registration at GP and if a clinical concern arises at any
  time (e.g. unexpected post-operative long-standing ileus) [C]. Screening
  should be repeated weekly for inpatients or outpatients if there is
  clinical concern.
- *Method of screening*—includes a thorough clinical and laboratory
  assessment by appropriately trained health care professional (Box 22.3)
  [D]. The Malnutrition Universal Screening Tool (MUST) (BMI + degree of
  unintentional weight loss + effect of acute disease) has been developed by
  British Association for Parenteral and Enteral Nutrition (BAPEN) to ensure
  a reliable, thorough, and reproducible technique for screening.

Nutritional support—requirements

- Nutritional support should be considered for all patients who have eaten little or nothing for 5d or likely not to do so. It should also be considered in patients with poor absorption or increased metabolism.
- The usual nutritional support should include adequate calories (total energy 25–35kcal/kg/d), protein (0.8–1.5g protein/kg/d), fluid (30–35mL fluid/kg), and electrolytes, micronutrients, minerals, and fibre where appropriate [D]. A typical 70-kg man requires 1,800cals (9gN$_2$) at rest, 2,100 cals (11gN$_2$) on activity, 2,300 cals (14gN$_2$) when septic, and 2,500 cals (17gN$_2$) when suffering from severe burns.

Perioperative nutritional support

- Oral preoperative carbohydrate treatment (instead of overnight fasting) the night before and 2h before surgery should be administered [B]. Preoperative carbohydrates can be considered in patients undergoing major surgery.
- Oral intake, including clear liquids, shall be initiated within hours after surgery in most patients [A]. In general, oral nutritional intake shall be continued after surgery without interruption [A]. If enteral feeding is indicated, this should be initiated within 24h after surgery. [A] Start at low rate then increase to full requirement within 5–7d. where long-term enteral feeding is needed (>4wk such as head injury), consider percutaneous tube.
- If the energy and nutrient requirements cannot be met by oral and enteral intake alone (<50% of caloric requirement) for more than 7d, a combination of enteral and parenteral nutrition is recommended (GPP) [A].
- Parenteral glutamine and omega-3-fatty acids supplementation may be considered in patients who cannot be fed adequately enterally and, therefore, require total PN [B]. Patients undergoing major cancer surgery should be considered for supplementary specific formula enriched with immunonutrients (arginine, omega-3-fatty acids, ribo- nucleotides) [B].
- Patients with severe malnutrition should receive nutritional therapy prior to major surgery [A] even if operations including those for cancer have to be delayed. A period of 7–14d may be appropriate. This should be preferably provided BEFORE hospital admission to reduce costs and hospital-acquired infection. Oral or enteral route are always preferable.

Nutritional support—oral

- *Patient selection*—should be offered to all patients at risk or in existing malnutrition, providing the patient's swallowing function is intact and efficient [D]. Patients with impaired swallowing function should be referred to the swallowing assessment service [D].
- *Method of support*—provide normal diet and fluid, with adequate quality and quantity, appropriate feeding aids, and encouraging environment to eat. Modification of diet and fluid should be considered in individual cases (e.g. multivitamins, modified oral nutrition, mineral supplements) [D].
- *Efficiency*—nutrition supplements can decrease the infection rate (ARR ×10%) and length of hospital stay (by 2d) when compared to no supplements. However, the quality of available trials is low and insufficient to conclude solid recommendations.

Nutritional support—enteral

- *Patient selection*—should be offered to all patients at risk or in existing malnutrition who have inappropriate (or unsafe) oral route, but intact GI tract [B]. All patients undergoing major abdominal procedures should be considered for preoperative enteral nutrition support (preferably with immune-modulating substrates such as arginine, omega-3 fatty acids, and nucleotides) for 5–7d (but not within 48h of surgery) [A].
- *Method of support*—special diet and fluid can be delivered preferably via a tube to the stomach (NG feeding tube, gastrostomy) [A], or to the duodenum or jejunum if stomach tube is inappropriate [D]. Confirmation of tube position is necessary [D]. Feeding can be delivered in boluses (gastric tube) or continuously (gastric or enteral tubes) over 16–24h [B].
- *Efficiency*—enteral nutrition (using a tube) can decrease the infection rate (ARR ×11%), but has no significant effect on the length of hospital stay when compared to no artificial nutrition. When compared to parenteral nutrition, patients on enteral nutrition have decreased infections rate (ARR ×11%), decreased complication rate (ARR ×6% for major complications), and shorter length of hospital stay (by ~1.7d).

Nutritional support—parenteral

- *Patient selection*—should be offered to all patients at risk or in existing malnutrition who have inappropriate (or unsafe) oral route and disrupted (inaccessible, non-functional, or leaking) GI tract [D].
- *Method of support*—best delivered via a dedicated central catheter. This can be inserted via peripheral access (for short-term feeding <14d) [B], non-tunnelled subclavian line (feeding requirement <30d) [B], or via a tunnelled subclavian line (feeding requirement >30d) [D]. Feeding is best delivered continuously (or cyclical if nutritional requirement exceeds 2wk) [D].
- *Efficiency*—when compared to enteral nutrition, patients on parenteral nutrition have increased infections rate, increased complication rate, and longer length of hospital stay. Parenteral nutrition should therefore be used judiciously to maximize benefits and minimize risks.

Further reading

National Institute for Health and Clinical Excellence (2017). Nutrition support in adults: oral nutrition support, enteral tube feeding and parenteral nutrition. Available from: http://www.nice.org.uk/CG32.

National Institute for Health and Clinical Excellence (2012) Quality standard for nutrition support in adults (QS24) Avalable from: http://www.nice.org.uk/guidance/qs24

European Society for Clinical Nutrition and Metabolism – ESPEN (2017). Guidelines on enteral nutrition: non-surgical oncology.

European Society for Clinical Nutrition and Metabolism (2009)

Arends J, Bodoky G, Bozzetti F et al. (2006). ESPEN guidelines on enteral nutrition: non-surgical oncology. Clin Nutr 25, 245–59.

Council of Europe Resolution Food and Nutritional Care in Hospitals (2003). 10 key characteristics of good nutritional care in hospitals. Available from: http://www.bapen.org.uk/pdfs/coe_leaflet.pdf.

British Association for Parenteral and Enteral Nutrition. Available from: http://www.bapen. org.uk/.

American Society for Parenteral and Enteral Nutrition (2004). Nutrition requirements: safe practices for parenteral nutrition. Available from: http://journals.sagepub.com/doi/abs/10.1177/0148607104028006S39

Cerra FB, Benitez MR, Blackburn GL (1997). Applied nutrition in ICU patients. A consensus statement of the American College of Chest Physicians. Chest 111, 769–78.

Elia M, ed. (2003). The 'MUST' report. Nutritional screening for adults: a multidisciplinary responsibility. Development and use of the 'Malnutrition Universal Screening Tool' ('MUST') for adults. A report by the Malnutrition Advisory Group of the British Association for Parenteral and Enteral Nutrition, BAPEN, Redditch, UK.

Margenthaler J, Herrmann V (2002). Nutrition. In: The Washington manual of surgery, 3rd ed, Lippincott Williams & Wilkins.

Rubinson L, Diette GB, Song X, Brower RG, Krishnan JA (2004). Low caloric intake is associated with nosocomial bloodstream infections in patients in the medical intensive care unit. Crit Care Med 32, 350–7.

Haydock DA, Hill GL (1986). Impaired wound healing in surgical patients with varying degrees of malnutrition. JPEN J Parenter Enteral Nutr 10, 550–4.

Albina JE (1994). Nutrition and wound healing. JPEN J Parenter Enteral Nutr 18, 367–76.

Koretz RL, Avenell A, Lipman TO, Braunschweig CL, Milne AC (2007). Does enteral nutrition affect clinical outcome? A systematic review of the randomized trials. Am J Gastroenterol 102, 412–29.

Part 3

Oesophagus

Gastro-oesophageal reflux disease (GORD)*

Basic facts *210*
Recommended initial approach *212*
Recommended secondary investigations *214*
Recommended treatment of resistant cases *216*
Newer interventional techniques *218*
Further reading *220*

Key guidelines
- NICE (2014). Dyspepsia and gastrooesophageal reflux disease.
- NICE (2017). Suspected cancer: recognition and referral.
- American College of Gastroenterology (2013). Diagnosis and management of gastroesophageal reflux disease.

---

* The guidelines on this chapter have been sourced and summarized from different UK, Europe, and international government sources, professional organizations, and medical specialty societies. Leading guidelines have been listed in the further reading section at the end of this chapter.

Basic facts

- *Definition*— gastro-oesophageal reflux disease (GORD) is the sensation of stomach contents returning past the oesophageal sphincter, prolonging acid and pepsin exposure in the lower oesophagus and affecting patient well-being. Gastro-oesophageal acid reflux is a normal physiologic process; GORD occurs when symptoms or complications result from the reflux episodes.
- *Incidence*—about 7% of the population in Europe and USA experience heartburn on a daily basis, over 25% of them have symptoms suggestive of GORD. Oesophagitis affects 7–16% of GORD patients.
- *Risk factors*—loss of the 'high pressure zone' at the gastro-oesophageal junction (GOJ) (the antireflux barrier) is a universal 'denominator' for almost all physiological or pathological episodes. Most patients (>60%) have mechanically defective lower oesophageal sphincter (LOS) function, most commonly caused by anatomical disruption of the GOJ, often associated with a hiatus hernia (Box 23.1).
- *Clinical presentation*—symptoms have low predictive power in estimating disease severity, underlying pathology, or the presence of complications (including Barrett's oesophagus). This applies to 'ALARM' symptoms as well. (Boxes 23.2 and 23.3).

Box 23.1 Risk factors for GORD

Obesity—significant risk factor (OR ×2.15) for GORD, erosive oesophagitis, and oesophageal adenocarcinoma, but association remains vague.

Social and dietary habits—insufficient evidence on the precise role of each factor. Possible implication of smoking, alcohol, dietary fat, mints, onions, citrus fruits, tomato, chocolate, and caffeine. Lifestyle changes are recommended for prevention (see below).

Medications—calcium channel blockers and anticholinergics can relax the LOS and promote GORD. Research data is limited for definite conclusions.

Genetics—suggested by twin studies.

Box 23.2 GORD symptoms and signs

Heartburn—retrosternal burning discomfort triggered or aggravated by bending over or lying flat, and radiating occasionally to the neck.

Regurgitation—sudden and effortless return of gastric or oesophageal contents into the pharynx, giving a sour or bitter taste ('acid brash').

Dysphagia—difficulty swallowing in long-standing GORD. Might result from severe chronic oesophageal inflammation, impaired peristalsis, or development of strictures.

GORD-associated chest pain—may mimic cardiac ischaemia, lasts minutes to hours, and resolves spontaneously or with antacids. Usually postprandial and may be aggravated by emotional stress.

Water brash or hypersalivation—patient foams at the mouth, producing salivary secretions as much as 10mL of saliva per minute.

Globus sensation—constant feeling of a lump on throat.

Odynophagia—painful swallowing.

Box 23.3 'ALARM' Upper GI symptoms and signs

Dysphagia, upper abdominal mass, enlarged liver, or a gastrointestinal bleeding.

Age >40y with jaundice;.

Aged >55y with weight loss and any of upper abdominal pain, reflux or dyspepsia.

Age >60y with weight loss and any of abdominal pain, nausea, vomiting, diarrhoea, constipation, back pain, or new-onset diabetes.

Recommended initial approach

- *General concepts*—investigations should follow a stepwise approach and sound clinical judgment (Fig. 23.1). 'ALARM' symptoms (Box 23.3) require urgent referral for investigation with endoscopy (2wk rule) (Box 23.4) [B].
- *Simple reflux-like disease*—requires no specific initial investigations [A].
  - *Initial advice*—begin with a comprehensive review of medications, practical lifestyle advice (healthy eating, weight reduction, and smoking cessation) [B], and proper advice to avoid known precipitants that provoke reflux symptoms (e.g. chocolate and caffeine) [C]. Consider psychological therapies to reduce dyspeptic symptoms in individual people (NICE 2014).
  - *Over-the-counter antacids*—useful in reducing the number of days with reflux symptoms and the median symptom score when compared with placebo, but have no significant effect on healing rate. Useful as patient-directed therapy for mild GORD [C].
  - Proton pump inhibitors (PPIs) (or Histamine2receptor inhibitors (H2RA) if inadequate response to PPI)—consider for 1mo in persistent mild to moderate symptoms [A]. PPIs promote healing in ~75% of patients with oesophagitis (NNT=2), reduce relapse at 6–12mo in ~35% of patients, and eliminate symptoms in 50% of patients with endoscopically negative reflux disease.
  - *Helicobacter (H.) pylori* 'test and treat'—consider as alternative initial step in investigating dyspepsia of unknown cause [A]. Patients with proven GORD do not require this testing initially. Leave a 2-wk washout period after PPI usage before testing for *H. pylori* with a breath test or a stool antigen test.
- *Recurrent mild symptoms*—encourage patients to step down the PPI or (H2RA) to the lowest dose necessary to control the symptoms, and to use treatment on an 'as-needed' basis following good control [B]. Avoid long-term continuous use.
- *Special precautions*—further actions may be required in patients with complicated oesophagitis, history of bleeding ulcer, and regular NSAIDs therapy.

Box 23.4 Referral to a specialist service (consider for endoscopy)

Patients of any age with ALARM symptoms.

Patients of any age with new onset of unexplained dyspepsia or reflux symptoms that have not responded to acid suppression treatment [B].

Persistent symptomatic GORD despite adequate investigations and treatment (including *Helicobacter pylori* 'test and treat') in primary care (e.g. frequent relapses, severe symptoms) [B].

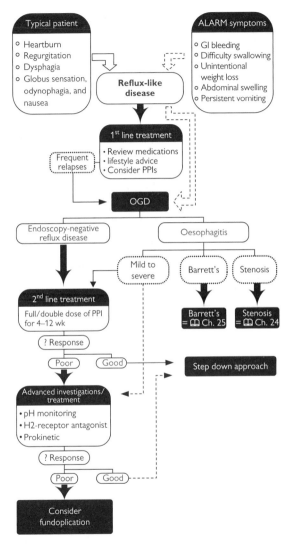

Fig. 23.1 GORD recommended approach.

Recommended secondary investigations

- *Endoscopy*—very reliable in detecting and stratifying pathological changes (Box 23.4). Absence of endoscopic features of GORD does not exclude the diagnosis or indicate an easy-to-control case. Inter-observer variability exists and may affect the reliability of the investigation. Commonly used classification systems are the Savary–Miller and Los Angeles classifications (Table 23.1).
  - *Endoscopy-negative reflux disease*—refers to patients with established reflux symptoms and normal endoscopic findings. Up to 75% of those patients have histological evidence of oesophageal injury and respond significantly to acid suppression.
  - *Reflux oesophagitis*—is confirmed by finding inflammatory features in the oesophagus by endoscopy or biopsy.
- *Double contrast barium meal studies*—are of limited use in current modern practice. May be helpful for investigating complicated GORD cases (sensitivity reaches over 80%). Should be tailored to individual patient's needs. Has relatively low sensitivity (25%) and specificity (50%) compared to endoscopy in mild forms of GORD. Biopsies cannot be taken for suspicious lesions.
- *Ambulatory oesophageal pH studies*—consider in all patients with persistent symptoms who have no evidence of mucosal damage and have failed to respond to acid suppression management [C]. The test is reproducible, sensitive, and specific (96%) to confirm or exclude the presence of GORD.
  - *Prospects*—two other modalities have potential significant impact on GORD approach:
    1. Combined impendence and acid testing—allow for accurate measurement of acidity and volume of reflux.
    2. Tubeless telemetric acid monitoring—decreases patient's discomfort and allows for a longer monitoring period.
- *Oesophageal manometric testing*—has minimal role in making or confirming the suspected diagnosis of GORD [C]. Used mainly to assess the structural integrity of the LOS, to investigate and diagnose any motility disorder, to assess the accurate location of the upper border of the LOS for correct positioning of the pH electrode in ambulatory pH monitoring, and proper planning of antireflux surgery.

Table 23.1 Savary–Miller classification of reflux disease.

Grade I	One or more non-confluent reddish spots (± exudate).
Grade II	Distal oesophagus non-circumferential erosive and exudative lesions that may be confluent.
Grade III	Circumferential distal oesophagus erosions covered with haemorrhagic and pseudomembranous exudates.
Grade IV	Chronic complications—including deep ulcers, stenosis, or scarring with Barrett's metaplasia.

Reproduced from Monnier P, Savary M. Contribution of endoscopy to gastroesophageal reflux disease. *Scand J Gastroenterol.* 1984;19(Suppl 106):26 with permission from Taylor and Francis.

Recommended treatment of resistant cases

Medical treatment

- *PPI therapy*—offer further PPI at full dose for 4–8wk [A]. Consider PPIs at a double dose for further 4wk in resistant or recurrent cases [C*].
- *H2–receptor antagonist (H2RA) (prokinetics not recommended)*—consider for patients with inadequate response to PPIs [B].
- *Refractory cases*—check compliance, tolerability of treatment, and confounding factors. If symptoms recur after initial treatment, offer a PPI at the lowest dose possible to control symptoms. Consider advanced investigations (pH monitoring) and surgery if appropriate.

Antireflux surgery

- *Indications*—antireflux surgery cannot be recommended for every patient with recurrent symptoms. Where indicated, surgery has shown significant improvement in quality of life compared to medical therapy, and is as effective as medical therapy for carefully selected (and medically responding) patients when performed by an experienced surgeon.
  - Surgery should be considered in patients with confirmed acid reflux, adequate response to acid-suppression therapy, but who do not wish to continue on this therapy or who are intolerant. Other indications include morbid obesity and large hiatus hernia. Surgery is generally not indicated for poor respondents to PPI.
  - In the absence of a PPI response, surgery is unlikely to be effective even with an abnormal pH study.
- *Benefits and risks*—see Box 23.5.

Box 23.5 Antireflux surgery—benefits and risks

Main benefits.

- Symptom relief—significant improvement in oesophagitis and heartburn symptoms (about 85–90% of patients at 3y and ~80% at 5y). Studies are heterogeneous with ORs for improvement (compared to medical treatment) ranging from 1.2 to 200, and NNT ranging from 1.2 to 58.
- High patient satisfaction—up to 95% for Nissen fundoplication when performed by experienced surgeons.

Main risks.

- Recurrence of symptoms—about 62% of patients will require further acid-suppressant medications at 10y to control symptoms.
- Operative morbidity—including significant increase in early satiety, inability to belch, and inability to vomit.
- Operative mortality—small (0.1–0.5%) but significant.

- *Selection of surgical technique.*
  - Types of surgical techniques—different types available. Fundoplication procedure introduced by Nissen in 1956 or its variants is the most commonly used antireflux operation in the world. Nissen fundoplication is performed by mobilizing the lower oesophagus and wrapping the fundus of stomach around the mobilized area.
  - Fundoplication can be total or partial, in anterior or posterior positions, and can be performed using open or laparoscopic techniques. Other surgical techniques include posterior and anterior partial fundoplication, Hill's procedure, Collis procedure, and Angelchik prosthesis.
- *Choice of surgical technique*—the choice depends on the efficiency and complication rate of each technique as well as the individual patient case.
  - Laparoscopic Nissen fundoplication (the gold standard procedure) has fewer overall complications and shorter recovery compared to open approach. There is no significant difference in recurrence rate of GORD or relief of heartburn [A].
  - Nissen fundoplication and posterior partial fundoplication have no significant difference in post-operative dysphagia or recurrent GORD rate [B].
  - Partial and anterior fundoplication have less post-operative wind-related complications compared to total fundoplication.
  - Dysphagia is less common in anterior partial fundoplication [B].
  - There is no difference in the outcome whether vagus nerves were included or excluded, and whether short gastric arteries were divided or left intact.

Newer interventional techniques

The usage of current endoscopic therapy or transoral incisionless fundoplication cannot be recommended as an alternative to medical or traditional surgical therapy [moderate level of evidence] (Box 23.6).

Box 23.6 Alternative antireflux techniques

Endoluminal gastroplication.

- Technique – outpatient procedure. Using a standard endoscope and endoscopic sewing device, a plication (or pleat) is created at the LOS.
- Safety—no major safety concerns according to current available evidence.
- Efficiency—unknown. Procedure is at the early stages of development.
- Terms of use—special arrangements should be undertaken for clinical governance, patient consent, audit, and review of all outcome results by a dedicated team.

Endoscopic injection of bulking agents.

- Technique—patient sedated. Using a standard endoscope and fluoroscopic control, a needle catheter (filled with a bio-compatible polymer and solvent) is introduced into the GOJ. The polymer is injected (or implanted) into the GOJ (often four injections), along the muscle layer or deep submucosal layer of the cardia.
- Safety—no major safety concerns, but side effects have been reported (chest pain in 50–90% of patients, dysphagia, fever, nausea). Current evidences are insufficient to support the use of this procedure without special arrangements in the unit.
- Efficiency—unknown as the procedure is at the early stages of development.

Endoscopic radiofrequency ablation (NICE 2014).

- Can be used within a proper governance framework.

Endoscopic augmentation of the LOS using hydrogel implants

- Performed under sedation by using a special delivery system to apply suction on the GOJ mucosa and implant a hydrogel prosthesis. The prosthesis absorbs water and takes its full shape within 24h. Current evidence raises concerns on the safety of this procedure, and its use is therefore NOT recommended outside of a strict clinical governance setting by well-trained endoscopists.
- Laparoscopic insertion of a magnetic bead band for GORD (NICE 2012). Can be used within a proper governance framework.

Expert comments

GORD is a very common problem, in many instances related to life-style, and particularly, the rise in obesity which raises the intra-abdominal pressure leading to reflux of the gastric contents and acid into the oesophagus. This may also be related to the rise in detection of Barrett's oesophagus and oesophageal adenocarcinoma. Barrett's oesophagus is probably a protective mechanism, and may reduce the symptoms of GORD and delay the diagnosis of cancer.

First-line treatment should be attention to lifestyle, including weight and smoking.

For infrequent episodes of reflux, antacid treatment provides effective symptomatic relief.

H2–receptor antagonists reduce the acidity of the gastric secretions and are effective treatments, but the most effective medical treatment of GORD is the PPI class of drugs. These provide effective acid suppression throughout the day, and especially at night when the added effect of gravity exacerbates GORD symptoms. As such, PPI therapy should be first-line for symptomatic reflux disease. The neutralized gastric secretion does not cause the heartburn pain of GORD.

Prokinetic drugs help to reduce the exposure of the oesophagus to gastric secretion. Metoclopramide is probably the most effective, but has a wider side-effect profile than the acid suppression treatments. Similarly, cisapride is an effective medication, but was withdrawn because of cardiac arrhythmias.

It seems unlikely that more effective acid suppression drugs will be developed. Drugs, which selectively work on a dysfunctional LOS, may be developed in future years.

Laparoscopic fundoplication with relatively minor variations in technique is the gold standard surgical treatment of GORD refractory to medical treatment or in younger patients where lifelong medical treatment is not desired.

Therapeutic endoscopic treatments are intuitively attractive in avoiding the risks of major surgery. Endoscopic treatments consist of three basic principles, namely suturing the mucosa at the GOJ to create a valve which prevents reflux, radiofrequency ablation at the GOJ to create scarring and achieve the same aim, and the injection of polymers at the GOJ. All the techniques remain experimental, and generally are less effective than conventional surgery with a greater risk of recurrent disease. Innovation continues to contribute to this field; however, these techniques have not become mainstream treatment. Hybrid techniques utilizing NOTES (Natural Orifice Transluminal Endoscopic Surgery), surgery conventionally performed through incisions being performed through natural orifices (mouth, anus, vagina), may stimulate advances in effective antireflux surgery. *Mr David Corless*

Further reading

National Institute for Health and Clinical Excellence (2014). Gastro-oesophageal reflux disease and dyspepsia in adults:investigation and management. Available from: http://guidance.nice.org.uk/CG184.

National Institute for Health and Clinical Excellence (2013). Endoscopic radiofrequency ablation for gastro- oesophageal reflux disease.

Available from: https://www.nice.org.uk/guidance/ipg461/resources/endoscopic-radiofrequency-ablation-for-gastrooesophageal-reflux-disease-1899869865904069

DeVault KR, Castell DO; American College of Gastroenterology (2013). Updated guidelines for the diagnosis and treatment of gastroesophageal reflux disease. Am J Gastroenterol 100, 190–200.

Richter JE (1996). Typical and atypical presentations of gastroesophageal reflux disease. The role of oesophageal testing in diagnosis and management. Gastroenterol Clin North Am 25, 75–102.

Dent J, El-Serag HB, Wallander MA, Johansson S (2005). Epidemiology of gastro-oesophageal reflux disease: a systematic review. Gut 54, 710–7.

Moayyedi P, Delaney B, Forman D (2005). Gastro-oesophageal reflux disease. Clin Evid 14, 567–81.

Corley DA, Kubo A (2006). Body mass index and gastroesophageal reflux disease: a systematic review and meta-analysis. Am J Gastroenterol 101, 2619–28.

Lagergren J, Bergström R, Adami HO, Nyren O (2000). Association between medications that relax the lower oesophageal sphincter and risk for oesophageal adenocarcinoma.Ann Intern Med 133, 165–75.

Romero Y, Cameron AJ, Locke GR 3rd et al. (1997). Familial aggregation of gastroesophageal reflux in patients with Barrett's oesophagus and oesophageal adenocarcinoma. Gastroenterology 113, 1449–56.

Ott DJ, Gelfand DW, Chen YM, Wu WC, Munitz HA (1985). Predictive relationship of hiatal hernia to reflux oesophagitis. Gastrointest Radiol 10, 317–20.

Wright RA, Hurwitz AL (1979). Relationship of hiatal hernia to endoscopically proved reflux oesophagitis. Dig Dis Sci 24, 311–3.

Reginald V, Lord N, Demeester TR. Reflux disease and hiatus hernia In: Oxford Textbook of Surgery. Chapter 22.2.1. 2nd edition, Oxford University Press, Oxford.

Reginald V, Lord N, Demeester TR (2001). Reflux disease and hiatus hernia. In: Oxford Textbook of Surgery, 2nd ed, Oxford University Press, Oxford.

Dent J (2007). Microscopic oesophageal mucosal injury in non-erosive reflux disease. Clin Gastroenterol Hepatol 5, 4–16.

Nichols JH, Taylor D, Varnholt H, Williams L (2006). pH testing. In: Laboratory medicine practice guidelines: evidence-based practice for point-of-care testing, pp. 120–5, National Academy of Clinical Biochemistry (NACB), Washington DC.

Pandolfino JE, Kahrilas PJ; American Gastroenterological Association (2005). American Gastroenterological Association medical position statement: clinical use of oesophageal manometry. Gastroenterology 128, 207–8.

Allgood PC, Bachmann M (2000) Medical or surgical treatment for chronic gastro-oesophageal reflux? A systematic review of published evidence of effectiveness. Eur J Surg 166, 713–21.

Dassinger MS, Torquati A, Houston HL, Holzman MD, Sharp KW, Richards WO (2004). Laparoscopic fundoplication: 5-year follow-up. Am Surg 70, 691–4.

Hagedorn C, Lönroth H, Rydberg L, Ruth M, Lundell L (2002). Long-term efficacy of total (Nissen–Rossetti) and posterior partial (Toupet) fundoplication: results of a randomized clinical trial. J Gastrointest Surg 6, 540–5.

Watson D, Jamieson G (2006). Treatment of gastro-oesophageal reflux disease. In: Oesophagogastric surgery: a companion to specialist surgical practice, 3rd ed. Elsevier, London. Saunders Ltd Publications.

National Institute for Health and Clinical Excellence (2005). Endoluminal gastroplication for gastro-oesophageal reflux disease. Available from: https://www.nice.org.uk/guidance/ipg404

National Institute for Health and Clinical Excellence (2009). Endoscopic radiofrequency abla- tion for gastro-oesophageal reflux disease. Available from: https://www.nice.org.uk/guidance/ipg461

Monnier P, Savary M (1984). Contribution of endoscopy to gastroesophageal reflux disease. Scand J Gastroenterol 19 (Suppl. 106), 26.

National Institute for Health and Clinical Excellence (2007). Endoscopic augmentation of the lower oesophageal sphincter using hydrogel implants for the treatment of gastro-oesophageal reflux disease. Available from: http://www.nice.org.uk/Guidance/IPG222.

NICE (2017). Suspected cancer: diagnosis and referral. July 2017.

Wileman SM, McCann S, Grant AM et al. Medical versus surgical management for gastro-oesophageal reflux disease (GORD) in adults. Cochrane Database Syst Rev 2010, CD003243.

Ingestion of foreign bodies*

Basic facts *222*
Recommended investigations *224*
Recommended management *226*
Further reading *227*

Key guidelines

- American Society for Gastrointestinal Endoscopy (2011). Guideline for the management of ingested foreign bodies and food impactions.
- European Society of Gastrointestinal Endoscopy (ESGE) Clinical Guideline (2016). Removal of foreign bodies in the upper gastrointestinal tract in adults.

---

* The guidelines on this chapter have been sourced and summarized from different UK, Europe, and international government sources, professional organizations, and medical specialty societies. Leading guidelines have been listed in the further reading section at the end of this chapter.

Basic facts

- *Incidence*—relatively common event; about 4% of children in the USA swallow a coin during their childhood.
- Risk factors—common sources are coins in children and meat bolus in adults (Box 24.1).
- *Clinical presentation*—varies between different age groups (Box 24.2).

Box 24.1 Risk factors for ingestion of foreign bodies

Age—more common in patients between 6mo and 5y.

Underlying conditions—more common in the presence of oesophageal carcinoma, strictures, diverticulum, post-gastrectomy, hiatus hernia, and achalasia.

Special groups—more common among mental illness patients, prisoners, and persons involved in smuggling of illicit drugs.

Impaction, perforation, or obstruction often occurs at GI angulations or narrowing, Hence, patients with previous GI tract surgery or congenital gut malformations are at increased risk.

Common sources—coins in children and meat bolus in adults. Fish or chicken bones, wood, plastic, glass, and other objects are familiar as well.

Box 24.2 Clinical presentation

Clinical presentation.
- Fully sensible adults and older children—may give clear history and point to the location of maximum discomfort.
- Younger children and mentally impaired adults—may not recognize the incident and present late with non-specific symptoms and signs.
- Most common symptoms—acute dysphagia, inability to swallow, hypersalivation, retrosternal fullness, regurgitation of undigested food, and odynophagia.
  - Oropharyngeal foreign bodies—sensation of trapped, well-localized object (usually bones and toothpicks) in the throat. May be associated with mild to severe discomfort, inability to swallow, and occasional compromise of airways.
  - Oesophageal foreign bodies—sudden onset of severe dysphagia following the event in fully conscious patients.

Physical examination.
- May reveal swelling, erythema, tenderness, or crepitus in the neck if oropharyngeal or proximal oesophageal perforation occurred. Abdomen should be carefully examined for evidence of peritonitis or small bowel obstruction.

Recommended investigations

- *Biplane radiographs*—can identify most true foreign objects, steak bones, and free mediastinal or peritoneal air. Lateral view helps in confirming the location in oesophagus and revealing the presence of more than one coin. Some objects like fish or chicken bones, wood, plastic, most glass, and thin metal objects may not be readily seen. Plain radiography is recommended to assess the presence, location, size, configuration, and number of ingested foreign bodies if ingestion of radiopaque objects is suspected or type of object is unknown [Strong recommendation – S].
- *CT scan*—indicated if symptoms are not specific and foreign body is still suspected. CT scan is recommended in patients with suspected perforation or other complications that may require surgery [S]. Handheld metal detectors and cautious endoscopy can also be used.
- *Contrast examination*—should not be performed routinely due to the risk of aspiration and coating of the foreign body which may compromise subsequent endoscopic removal (Fig. 24.1) [S].

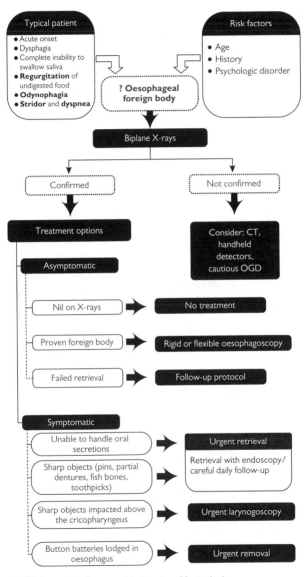

Fig. 24.1 Algorithim for approaching ingestion of foreign body.

Recommended management

- Ensure that airways are clear and secured.

Natural history—most will pass through the bowel with faeces (those that reach the stomach have 80–90% chance of passing through). Some may become lodged and cause damage to the GI tract.

- *Factors affecting treatment options and timing for a procedure*—age, severity of clinical condition, anatomical location, size and shape of ingested material, and technical skills of the endoscopist.
- Consult with an otorhinolaryngologist for foreign bodies at or above the level of cricopharyngus.
- *Asymptomatic patient with negative radiographs*—no specific treatment required. The foreign body may have passed out of the oesophagus. Asymptomatic patients with ingestion of blunt and small objects (except batteries and magnets) can be observed without the need for endoscopy [S]. Packets of drugs should also be observed and not retrieved endoscopically [S].
- *Pharmacological therapy*—using glucagon 1.0mg IV has been advocated to treat food boluses to cause relaxation of the lower oesophagus but should not delay definitive endoscopic management (Fig. 24.1).
    - *Obstructing objects and sharp-pointing objects*—should be retrieved within 6h (preferably within 2h). Incompletely obstructing large foreign bodies should be retrieved within 24h [S]. Food boluses should be pushed rather than pulled if safe and possible [S].
    - *Failed retrieval*—objects may be advanced into the stomach for easier grasping. If unable to retrieve from stomach, treat conservatively as outpatient. Advise patient on regular diet and observation of stool. If patient remains asymptomatic, weekly radiographs are recommended to follow the progression of small blunt objects.
    - *Lodged objects*—objects failed to leave stomach within 3–4wk should be removed endoscopically. Objects remaining in the same location (after passing the stomach) for more than 1wk should be removed surgically.
- *Sharp objects*—include chicken and fish bones, straightened paperclips, toothpicks, needles, bread bag clips, and dental bridgework. Many are not visible on X-ray and should be carefully investigated by laryngoscopy or oesophago-gastro-duodenoscopy (OGD).
    - Sharp objects must be retrieved or carefully followed up by daily radiographs. The risk of developing complications is >35%.
    - Objects failing to progress in three consecutive days may require surgical intervention.
- *Disc battery ingestion*—high risk of causing liquefaction necrosis and perforation of oesophagus, with possible death. Disc batteries should be retrieved immediately using a basket or a net.
- *Magnets*—should be removed due to the potential for pressure necrosis, perforation, or volvulus if other magnets or metal objects have been ingested and the attractive forces between these objects trap small bowel between them.

Further reading

Removal of foreign bodies in the upper gastrointestinal tract in adults: European Society of Gastrointestinal Endoscopy (ESGE) Clinical Guideline (2016).

Committee ASoP, Ikenberry SO, Jue TL, et al. Management of ingested foreign bodies and food impactions. (2011) Gastrointest Endosc 73, 1085–1091.

Conners GP, Chamberlain JM, Weiner PR (1995). Paediatric coin ingestion: a home-based survey. Am J Emerg Med 13, 638–40.

Li ZS, Sun ZX, Zou DW, Xu GM, Wu RP, Liao Z (2006). Endoscopic management of foreign bodies in the upper GI tract: experience with 1,088 cases in China. Gastrointest Endosc 64, 485–92.

PatientPlus. Swallowed foreign bodies. Available from: http://www.patient.co.uk/showdoc/ 40024855/.

Cheng W, Tam PK (1999). Foreign body ingestion in children: experience with 1,265 cases. J Pediatr Surg 34, 1472–6.

Vicari JJ, Johansson JF, Frakes JT (2001). Outcomes of acute oesophageal food impaction: success of the push technique. Gastrointest Endosc 53, 178–81.

Webb WA (1995). Management of foreign bodies of the upper gastrointestinal tract: update. Gastrointest Endosc 41, 39–51.

Vizcarrondo FJ, Brady PG, Nord HJ (1983). Foreign bodies of the upper gastrointestinal tract. Gastrointest Endosc 29, 208–10.

Litovitz T, Schmitz BF (1992). Ingestion of cylindrical and button batteries: an analysis of 2,382 cases. Pediatrics 89(4 Pt 2), 747–57.

Gordon AC, Gough MH (1993). Oesophageal perforation after button battery ingestion. Ann R Coll Surg Engl 75, 362–4.

Achalasia*

Basic facts 230
Recommended investigations 232
Recommended treatment 234
Further reading 235

Key guidelines

- ACG Clinical Guidelines: Diagnosis and Management of Achalasia (2013).
- Management of Achalasia: Surgery or Pneumatic Dilatation (GUT 2010).
- The Society for Surgery of the Alimentary Tract (2006). Patient care guidelines: oesophageal achalasia..
- Kahrilas PJ et al. (2015). The Chicago Classification of esophageal motility disorders, v3.0.
- Kahrilas PJ et al. (2017). Expert consensus document: Advances in the management of oesophageal motility disorders in the era of high-resolution manometry: a focus on achalasia syndromes.

* The guidelines on this chapter have been sourced and summarized from different UK, Europe, and international government sources, professional organizations, and medical specialty societies. Leading guidelines have been listed in the further reading section at the end of this chapter.

Basic facts

- *Definition*—primary oesophageal motility disorder, characterized by failure of the lower oesophageal sphincter (LOS) to relax in response to swallowing and by the absence of peristalsis in the oesophageal body.
- *Incidence*—about 0.5–1.0 cases/100,000 population per year.
- *Pathogenesis*—poorly understood. Possibly results from the dysfunction of inhibitory neurons containing nitric oxide and vasoactive intestinal polypeptide in the distal oesophagus. Unknown aetiology.
- *Clinical presentation*—slow progressive dysphagia (almost all patients) and regurgitation (60%). This occurs more often in supine position, with higher risk of aspiration of undigested food. Other findings include weight loss (60%), chest pain (40%) usually at the time of meal, nocturnal regurgitation, and pneumonia.

Recommended investigations

- *Routine blood tests*—iron deficiency anaemia may be detected.
- *Plain chest radiograph*—may show widening of the mediastinum and posterior mediastinal air–fluid level. Signs of chronic aspiration may show on lung fields.
- *Upper GI endoscopy and/or barium swallow*—are the initial investigations of choice, and should be performed urgently for patients with dysphagia (one of the 'ALARM' symptoms) [B].
  - *Endoscopy*— recommended to all patients. Endoscopy can detect complications and reliably rule out cancer. Retention oesophagitis may be found. Passage of the scope through the LOS often produces a characteristic 'pop' sensation.
  - *Barium swallow*—over 85% of cases have the characteristic dilated oesophagus with narrowing at the gastro-oesophageal junction (bird's beak deformity).
  - *Disease severity*—can be determined by the oesophageal diameter (<4cm, 4–6cm, >6cm), amount of retained food, and degree of peristalsis.
- *Oesophageal manometry*—confirms the diagnosis.
- *Classic findings*—absence of oesophageal peristalsis, and hypertensive or normotensive LOS that fails to relax completely in response to swallowing.
- *Differential diagnosis*—Chagas' disease and pseudoachalasia accompanying carcinoma (Fig. 25.1).

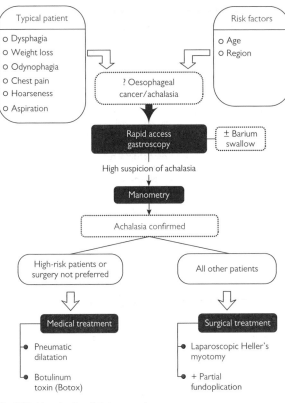

Fig. 25.1 Algorithm for achalasia approach.

Recommended treatment

- *Main goals*—palliative. Mainly to eliminate the outflow resistance at the gastro-oesophageal junction.
- *Minimally invasive surgery or graded pneumatic dilatation*—are recommended as initial treatment of choice where experience exists (high volume centres).
  - Technique—laparoscopic Heller's myotomy with a partial fundoplication is the surgical treatment of choice. A generous myotomy of the lower oesophagus should be performed and extended (2–3cm) onto the gastric wall.
- *Pneumatic dilatation*—above 75% success rate. Advantages include relatively low cost and avoidance of general anaesthesia. Possible complications include gastro-oesophageal reflux (25–35% of patients) and perforation (up to 5% of patients).
- *Medical treatment*—use only in patients unable (or unwilling) to undergo standard treatment. Options include calcium channel blockers and nitrates (50% initial success).
- *Intrasphincteric injection of botulinum toxin*—only in patients not suitable for above.
  - Advantages—about 60% success rate initially in relieving symptoms, but recurs within a year in the majority of patients.
  - Disadvantages—may cause inflammatory reaction at the gastro-oesophageal junction and obliterates anatomic planes. Less effective in recurrent cases.
- *Oesophagectomy*—can be required for patients with 'end stage' achalasia consisting of megaoesophagus or sigmoid oesophagus and who have failed management with myotomy or PD. Gastric interposition is the conduit of choice.
- *Surveillance endoscopy*—should not be offered to patients on the pure reason of increased risk for developing both squamous and adenocarcinoma of oesophagus but only after disease present for 10–15y with 3 yearly intervals between.
- *Future therapies*—hybrid techniques incorporating an endoscopic approach with principles of NOTES (natural orifice transluminal endoscopic surgery) termed POEM (peroral esophageal myotomy), metallic stents crossing the GOJ without reflux and neuronal stem cell transplants (Fig. 25.1).

Further reading

Vaezi MF, Pandolfino JE, Vela MF. ACG clinical guideline: diagnosis and management of achalasia. The American journal of gastroenterology 2013;108:1238-49

Stavropoulos SN, Friedel D, Modayil R, Iqbal S, Grendell JH. Endoscopic approaches to treatment of achalasia. Therapeutic advances in gastroenterology 2013;6:115-35.

Richter JE, Boeckxstaens GE. Management of achalasia: surgery or pneumatic dilation. Gut 2011;60:869-76.

The Society for Surgery of the Alimentary Tract (2006). SSAT patient care guidelines: oesophageal achalasia. Available from: https://www.ncbi.nlm.nih.gov/pubmed/18062073

Morris PJ, Wood WC (2000). Oxford Textbook of Surgery, 2nd ed, Oxford University Press, Oxford.

Clinical Knowledge Summaries. Gastrointestinal (upper) cancer—suspected. Available from: https://cks.nice.org.uk/gastrointestinal-tract-upper-cancers-recognition-and-referral

Kumar V, Abbas AK, Fausto N (2004). Pathologic basis of disease, 7th ed, Saunders, London.

Kahrilas, P. J. et al. The Chicago Classification of esophageal motility disorders, v3.0. Neurogastroenterol. Motil. 27, 160–174 (2015).

Kahrilas PJ et al. Expert consensus document: Advances in the management of oesophageal motility disorders in the era of high-resolution manometry: a focus on achalasia syndromes. Nature Reviews Gastroenterology & Hepatology (2017). doi:10.1038/nrgastro.2017.132

Oesophageal cancer

Basic facts *238*
Recommended investigations *240*
Recommended initial assessment/staging *242*
Recommended advanced staging *244*
Recommended treatment *246*
Recommendation for chemoradiotherapy *248*
Recommendation for palliative treatment *249*
Further reading *250*

Key guidelines

- Association of Upper Gastrointestinal Surgeons of Great Britain and Ireland, British Society of Gastroenterology, British Association of Surgical Oncology (2011). Guidelines for the management of oesophageal and gastric cancer.
- Oesophageal Cancer: ESMO Clinical Practice Guidelines (2016).
- NICE (2014). Gastric-oesophageal reflux disease and dyspepsia in adults: investigation and management.
- NICE (2017). Suspected cancer: recognition and referral.
- NCCN guidelines. Esophageal and esophagogastric junction cancers.

Basic facts

- *Incidence*—thirteenth most common cancer in the UK (23 people every day). Most cases occur in over 60y. Most common types are squamous cell carcinoma (SCC) and adenocarcinoma (ACA). The male to female ratio is 3:2 for SCC and 5–10:1 for ACA.
- *Risk factors*—almost 90% of cases are linked to major lifestyle and other risk factors. Risk factors for SCC include geographic location (more common in China and South Africa), people of African-American origin, excessive smoking (OR × 4–17), excessive alcohol consumption (OR × 2–10), and other factors (caustic oesophageal injury, etc.). Risk factors for ACA include long-standing reflux oesophagitis (RR × 2), and Barrett's oesophagus (OR × 44). Diet deficient in vegetables, fruit, dairy products, and diet with low contents of vitamin A, C, and riboflavin may have a role in the development of SCC.
- *Clinical presentation*—transient 'sticking' of apples, meat, or bread may precede frank dysphagia (once lumen diameter is <13mm). Odynophagia, reflux oesophagitis, deep chest pain, cough, hoarseness, aspiration pneumonia, lymphadenopathy, unexplained anaemia (in chronic GI bleeding), anorexia, and hepatomegaly.

Recommended investigations

- *Upper GI endoscopy*—the first investigation of choice to confirm diagnosis and obtain sufficient tissue biopsies (Box 26.1) [B].
  - *Referral guidelines*—patients with dysphagia or any other 'ALARM' symptoms (see ➜ Chapter 23, p.212) should be investigated urgently using upper GI endoscopy [B].
  - *Barium studies*—can be considered as the primary investigation if endoscopy is inappropriate [C].
  - High resolution endoscopy, chromoendoscopy, spectroscopy, narrow band imaging, and autofluorescence imaging are under evaluation and their roles are not yet defined [C].
- *Pathologic confirmation*—multiple (>6) biopsies should always be obtained from suspicious lesions [B].
  - *Biopsy detection rate*—ranges from 93% for one biopsy to 98% for seven biopsies.
  - *Cytology*—complements histology and can increase accuracy to 100% (Fig. 26.1).

Box 26.1 Endoscopy for oesophageal cancer

- *Preparation*—withhold antacids and anti-secretory treatment if possible until after endoscopy to avoid any misdiagnosis.
- *Findings*.
  - *Early oesophageal cancer*—may appear as a superficial plaque or ulceration.
  - *Advanced cancer*—may appear as an ulcerated mass, diffuse ulceration, stricture, or circumferential lesion.

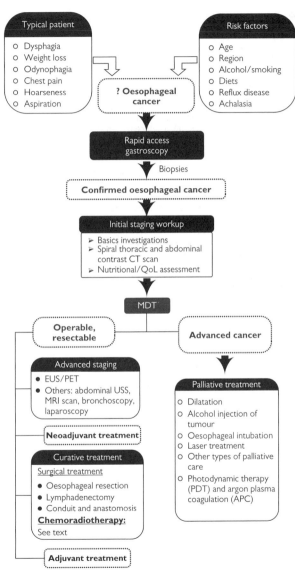

Fig. 26.1 Algorithm for approaching the oesophageal cancer patient (QoL = Quality of Life).

Recommended initial assessment/staging

- Please see Fig. 26.1.
- *Basic investigations*—baseline haematological and biochemical profile, ABGs, pulmonary function tests (PFTs), CXR, and ECG [B].
- *Spiral thoracic and abdominal contrast CT scan.*
  - *Indications*—first staging investigation of choice to evaluate the presence of metastatic disease [B].
  - *Technique*—thin (2.5–5mm) slices and gastric distension with 600–800mL of water are recommended.
  - *Accuracy*—>85% accurate in detecting mediastinal or liver involvement.
  - *TNM staging*—see Box 26.2.
- *Nutritional assessment.*
  - *Effect on surgery*—risk increases in patients with BMI <18.5, BMI
  - <90% of predicted value, recent weight loss of >20%, and low serum albumin (see Chapter 22). Obesity increases the risk as well.
  - *Optimization*—essential part of perioperative care. Nutritional support (enteral or parenteral) should be considered on all patients in the pre- and post-operative period [B].
- *MDT discussion*—essential requirement prior to commencing any definitive staging or treatment [C]. Decisions are taken in the context of predicted prognosis and expected effect of any investigation or treatment intervention on quality of life.
- *Breaking bad news*—should be done in a professional and effective way. The role of an Upper GI Clinical Nurse Specialist is essential.
  - *Recommended points to discuss*—confirmation of diagnosis, available treatment options, expected perioperative period experience, contact details, and sources for further information (including patient support groups). Discussion should be documented and communicated to other members of the team (e.g. GP, oncologists, and cancer care nurses).
- *Advanced staging*—only required if the patient is a good candidate for surgical resection.

Recommended advanced staging

- *Patient selection*—all patients without evidence of metastatic disease on CT scan who are eligible for curative surgery should undergo endoscopic ultrasonography if available [B] (Fig. 26.1).
- *Endoscopic ultrasonography (EUS)*—this is recommended for all oesophageal, oesophago-gastric junction, and selected gastric cancer [B].
  - EUS is superior to CT scan for local staging and more accurate in predicting resectability. EUS can identify the five-layered structure of oesophageal wall (T staging), provide accurate and reliable N staging (features like well-defined margins of nodes over 1cm in diameter, rounded, and hypoechoic nodes are likely to correlate well with malignant infiltration). It can demonstrate the presence of small volumes of ascites (M staging).
- *Other recommended investigations.*
  - *Positron emission tomography (PET)*—is superior to CT scan or EUS in detecting distant metastasis and should be used in combination with CT and EUS [B]. PET scan can change the management plan in 5–20% of cases, and has become an essential part of advanced staging in many cancer centres.
  - *Transabdominal USS*—indicated if treatment options are limited and good clinical evidence of liver metastasis exists. Confirmation of disease extent is required before commencing palliative treatment [C].
  - *MRI scan*—has no advantages over spiral CT scan in most cases. Usually used in certain individual cases such as allergy to IV contrast or the need for specific extra details [C].
  - *Bronchoscopy*—recommended if CT scan and EUS raise suspicion of bronchotracheal involvement [D]. Bronchoscopy may be inconclusive.
  - *Laparoscopy*—recommended in the perioperative period for suspicious peritoneal spread on CT scan or EUS, and for cancers at the gastro-oesophageal junction [C].

  TNM staging—see Table 26.1 and Box 26.2.

Table 26.1 TNM staging 7th Edition for Oesophageal Cancer.

T–primary tumour	
Tis	Carcinoma in-situ / high grade dysplasia
T1	Invasion reaching the lamina propria or submucosa
	T1a lamina propriae or muscularis mucosae
	T1b submucosa
T2	Invasion reaching the muscularis propria
T3	Invasion reaching the adventitia
T4	T4a resectable cancer invades adjacent structures such as pleura, pericardium, diaphragm
	T4b unresectable cancer invades adjacent structures such as aorta, vertebral body, trachea
N—regional lymph nodes	
N0	No evidence of regional lymph node involvement
N1	1 to 2 positive regional lymph nodes
N2	3 to 6 positive regional lymph nodes
N3	7 or more positive regional lymph nodes
M—distant metastasis	
M0	No evidence of distant metastasis
M1	Distant metastasis

A tumour where the epicentre is within 5cm of the oesophagogastric junction and it extends into the oesophagus is classified and staged according to the oesophageal scheme.

Data from Rice TW, Blackstone EH, Rusch VW. 7th edition of the AJCC Cancer Staging Manual: esophagus and esophagogastric junction. *Annals of Surgical Oncology* 17, 1721–4.

Recommended treatment

General approach

- Endoscopic resection (*mucosal resection and endoscopic submucosal dissection*) should be considered for early cancer (pT1sm1; <500 μm invasion, L0, V0, G1/2, <20mm diameter, no ulceration) [B] (Fig. 26.1).
- Endoscopic en-bloc resection should be considered for higher risk but localized tumors (L0, V0, no ulceration, grading G1/G2, infiltration grade m1/m2) [A].
- Radical surgery should be recommended for patients with localized tumours, who are fit enough to tolerate major surgery where surgery takes place in high volume cancer centres [B]. Combination therapy should be considered for T2 tumours. Other therapeutic modalities in the context of controlled trials should be offered to advanced cancer patients [D].

Standards for surgical resection

- *Preoperative preparation*—should include psychological preparation, thromboembolic and antibiotic prophylaxis, and blood cross-matching. Full communication with anaesthetist familiar with the complexity of one lung ventilation and epidural anaesthesia is recommended [C]. Depending on local protocols, an ICU or HDU bed should be booked prior to surgery.
- *Operative approach*—most widely used technique is the two-phase Lewis–Tanner (laparoscopic or open).
  - *Summary of technique*—the tumour is resected through laparotomy/laparoscopy and right thoracotomy/thoracoscopy, followed by construction of a gastric tube and performing of oesophagogastric anastomosis. A third cervical phase may be added in the case of proximally situated tumours in order to achieve appropriate degree of longitudinal clearance.
  - *Efficiency*—there is no evidence favouring one method of resection over another [A]. All types of operations should ensure adequate oncological standards (see below) [B].
  - *Growing interest in minimal access*—growing uptake presently in minimal access techniques to replace conventional open surgery. Evidence for minimal access technique is still limited [C]. Effectiveness and cost effectiveness of minimal access therapy yet to be demonstrated. Specific complications include gastric tube necrosis (up to 13%).
- *Oncological standards*.
  - *Main objectives*—adequate free-of-tumour longitudinal and radial resection margins, with appropriate lymphadenectomy [B].
  - *Proximal extent of resection*—should ideally be 10cm above the macroscopic tumour and 5cm distal to it [D*].
- *Outcome measures*—anastomotic leakage rate <5%, Curative (R0) resection rates >30%, and overall in-hospital mortality <10% [B].
- *Pathology report*—should follow the pathologic report minimum dataset (Box 26.3) [B].

Box 26.2 TNM staging on CT scan.

- *T staging.*
  - *T1 to T3*—unreliable in differentiating T1 from T2 cancers or in accurate estimation of microscopic invasion in T3.
  - *T4*—can be identified by finding:
  - Intimate contact between tumour and contiguous organs
  - Focal loss of intervening fat plane
  - Clear CT scan evidence of direct organ invasion.
- *N staging.*
  - Accuracy—node involvement can be identified in 38–70% of cases.
  - Criteria—node size is the main criterion used for identification and still of low accuracy (48% sensitivity and 93% specificity if size >8mm was considered abnormal in coeliac axis).
- *M staging.*
  - Accuracy—metastatic disease can be detected in 75–80% of 'truly positive' cases using newer techniques. Can only detect 50% of lesions with size <1cm.

Data from Rice TW, Blackstone EH, Rusch VW. 7th edition of the AJCC Cancer Staging Manual: esophagus and esophagogastric junction. *Annals of Surgical Oncology* 2010;17:1721–4.

Box 26.3 Pathologic report minimum dataset

- Type of tumour.
- Depth of invasion.
- Resection margins involvement.
- Vascular invasion.
- Presence of Barrett's metaplasia.
- Number of nodes resected and number containing metastatic tumour.

Recommendation for chemoradiotherapy

- *SCC*—chemoradiation is the treatment of choice for localized SCC in the proximal oesophagus [A]. Localized SCC of the middle or lower third of the oesophagus may be treated with chemoradio-therapy alone or chemoradiotherapy plus surgery [A].
  - Patients with locally advanced SCC benefit from preoperative chemotherapy or, most likely to a greater extent, from preoperative CRT, with higher rates of complete tumour resection and better local tumour control and survival [A].
- *ACC*—perioperative chemotherapy (combined preoperative and postoperative) conveys a survival benefit and is the preferred option for type II and III oesophago-gastric junctional adenocarcinoma [A].
  - Perioperative chemotherapy with regimens containing a platinum and a fluoropyrimidine for a duration of 8–9wk in the preoperative or preoperative chemoradiotherapy should be considered standard [A].

Recommendation for palliative treatment

- *General approach*—appropriate palliative treatment plan should be formulated at the MDT meeting for patients with inoperable cancers. A direct involvement of the palliative care team is recommended.
- *Options.*
  - *Dilatation*—indicated only for patients with predicted extremely short lifespan (4wk or less) who find difficulties in swallowing saliva. Consider also as a very short-term measure to relieve dysphagia while awaiting a more definitive treatment [B].
  - *Alcohol injection of tumour*—there is no indication for local ethanol injection for symptom palliation [B].
  - *Oesophageal intubation*—the treatment of choice for palliation of firm stenosing tumours lying more than 2cm from the cricopharyngeus:
    —Expandable metal stents preferable to plastic tubes—lower complication rate and shorter length of hospital stay.
    —Malignant tracheo-oesophageal fistulas or oesophageal perforation—use covered expandable metal stents or cuffed plastic tubes as the treatment of choice.
  - *Laser treatment*—indicated for exophytic tumours (or tumour over-growth following intubation) to relieve dysphagia [A].
  - *Other types of palliative care*—adjunctive external beam radiotherapy [B] or brachytherapy [A] and chemoradiation in patients with locally advanced metastatic cancer with good performance status.
  - Single-dose brachytherapy may be a preferred option even after external RT, since it provides better long-term relief of dysphagia with fewer complications than metal stent placement [B].
  - *Photodynamic therapy (PDT) and argon plasma coagulation (APC)* [B].
  - Follow up—there is currently no solid evidence evaluating follow up strategies. Local policies with MDT discussions should be followed.

Further reading

Allum WH, Griffin SM, Watson A, Colin–Jones D, et al. Association of Upper Gastrointestinal Surgeons of Great Britain and Ireland, British Society of Gastroenterology, British Association of Surgical Oncology (2011). Guidelines for the management of oesophageal and gastric cancer. Gut 2011;60:1449-72.

National Institute for Health and Clinical Excellence (2014). Dyspepsia and gastro-oesophageal reflux. Available from: http://guidance.nice.org.uk/CG184.

Oesophageal Cancer: ESMO Clinical Practice Guidelines (2016)

NICE (2017). Suspected cancer: recognition and referral.

Barrett's oesophagus[*]

Basic facts *252*
Recommended investigations *254*
Recommended treatment *256*
Further reading *258*

Key guidelines

- British Society of Gastroenterology (2013). Guidelines on the diagnosis and management of Barrett's oesophagus. (with update 2017).
- Barrett's Dysplasia and Cancer Task Force (2012). Consensus statements for management of Barrett's dysplasia and early stage esophageal adenocarcinoma.
- Endoscopic management of Barrett's oesophagus. ESGE position statement 2017.

---

[*] The guidelines on this chapter have been sourced and summarized from different UK, Europe, and international government sources, professional organizations, and medical specialty societies. Leading guidelines have been listed in the further reading section at the end of this chapter.

Basic facts

- *Definition*—a condition that complicates chronic gastro-oesophageal reflux disease (GORD), in which any portion of the normal squamous lining of oesophagus is replaced by 'any' length of a histologically confirmed metaplastic columnar epithelium of intestinal type, visible macroscopically above the gastro-oesophageal junction (GOJ). Barrett's oesophagus has recently been referred to as 'columnar-lined oesophagus (CLO)'. Short segment Barrett's refers to CLO with intestinal metaplasia that is less than 3cm in length.
- *Incidence*—in a catchment population of 250,000, the annual incidence is around 30 new cases per year. Mean age at the time of diagnosis is 55. Male to female ratio is 2:1.7 CLO is found in 12% of patients undergoing endoscopy for GORD and 36% of patients with confirmed oesophagitis.
- *Clinical presentation*—similar to chronic GORD. Heartburn, dysphagia, and bleeding are seen in 50, 75, and 25% of CLO patients, respectively. CLO is found more frequently in patients with severe and recurrent symptoms. The metaplastic intestinal columnar metaplasia of Barrett's oesophagus causes no symptoms.
- *Malignancy potential*—summarized in Box 27.1.

Box 27.1 Malignancy potentials of CLO

- *Development*—GORD usually precedes CLO for up to 10y. About 30% of CLO patients develop ulcerations and strictures. Up to 5% of them develop dysplasia.
  - *Low-grade dysplasia*—progresses in 10–50% of patients into high-grade dysplasia within 2–5y.
  - *High-grade dysplasia*—will have a focus of invasive adenocarcinoma in 40–50% of cases at the time of diagnosis.
- *Risk factors for malignancy*—male patients, age >45, CLO segment >8cm, long duration of reflux symptoms, onset of GORD at early age, persistent GORD, presence of mucosal damage (ulceration and stricture), and possibly family history.
- *Overall malignancy risk*—30-fold above general population. The incidence of adenocarcinoma is 1–1.5% per year.

Recommended investigations

Upper GI endoscopy

- *Anatomical landmarks*—see Box 27.2.
- *Endoscopic reporting*—should use a minimum dataset including the length using Prague criteria (circumferential extent (C), maximum extent (M) of endoscopically visible columnar-lined oesophagus in centimetres and any separate islands above the main columnar-lined segment noted) [B].
- *Current diagnostic criteria*.
  - If the Z-line is located proximal to the GOJ line, a columnar-lined segment of oesophagus is diagnosed.
  - If biopsy specimens from this segment shows native oesophageal structures juxtapositioned to metaplastic glandular mucosa (whether intestinalized or not), Barrett's oesophagus (CLO) is diagnosed [C].
  - Histologic 'corroboration' (non-typical special histology) also represents high diagnostic possibility for CLO [C].
  - In long segment CLO, the distance between Z-line and GOJ is ≥3cm; in short segment CLO, the distance is <3cm.
- *Accuracy and reliability*—see Box 27.3.

Recommended biopsy protocols

- No optimal protocol has been established. Most widely recommended protocol is to take quadrantic biopsies at 2cm intervals in the columnar segment together with biopsies of any visible lesion [C].
- *PET-CT, EUS, and chromoscopy*
  - Before endoscopic resection, the routine use of CT, PET-CT, or EUS cannot be recommended [B]. Individualized decisions should be made at the MDT discussion.

Box 27.2 Upper GI endoscopy—anatomic landmarks

- *GOJ*—imaginary line where the proximal limits of gastric folds are seen on retroflexing the endoscope and minimal air insufflation.
- *Squamo-columnar junction (Z-line)*—the line where columnar epithelium (reddish, velvet-like area) joins the squamous epithelium (pale, glossy appearance area).
- *Lower oesophageal sphincter (LOS)*—difficult to reliably identify by endoscope and is not used for diagnosis purposes.

Box 27.3 Upper GI endoscopy—accuracy and reliability

- *Accuracy*—overall sensitivity and specificity of endoscopy with biopsy is ~80%. Positive predictive value (correct correlation between detected CLO cases on endoscopy and definition) is ~35%. Negative predictive value (correct exclusion of CLO in negative endoscopy) is >95%.
- *Reliability*—determined by the length of involved mucosa. Highly accurate and reliable if traditional Barrett's oesophagus definition with long segment CLO (>3cm) is used. Unreliable enough if short segment CLO is added to the definition.

Recommended management

General principles

- Management involves three main components: management of GORD, endoscopic screening for GORD patients, and treatment of proven CLO with and without dysplasia.

Management of GORD

- See Chapter 23 pp.210–220

Endoscopic screening to detect CLO

- Not currently recommended for all patients with chronic heartburn [C]. Screening can be considered in patients with chronic GORD symptoms and multiple risk factors (at least three of age 50 years or older, white race, male sex, and obesity), especially with +ve family history [C].

Recommended management of non-dysplastic CLO

- *Reflux symptoms control*—should follow the same GORD treatment principles (many have few or no symptoms). The absence of symptoms is not a reliable indicator for effective treatment [B].
- *Proton pump inhibitors (PPIs)*—may require up to four times the standard daily dose to control symptoms and promote healing. Doses up to the maximal manufacturers' recommendations should be considered.
- *Poorly controlled CLO (poor symptom control and/or poor healing)*—requires further assessment using pH monitoring [C].
- *Surgical fundoplication*—indications should follow the same GORD approach. Surgical management is often more required in CLO patients (high-dose PPI therapy, higher incidence of hiatus hernia and LOS failure, reflux of duodenal contents). Fundoplication is currently NOT recommended on the sole basis of finding CLO in GORD patients [B].
- *Endoscopic ablation*—effective in achieving squamous re-epithelialization, but remains experimental [C].

Management of dysplastic CLO

- *Indefinite dysplasia*—a misleading diagnosis. Diagnosed if histologic changes suggest dysplasia, but definite diagnosis cannot be made due to inflammatory reaction. Treat aggressively with PPI and re-investigate early with new biopsies. If no definite dysplasia was detected in 6-month's follow-up, treat as 'CLO with no dysplasia' [C].
- *Low-grade dysplasia (LGD)*.
  - Treat aggressively with intensive acid suppression for 2–4mo, then re-biopsy [C].
  - *Persistent low-grade dysplasia*—surveillance follow-up on 6-monthly bases. If regressed in two consequent occasions, increase surveillance to 2–3 yearly [C].
  - Ablation therapy should be offered once LGD is detected (2015 guidelines) [A]. If ablation is not undertaken, 6-monthly surveillance is recommended [C].

- *High-grade dysplasia (HGD)*—if persistent after intensive acid suppression
  - Confirm diagnosis by two expert pathologists, using high-resolution endoscopy (HRE) [B]. Visible lesions are malignant till proven otherwise [C] (using Paris classification is recommended).
  - Endoscopic resection (ER) is preferred for all visible dysplastic lesions and T1a adenocarcinoma over surgery or endoscopic surveillance [B]. This should be carried out in high volume centres who can offer both endoscopic and surgical procedures.
  - The cap and snare technique with submucosal injection and the band ligation technique without submucosal injection are considered to be equally effective [A].
  - Consider endoscopic ablation or mucosal resection for unfit patients with good prognosis T1b adenocarcinoma [C]. This is not to be considered curative [C].
  - Ablative therapy for flat HGD and residual Barrett's after ER is recommended [A].
- *Circumferential epithelial radiofrequency (RF) ablation.*
  - RF beam is used to obliterate a thin layer of oesophageal epithelium (containing CLO) for a few cm in length using endoscopy.
  - The 12mo follow-up studies showed an overall efficiency of up to 69% with low transient morbidity.
  - Radiofrequency ablation (RFA) has currently a better safety and side-effect profile and comparable efficiency [A].
- *Photodynamic therapy for high-grade dysplasia.*
  - A photosensitizing agent is administered, and then activated using light beam to selected areas (containing CLO) to generate highly reactive oxygen molecules, leading to necrosis of the area.
  - Follow-up studies showed an overall efficiency of 77–98% in downgrading the dysplasia, and 42–98% in eliminating the CLO. Strictures occurred in about a third of patients and photosensitivity (skin reaction) occurred in a third of them.
  - The procedure has enough evidence to support its use in the clinical practice. This should be done within a proper clinical governance framework as per NICE guidance.
- Surgical management for early Barrett's neoplasia—is only considered where neoplasia has extended into submucosa [B].
- There is not yet sufficient evidence to advocate acid-suppression drugs as chemopreventive agents [C].

Further reading

British Society of Gastroenterology (2017). Guidelines on the diagnosis and management of Barrett's oesophagus. Available from: http://gut.bmj.com/content/early/2017/04/07/gutjnl-2017-314135#BIBL

Barrett's Dysplasia and Cancer Task Force (2013). Consensus statements for management of Barrett's dysplasia and early stage esophageal adenocarcinoma, based on a Delphi process. Gastroenterology 2012;143:336–346 Available from: http://www.gastrojournal.org/article/S0016-5085(12)00614-2/pdf

National Institute for Health and Clinical Excellence (2010). Ablative therapy for the treatment of Barrett's oesophagus. Available from: https://www.nice.org.uk/guidance/cg106/resources/guidance-barretts-oesophagus-pdf

National Institute for Health and Clinical Excellence (2010). Epithelial radiofrequency ablation for Barrett's oesophagus. Available from: https://www.nice.org.uk/guidance/ipg344

National Institute for Health and Clinical Excellence (2014). Endoscopic radiofrequency ablation for Barrett's oesophagus with low grade dysplasia or no dysplasia. Available from: https://www.nice.org.uk/guidance/ipg496

National Institute for Health and Clinical Excellence (2010). Photodynamic therapy for Barrett's oesophagus. Available from: https://www.nice.org.uk/guidance/ipg350

Weusten Bas et al. Endoscopic management of Barrett's esophagus: European Society of Gastrointestinal Endoscopy (ESGE) Position Statement. Endoscopy 2017; 49(02): 191–198 DOI: 10.1055/s-0042-122140

Management of oesophageal variceal haemorrhage

Basic facts 260
Recommended prophylaxis against first bleeding 262
Recommended treatment for active bleeding 264
Recommended prevention of re-bleeding 266
Further reading 266

Key guidelines

- NICE (2016). Acute upper gastrointestinal bleeding in over 16s: management.
- Tripathi D, Stanley AJ, Hayes PC et al (2015) UK guidelines on the management of variceal haemorrhage in cirrhotic patients.
- American Association for the Study of Liver Diseases, American College of Gastroenterology (2007) Prevention and management of gastro-oesophageal varices and variceal haemorrhage in cirrhosis.
- World Gastroenterology Organisation Global Guidelines (2014). Oesophageal varices.
- National Institute for Health and Clinical Excellence (2011). Stent insertion for bleeding oesophageal varices.
- Scottish Intercollegiate Guidelines Network (2008). Management of acute upper and lower gastrointestinal bleeding.
- American Society for Gastrointestinal Endoscopy (2014). The role of endoscopy in the management of variceal bleeding.

Basic facts

- *Incidence*—at the time of diagnosis, around 30% of patients with cirrhosis have oesophageal varices, reaching 90% after approximately 10 years. Varix bleeding is the source of upper GI bleeding in 50–90% of cases in cirrhosis patients.
- *Pathogenesis*—varices develop as a decompression mechanism of hypertensive portal vein to return the blood to systemic circulation. They become apparent when the pressure gradient between portal and hepatic veins rises over 12mmHg. The average pressure gradient in bleeding varices is 20mmHg.
- *Consensus definitions*—see Box 28.1.
- *Predicting 'at risk' patients.*
  - *Severity of liver dysfunction*—as estimated by Child classification. Bleeding occurs more frequently in severe cases.
  - *Patient history*—risk increases in active alcoholics, patients with previous history of variceal bleeding, and patients with ascites.
  - *Variceal pressure*—Those with hepatic venous pressure gradient>20mmHg within 24 h of variceal haemorrhage are at higher risk for recurrent bleeding within the first week of admission, and higher risk of failure to control bleeding.
  - *Variceal size*—correlates well with the risk of bleeding. Varices can be small (straight), enlarged (tortuous varices occupying less than one third of the lumen), and large (coil-shaped, occupying more than one third of the lumen).
  - *Variceal location*—isolated gastric varices in fundus bleed more commonly than both gastro-oesophageal varices and isolated gastric varices in other sites.
  - *Appearance of varices*—risk increases with the presence of red wale marks (longitudinal red streaks on the varices), cherry red spots (discrete red cherry colour spots overlying the varices), haematocystic spots (raised discrete red spots overlying the varices), and diffuse erythema (diffuse red colour of the varices).
  - Presence of coagulopathy at initial bleeding episode.

Box 28.1 Consensus definitions in variceal bleeding

- *Time zero*—the time of first admission to a medical care centre.
- *Acute bleeding episode*—occurs when the bleeding events take place in the interval of 48h from time zero. Any bleeding during this time should be considered to reflect a failure of therapy rather than a re-bleeding event.
- *Clinically significant bleeding*—bleeding that requires a transfusion of ≥2 units of blood within 24h of time zero concurrently with a systolic BP of <100mmHg, a postural systolic change of >20mmHg, and/or a pulse rate of >100bpm at time zero.
- *Failure of therapy*—occurs in two time frames.
  - *0–6h*—transfusion requirement of >4 units and persistent systolic BP <70mmHg, inability to increase BP by 20mmHg, and/or persistent pulse rate >100bpm.
  - *Over 6h from time zero*—one or more events of haematemesis with increased pulse rate by 20bpm, drop in systolic BP of >20mmHg and the need for a transfusion of ≥2 units of blood to keep Hb at around 9g/dL
- *Early re-bleeding*—occurs when the bleeding event occurs after 48h from the initial haemostasis counted from time zero, but less than 6wk.

Recommended prophylaxis against first bleeding

- *Screening OGD*—recommended for all patients when diagnosis of cirrhosis is made [C].
- *Cirrhotic patients with no varices*—repeat OGD at 23y interval [A].
- Selective B-blockers are not recommended [B].
- *Cirrhotic patients with small varices*—repeat OGD every 1–2y, depending on the presence or absence of signs of liver decompensation, the severity of cirrhosis, and the current use of B-blockers [A]. Non-selective B-blockers should be used for the prevention of first variceal haemorrhage in patients at very high risk [C]. Medium-risk patents can be considered for B-blockers, but long-term benefits remain unclear [B].
- *Cirrhotic patients with medium or large varices*—endoscopic variceal ligation (EVL) or B-blockers recommended in high-risk patients. In comparison with B-blockers, EVL reduces bleeding episodes/adverse events significantly, but does not affect mortality [A].
- *Other treatment modalities*—nitrates (either alone or in combination with B-blockers), shunt therapy, or sclerotherapy have no proven role in the primary prophylaxis of variceal bleeding [A].

Recommended treatment for active bleeding

- See Fig. 28.1

Active resuscitation [B]

- Protect airways in severe, uncontrolled bleeding or severe encephalopathy.
- Large bore peripheral IV lines or central line.
- Cross-match six units of blood and replace blood loss with packed cells. Monitor carefully to avoid overtransfusion which may increase the risk of rebound portal hypertension and induced re-bleeding. Maintain the haemoglobin levels at about 8g/dL.
- Give fresh frozen plasma if fibrinogen<1g/litre or prothrombin time>1.5 times normal.
- Replace platelets if the count drops below 50,000/mm3 within the first 48h.
- Monitor serum ionized calcium concentration in massive bleeding and replace as appropriate.

Risk assessment

- Use Blatchford score at first assessment and full Rockall score after endoscopy.

Prophylactic antibiotics

- Short-term (maximum 1wk) antibiotic prophylaxis should be used at presentation in any patient with cirrhosis and GI bleeding. Oral or
- IV fluoroquinolone (ciprofloxacin) is recommended [A].

Control of bleeding

- *OGD*—perform as soon as the patient is stable [A].
- *Terlipressin*—use in suspected variceal haemorrhage at presentation and stop at 5 days unless there is another indication for its use.
- *EVL*—first treatment of choice [A]. Proper ligation is effective in over 90% of cases in controlling bleeding.
- *Stent insertion for bleeding oesophageal varices*—may be used. A coated metal stent is inserted with the aim of compressing the bleeding varices. The stent is usually inserted with the aid of an endoscope and positioning should be confirmed radiologically, endoscopically, or by chest X ray. The stent is left in place for 2 weeks and then removed endoscopically.

Failure to control bleeding

- *Balloon Sengstaken tube tamponade*—use temporarily (maximum 24h) in patients with uncontrollable bleeding until further definitive therapy (transjugular intrahepatic portosystemic shunt (TIPS) or endoscopic therapy) is instituted [B].
- *TIPS*—consider in patients with difficult-to-control haemorrhage despite combined pharmacological and endoscopic therapy [B].

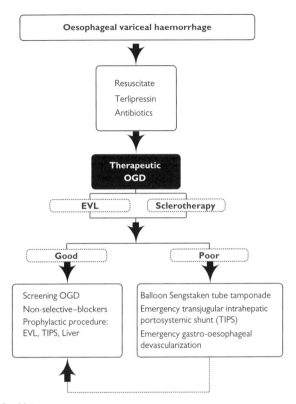

Fig. 28.1 Approach to oesophageal variceal haemorrhage.

Recommended prevention of re-bleeding

- See Fig. 28.1
- *In general*—prophylaxis should be applied to all patients after surviving the episode of active bleeding [A].
- *Combination treatment: EVL + B-blocker.*
  - *EVL*—first method of choice [A]. Apply a single band on each varix at weekly intervals until all varices are eradicated [B]. Monitor with regular OGD at 3mo after obliteration, then every 6–12mo thereafter [A].
  - *Endoscopic variceal sclerotherapy*—should be used if EVL is technically difficult or unavailable [B]. Use the same interval protocols as above to treat each varix.
  - *B-blocker*—can be used alone in mild cases. Measure variceal pressure during treatment to ensure a safe level below 12mmHg [A].
- *TIPS*—more effective than endoscopic procedures, but does not increase survival. Consider in individual cases where expertise is available [A].
- *Liver transplant*—should be considered for eligible patients [C].

Further reading

National Institute for Health and Clinical Excellence (2016). Acute upper gastrointestinal bleeding:management

World Gastroenterology Organisation Global Guidelines (2014). Oesophageal varices.

National Institute for Health and Clinical Excellence (2011). Stent insertion for bleeding oesophageal varices.

Scottish Intercollegiate Guidelines Network (2008). Management of acute upper and lower gastrointestinal bleeding.

American Society for Gastrointestinal Endoscopy (2014). The role of endoscopy in the management of variceal bleeding.

Jalan R, Hayes PC (2000). UK guidelines on the management of variceal haemorrhage in cirrhotic patients. Available from: http://gut.bmj.com/content/46/suppl_3/iii1

American Association for the Study of Liver Diseases, American College of Gastroenterology (2007).

Prevention and management of gastro-oesophageal varices and variceal haemorrhage in cirrhosis. D'Amico G, Garcia–Pagan JC, Luca A, Bosch J (2006). Hepatic vein pressure gradient reduction and prevention of variceal bleeding in cirrhosis: a systematic review. Gastroenterology 131, 1611–24.

Odelowo OO, Smoot DT, Kim K (2002). Upper gastrointestinal bleeding in patients with liver cirrhosis. J Natl Med Assoc 94, 712–5.

Tripathi D, Stanley AJ, Hayes PC et al. UK guidelines on the management of variceal haemorrhage in cirrhotic patients. Gut 2015;0:1–25. doi:10.1136/gutjnl-2015-309262 World Gastroenterology Global guidelines Esophageal varices January 2014

National Institute for Health and Clinical Excellence (2011) Stent insertion for bleeding oesophageal varices. Available from: http://www.nice.org.uk/nicemedia/pdf/IPG265Guidance.pdf.

Part 4

Stomach and duodenum

Chapter 29

Peptic ulcer disease*

Basic facts 270
Recommended investigations 272
Recommended treatment 276
Further reading 277

Key guidelines

- National Institute for Health and Clinical Excellence (2014). Gastro-oesophageal reflux disease and dyspepsia in adults: investigation and management.
- European Helicobacter Group (2012). Current concepts in the management of *Helicobacter pylori* infection: the Maastricht IV/Florence Consensus Report.
- University of Michigan Health System (2005). Peptic ulcer disease.
- ACG and CAG clinical guideline: Management of dyspepsia. 2017.
- ACG clinical guidelines: Treatment of *Helicobacter pylori* infection 2017.

---

* The guidelines on this chapter have been sourced and summarized from different UK, Europe, and international government sources, professional organizations, and medical specialty societies. Leading guidelines have been listed in the further reading section at the end of this chapter.

Basic facts

- *Definition*—abnormal gastrointestinal mucosal defect, caused by abnormal exposure to peptic juice, that extends through the muscularis mucosa layer, submucosa, or beyond.
- *Incidence*—about 10% of the population in Europe and USA suffer from an ulcer at some time in their life. Peptic ulcers are found in 10–15% of patients investigated by endoscopy for dyspepsia.
  - The prevalence of *H. pylori* infection varies internationally, with over 80% of Japanese and South American people infected, compared with rate approximate 40% in the UK and 20% in Scandinavia.
- *Risk factors*—three major risk factors attribute to 95% of cases: *Helicobacter (H.) pylori* infection, NSAIDs, and smoking (Box 29.1).
- *Clinical presentation*—may remain asymptomatic, presents with typical or atypical symptoms, or present initially with complications (perforation, bleeding, or obstruction in 20% of cases). Symptoms have poor sensitivity, specificity, and predictive value for the presence of either duodenal ulcer (DU) or gastric ulcer (GU). Only 50% of patients with DU would have the classic ulcer-like dyspepsia, and only 15–25% of patients with ulcer-like dyspepsia would have an underlying peptic ulcer disease (gastroduodenitis is found in 40% of such cases).
  - *DU*—the typical 'hunger' pain occurs 90min to 3h after a meal, frequently relieved by antacids or food, and awakes patient from sleep between midnight and 3 am (most discriminating symptom that occurs in about two thirds of DU patients).
  - *GU*—the pain typically precipitated by food, associated with nausea and weight loss (more commonly than DU). GU and DU patients can present with ill-defined burning or gnawing epigastric discomfort or ache.

Box 29.1 Risk factors for peptic ulcer

H. pylori infection—presents in virtually all patients with DU and in ~70% of GU. Eradication of *H. pylori* is associated with higher healing rate (92% vs 61% when *H. pylori* persists after treatment) and lower recurrence rate (21% vs 84% in 12mo).

NSAIDs—within 90min of taking 300–600mg of aspirin, nearly everyone develops acute injury consisting of intramucosal petechiae and erosions. GU and DU are found on endoscopy in 14–25% of NSAID users. The overall RR is 2.74 for serious gastrointestinal event.

Smoking—when associated with *H. pylori* infection (RR ×2.2).

Familial predisposition—first-degree relatives of patients with peptic ulcer have ~3-fold increase in prevalence of ulcer.

Blood group O—indirect genetic link.

High stress levels—RR ×3.2 in some, but not all studies.

Corticosteroid use

Others—no clear evidence exists for exact diet or alcohol relation.

Recommended investigations

- See Fig 29.1.
- *Initial approach*—should follow the general approach for dyspepsia (see Ch 23). Confirmation of peptic ulcer by endoscopy or barium studies is neither necessary nor practical for every patient with dyspepsia in the absence of ALARM symptoms [A]. Non-invasive *H. pylori* test is recommended as a first-line investigation in such patients.
- *Blood tests*—FBC, LFTs, and serum calcium are usually requested in patients with suspected peptic ulcer to exclude other diseases (e.g. liver disorders), and to identify patients with ALARM symptoms who require urgent endoscopy or other diagnostic testing.
- *H. pylori test*—can be performed using different techniques depending on the setting and stage of the treatment.
  - *Pre-treatment test* (before performing endoscopy)—best option is the carbon-13 urea breath test or stool antigen test (Box 29.2).
  - *Post-eradication testing*—best performed using a carbon-13 urea breath test only.
  - *Special precautions*—reduce false negative results by stopping PPIs and antibiotics 2wk and 4wk, respectively, before performing the *H. pylori* testing.
  - *Patients undergoing endoscopy*—use CLO test (Box 29.2).
- *Endoscopy*—the 'gold standard' investigation.
  - *Peptic ulcer appearance*—typically appears as mucosal defect with sharply demarcated edges and exposed underlying submucosa. Ulcer base is often clean and smooth, but can demonstrate eschar or ad-herent exudates in acute or bleeding cases. DU is more common in first part of duodenum.
  - *Other benefits*—can take biopsies for suspicious lesions and test for *H. pylori*.
  - *Accuracy*—correctly diagnose the peptic ulcers (positive and negative predictive values) in >95% of cases.
  - *Risks*—morbidity and mortality rates are low (1 in 200 and 1 in 2,000, respectively, in the UK).
- *Barium studies*—still used in some cases (e.g. patient refusing endoscopy) as first-line test for confirming peptic ulcer disease where appropriate.
- *Accuracy*—depends on the skills, techniques, and interests of the radiologist, and the ability of patient to cooperate. Single contrast studies can detect 50% of DUs. Double contrast studies can detect 80–90% of DUs. GU detection rate varies considerably depending on the technique used.

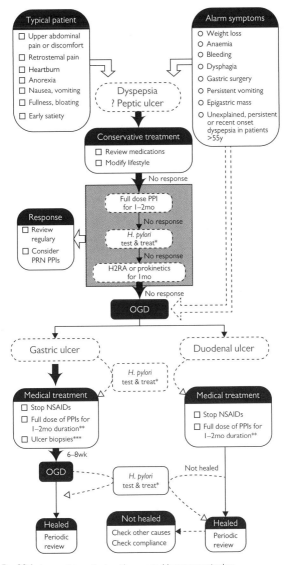

Fig. 29.1 Approach to patients with suspected/proven peptic ulcer.
* see text; ** or only eradication course if ulce not associated with NSAIDs use; *** see gastric cancer. Ch. 30.

Box 29.2 *H. pylori* test—laboratory options

Carbon-13 urea breath test

- *Preparation*—special arrangement for supervision required. Advise patients to keep fasting for a minimum of 6h before the test (if not diabetic where a special kit—diabact® UBT—should be used). Just before the test, patients should ingest citric acid or orange juice to slow gastric emptying.
- *Performing the test*—two or three breath samples are tested before ingestion of the carbon-13 tablet. Patient should then blow through a straw into a series of glass screw-topped tubes. Another breath test should be repeated 30min after carbon-13 ingestion.
- *Breath samples*—should be sent for analysis by mass spectrometry. Results are available in 724h.
- *Accuracy*—very high (95% sensitivity and specificity).

Stool antigen test

- Cheaper test and no separate appointment required. Very high accuracy (95% sensitivity and specificity).

Laboratory-based ELISA serology test.

- *Indications*—acceptable alternative if validated appropriately.
- *Accuracy*—sensitivity and specificity varies between different populations. Pay special precautions in interpreting results.

Campylobacter-like organism (CLO) test.

- *Indications*—patients undergoing endoscopy.
- *Technique*—take biopsies and use the rapid urease test pot.
- *Accuracy*—sensitivity and specificity are 85–90% and 98–100%, respectively.

Recommended treatment

- See Fig. 29.1.
- *General approach*—should be multimodal, including lifestyle adjustment, eradication of *H. pylori* infection, managing the NSAID, anti-secretory therapy, and/or surgery when indicated.
  - *Lifestyle adjustment*—advice for healthy eating, weight reduction, and smoking cessation.
  - *Healthy eating*—benefits the general health as well and should be encouraged. Advise against any identifiable precipitating factor (e.g. alcohol, caffeine, chocolate, fatty or spicy foods).
  - *Smoking*—in the pre-*H. pylori* era, smokers were more likely to develop ulcers and have recurrence. Smokers post-eradication of *H. pylori* have similar rate of ulcer relapse (73.6% for smokers vs 2% for non-smokers).
  - *Reflux symptoms*—advise on eating smaller meals, avoiding meals before going to sleep, and raising the bed head.
- *H. pylori eradication*—revolutionized the management and reduced the need for surgical intervention.
  - *Benefits*—reduced risk of bleeding, increased chance for complete healing, and reduced risk of NSAID-related complications.
  - *Recommended treatment*—one-week triple therapy regimen with a PPI and two antibiotics.
  - *Optimal regimes*—PAC regimen (double dose PPI + amoxicillin 1g + clarithromycin 500mg, all given twice a day) or the
  - PCM regimen (double dose PPI + clarithromycin 250mg + metronidazole 400mg, all given twice a day).
  - Eradication rate for both regimes—about 82%.

Second-line treatment

Offer people who still have symptoms after first-line eradication treatment for a week, twice daily course of treatment with PAC or PCM (whichever was not used as first line.

- In case of exposure to clarithromycin and metronidazole give quinolone or tetracycline.
- In case of allergy to penicillin offer PPI, metronidazole, and levofloxacin.
- In case of allergy to penicillin and previous exposure of quinolones give one week, twice daily regimen of: PPI, bismuth, metronidazole, and tetracycline.

- *PPI*.
  - *Benefits*—may be used as first-line treatment in dyspepsia, as part of eradication therapy for *H. pylori*, or as a stand-alone treatment for *H. pylori*-negative ulcers.
  - *Indications*—if the *H. pylori* test is negative, a course of full dose PPI for 1–2mo is recommended.
- *NSAID-induced ulcers*—stop NSAIDs where possible, test and treat *H. pylori*, and start on full dose PPI for 2mo. Re-test for *H. pylori* is necessary and treatment should be tailored accordingly to reduce the recurrence rate.

Further reading

National Institute for Health and Clinical Excellence (2014). Dyspepsia: managing dyspepsia in adults in primary care. Available from: http://guidance.nice.org.uk/CG184.

Kumar V, Abbas AK, Fausto N (2004). Robbins and Cotran Pathologic basis of disease, 7th ed. Saunders, London.

Johnson A (2001). Peptic ulcer. stomach and duodenum. In: Oxford Textbook of Surgery, 2nd ed. Oxford University Press, Oxford.

Kurata JH, Nogawa AN (1997). Meta-analysis of risk factors for peptic ulcer, non-steroidal anti-inflammatory drugs, *Helicobacter pylori*, and smoking. J Clin Gastroenterol 24, 2–17.

Marshall BJ, Goodwin CS, Warren JR (1988). Prospective double-blind trial of duodenal ulcer relapse after eradication of Campylobacter pylori. Lancet 2, 1437–42.

Hopkins RJ, Girardi LS, Turney EA (1996). Relationship between Helicobacter pylori eradication and reduced duodenal and gastric ulcer recurrence. Gastroenterology 110, 1244–52.

Laine L, Hopkins RJ, Girardi LS (1998). Has the impact of Helicobacter pylori therapy on ulcer recurrence in the United States been overstated? A meta-analysis of rigorously designed trials. Am J Gastroenterol 93, 1409–15.

Seager JM, Hawkey CJ (2001). ABC of the upper gastrointestinal tract: indigestion and non-steroidal anti-inflammatory drugs. BMJ 323, 1236–9.

Russell RI (2001). Non-steroidal anti-inflammatory drugs and gastrointestinal damage— problems and solutions. Postgrad Med J 77, 82–8.

Richy F, Bruyere O, Ethgen O (2004). Time-dependent risk of gastrointestinal complications induced by non-steroidal anti-inflammatory drug use: a consensus statement using a meta-analytic approach. Ann Rheum Dis 63, 759–66.

Räihä I, Kemppainen H, Kaprio J, Koskenvuo M, Sourander L (1998). Lifestyle, stress, and genes in peptic ulcer disease: a nationwide twin cohort study. Arch Intern Med 158, 698–704.

Hein HO, Suadicani P, Gyntelberg F (1997). Genetic markers for peptic ulcer. A study of 3,387 men aged 54 to 74 years: the Copenhagen Male Study. Scand J Gastroenterol 32, 16–21.

Sidebotham RL, Baron JH, Schrager J, Spencer J, Clamp JR, Hough L (1995). Influence of blood group and secretor status on carbohydrate structures in human gastric mucins: implications for peptic ulcer. Clin Sci (Lond) 89, 405–15.

Peters MN, Richardson CT (1983). Stressful life events, acid hypersecretion, and ulcer disease. Gastroenterology 84, 114–9.

Del Valle J (2005). Peptic ulcer disease and related disorders. In: Harrison's Principles of Internal Medicine, pp. 1747–62, 16th ed, McGraw-Hill Companies, Inc Publishing Group.

Pounder R (1989). Silent peptic ulceration: deadly silence or golden silence? Gastroenterology 96 (2 Pt 2 Suppl), 626–31.

Cotton PB, Shorvon PJ (1984). Analysis of endoscopy and radiography in the diagnosis, follow-up and treatment of peptic ulcer disease. Clin Gastroenterol 13, 383–403.

Levine MS (1995). Role of the double contrast upper gastrointestinal series in the 1990s. Gastroenterol Clin North Am 24, 289–308.

Eastwood GL (1997). Is smoking still important in the pathogenesis of peptic ulcer disease? J Clin Gastroenterol 25 (Suppl 1), S1–7.

Chan FK, Sung JJ, Lee YT et al. (1997). Does smoking predispose to peptic ulcer relapse after eradication of Helicobacter pylori? Am J Gastroenterol 92, 442–5.

Moayyedi PM et al. ACG and CAG clinical guideline:Management of dyspepsia. Am J Gastroenterol 2017; 112:988–1013; doi:10.1038/ajg.2017.154

Chey WD et al. ACG clinical guidelines: Treatment of Helicobacter pylori infection. Am J Gastroenterol 2017; 112:212–238; doi:10.1038/ajg.2016.563

Management of Helicobacter pylori infection- the Maastricht IV/ Florence Consensus ReportPeter Malfertheiner,Francis Megraud, Colm A O'Morain, John Atherton,Anthony T R Axon, Franco Bazzoli,Gian Franco Gensini,Javier P Gisbert, David Y Graham, Theodore Rokkas, Emad M El-Omar,Ernst J Kuipers,The European Helicobacter Study Group (EHSG)

Gut 2012;61:646e664. doi:10.1136/gutjnl-2012-302084

Gastric cancer[*]

Basic facts 280
Recommended investigations 282
Recommended initial assessment/staging 284
Recommended advanced staging 286
Recommended treatment 288
Further reading 292

Key guidelines

- Association of Upper Gastrointestinal Surgeons of Great Britain and Ireland, British Society of Gastroenterology and the British Association of Surgical Oncology (2011). Guidelines for the management of oesophageal and gastric cancer.
- NICE (2014) Gastro-oesophageal reflux disease and dyspepsia in adults: investigation and management.
- Gastric cancer: ESMO–ESSO–ESTRO Clinical Practice Guidelines for diagnosis, treatment and follow-up. 2013.
- Gastric cancer: ESMO Clinical Practice Guidelines for diagnosis, treatment and follow-up. 2016.
- Cancer Research UK. 2017.
- NICE (2017). Suspected cancer: Recognition and referral.
- NCCN guidelines: Gastric cancer.
- Japanese gastric cancer treatment guidelines 2014 (ver. 4).

---

[*] The guidelines on this chapter have been sourced and summarized from different UK, Europe, and international government sources, professional organizations, and medical specialty societies. Leading guidelines have been listed in the further reading section at the end of this chapter.

Basic facts

- *Incidence*—eleventh most common cancer in the UK and second most common cause of cancer mortality worldwide. Incidence rises steadily after the age of 40. Over 90% of cases are diagnosed after the age of 55. The male to female ratio is 1.7:1.
- *Risk factors*—over 75% of cases are related to major lifestyle or other specific risk factor (Box 30.1).
- *Clinical presentation*—over 85% of gastric cancers present initially with locally advanced or metastatic stage and poor resectability. Early gastric cancer presents with dyspepsia in 77% of cases and/or ALARM symptoms in 71% of cases. Dyspepsia in the general population is caused by cancer in only 1.6–4% of cases. Advanced cancers present with palpable lymph nodes, ascites, jaundice, and/or palpable abdominal or pelvic mass (Box 30.2).

Box 30.1 Risk factors for gastric cancer

Dietary factors—very important role. More common in persons consuming diet rich in complex carbohydrates (egg, fava beans), smoked, salted or pickled foods (24% of cases), cooking oil, and dried fish. Insufficient fruit and vegetables are responsible for 36% of cases in the UK.

Smoking and alcohol—smoking is responsible for 22% of cases in the UK. Evidence for linking alcohol consumption to stomach cancer is unclear.

Medical conditions.
- *H. pylori infection*—responsible for >30% of cases in the UK. Estimated relative risk (RR) 2–6.
- *Chronic atrophic gastritis*—with intestinal metaplasia. 11% develop gastric cancer.
- *Pernicious anaemia*—RR 2–3.
- *Benign gastric ulcer*—incidence ratio over 9y is 1.8.
- *Subtotal gastric resection*—RR 1.5–3.
- *Gastric polyps*—over 2cm in size.
- *Barrett's oesophagus*—precursor for proximal gastric cancers (gastric cardia and distal oesophageal cancer). Estimated risk is 0.2–2% per y.

Familial predisposition—small (2–4 fold) increased risk in patients with first-degree relative with gastric cancer.

Primary prevention—may be achieved by encouraging increased fruit and vegetables consumption (up to 5 servings/day) and *H. pylori* detection and eradication.

Box 30.2 Signs of advanced gastric cancer

Direct extension—palpable abdominal mass (poor prognostic sign, but not in itself an indication of inoperable disease).

Lymph node spread—periumbilical nodule (Sister Mary Joseph's node), left supraclavicular adenopathy (Virchow's node).

Peritoneal spread—enlarged ovary (Krukenberg's tumour), mass in the pelvic on rectal peritoneum examination (Blumer's shelf), ascites.

Liver metastasis—palpable liver mass, elevated serum alkaline phosphatase, jaundice.

Paraneoplastic manifestations—diffuse seborrhoeic keratoses (sign of Leser–Trelat), microangiopathic haemolytic anaemia, membranous nephropathy, hypercoagulable states (Trousseau's syndrome).

Recommended investigations

- *General approach*—should follow dyspepsia pathway (see
  ⊃ Chapter 23, p.212) as appropriate.
- *Upper GI endoscopy*—first investigation of choice to confirm diagnosis
  and obtain sufficient tissue biopsies [B].
  - *Endoscopic findings*—early gastric cancers appear as shallow ulcer,
    polypoid, flat, or plaque-like lesions. Advanced cancers appear typ-
    ically as an ulcerated mass or a large ulcer with irregular 'beaded'
    borders. The ulcer base is usually necrotic and shaggy.
- *Pathologic confirmation*—multiple (>six) biopsies should always be
  obtained from suspicious lesions, and read by two histopathologists, one
  with special interest in GI diseases [C].
  - *Biopsy detection rate*—ranges from 70% for one biopsy to 98%
    for seven biopsies. Using a combination of strip and bite bi-
    opsy techniques for suspicious diffuse types of gastric cancer is
    recommended.

Recommended initial assessment/staging

- *Basic investigations*—baseline haematological and biochemical profile, ABGs on air, PFTs, CXR, and ECG [B]. Check results and optimize as appropriate.
- *Spiral thoracic and abdominal contrast CT scan.*
  - *Indications*—first staging investigation to evaluate the presence of metastatic disease [B].
  - *Technique*—thin (5mm) slices and gastric distension with 600–800mL of water are recommended.
  - *Accuracy*—below 80% accuracy in identifying advanced disease in gastric cancer.
  - *TNM staging*—see Box 30.3.
- *Nutritional assessment.*
  - *Effect on surgery*—risk increases in patients with BMI <18.5, BMI <90% of predicted value, recent weight loss of >20%, and low serum albumin. Obesity increases the risk as well.
  - *Optimization*—essential part of the perioperative care. Nutritional support (enteral or parenteral) should be considered on all patients in the pre- and post-operative period [B].
- *MDT discussion*—essential requirement prior to commencing any definitive treatment [C]. Decisions are taken in the context of predicted prognosis and expected effect of any investigation or treatment intervention on quality of life.
- *Breaking bad news*—essential step to ensure adequate compliance. Should be done in a professional and effective way. The role of cancer care nurse is essential.
  - *Recommended points to discuss*—confirmation of diagnosis, available treatment options, expected perioperative period experi- ence, contact details, and sources for further information (including pa- tient support groups). Discussion should be documented and communicated to other members of the team (GP, oncologists, cancer care nurses, etc.).
- *Advanced staging*—only required if the patient is a good candidate for surgical resection.

Box 30.3 TNM staging on CT scan

T staging
- *T1 to T3*—unreliable in differentiating T1 from T2 cancers or in accurate estimation of microscopic invasion in T3, namely the differentiation between transmural extension and perigastric lymphadenopathy.
- *T4*—can be identified by finding:
  - Intimate contact between tumour and contiguous organs.
  - Focal loss of intervening fat plane.
  - Clear CT scan evidence of direct organ invasion.

N staging
- *Accuracy*—node involvement can be identified in 50–60% of cases.
- *Criteria*—node size is the main criterion used for identification and still of low accuracy (48% sensitivity and 93% specificity if size >8mm was considered abnormal in the coeliac axis). The number of involved lymph nodes is more important than the distance from the primary tumour in the current TNM classification system.

M staging
- *Accuracy*—metastatic disease can be detected in 75–80% of cases using newer techniques. Can only detect 50% of lesions with size <1.5cm.

https://cancerstaging.org/Pages/default.aspx

Recommended advanced staging

- *Patient selection*—all patients without evidence of metastatic disease on CT scan, who are eligible for curative surgery, should undergo endoscopic ultrasonography (EUS), if available [B].
- *EUS*—superior to CT scan for local staging of gastric cancer and more accurate in predicting resectability (Box 30.4).
- *Laparoscopy*—recommended for all gastric cancer patients following CT and EUS prior to consideration of radical resection.[C]
  - *Accuracy*—the only reliable method to detect peritoneal dissemination in apparently localized disease. Can result in 'upstaging' in 51% of patients.
- *Other recommended investigations.*
  - *Positron emission tomography (PET)*—is superior to CT scan or EUS in detecting distant metastasis.
  - *Transabdominal USS*—indicated if treatment options are limited and good clinical evidence of liver metastasis exists. Confirmation of disease extent is required before commencing palliative treatment [C].
  - *MRI scan*—has no advantages over spiral CT scan in most cases. Usually used in certain individual cases such as the allergy to IV contrast or the need for specific extra details [C].
  - *Tumour markers*—have no practical use.
  - *TNM staging*—Box 30.4

Box 30.4 TNM staging on EUS

T staging—can identify the different layer structure of stomach wall. Unable to delineate the omental reflections around the stomach clearly, and difficult or impossible to know if the carcinoma has penetrated the muscularis propria into the greater or lesser omenta (T2), but not breached the visceral peritoneum beyond (T3). Accuracy does not exceed 77% for staging the depth of invasion.

N staging—features like well-defined margins of nodes over 1cm in diameter, rounded, and hypoechoic nodes are likely to correlate well with malignant infiltration. Accuracy is 50% for nodal stage.

M staging—small volumes of ascites can be demonstrated (possible diffuse peritoneal spread).

https://cancerstaging.org/Pages/default.aspx

Recommended treatment

General approach

- *Endoscopic mucosal resection (EMR) and submucosal dissection (ESD)*—should be considered in early gastric cancer (T1, mucosal, and submucosal) if appropriate experience exists [B]. Indicated in well or moderately differentiated histology types, tumour of less than 30mm in size, or sm1, and in the absence of ulceration or any other invasive features.
- Surgical resection with curative intent should be offered to all patients who are medically fit for surgery and who have a potentially resectable cancer [D]. Complete surgical resection with resection of adjacent lymph nodes represents the best opportunity for long-term survival. Only a small proportion of patients will be deemed suitable for potential complete curative treatment, and less than a third will be able to have a curative resection.

Standards for surgical resection

- *Preoperative preparation*—should include psychological preparation, thromboembolic and antibiotic prophylaxis, and blood cross-matching.
- *Resection extent*—see Box 30.5.
- *Outlines of recommended surgical approach*—see Box 30.6.

Oncological standards

- *Main objectives*—to achieve a balance between macroscopic clearance and reduced morbidity. Well described by the Japanese classification for gastric cancer.
- *Margins of resection*—about or over 5cm from the gross tumour is currently recommended by most cancer centres. Transmural tumours (T4) may benefit from resection of adjacent organs if the patient is fit enough to tolerate radical surgery. No macroscopic residual disease should be allowed if possible.

Lymph node resection

- *Definitions*—see Box 30.7.
- *Extent of lymph node dissection*—see Box 30.8.
- *Reconstruction*—usually achieved with a Roux-en-Y or Billroth II gastrojejunostomy.

Laparoscopic gastrectomy for cancer

- Current evidence supports the use of this procedure by adequately trained laparoscopic surgeons for the management of operable gastric cancer patients. The procedure should only be performed within appropriate clinical governance setting. Benefits are confirmed mainly in distal gastrectomy. Patient selection should involve appropriate multidisciplinary team (MDT).
  - *Indications*—most gastric cancers amenable to open surgical treatment.
  - *Efficacy*—when performed by a well-trained surgeon in an appropriate centre, laparoscopic surgery has similar efficiency to open surgery in terms of resection margins, cancer-free survival rate,

Box 30.5 Stomach cancer resection—definitions

R0 (curative resection)—surgery with no macroscopic or microscopic residual cancer at the resection margins. Less than a third of patients can have curative resection.

R1—surgery with positive margins due to microscopic residual cancer.

R2—surgery with positive margins and gross (macroscopic) residual cancer.

Box 30.6 Stomach cancer resection—selection

Early or well-circumscribed cancers—EMR, ESD, or subtotal gastrectomy are recommended if the site of cancer allows a margin of >2cm proximally away from the cardia.

Infiltrative cancers—require 5cm clearance. Total gastrectomy is recommended if clearance is deemed impossible and the tumour is diffuse (with submucosal infiltration).

Junctional tumours—consider proximal oesophageal margin of 5cm. Lower cancers require total gastrectomy and abdominal lymphadenectomy.

Box 30.7 Lymph node dissection—definitions

D1 resection (limited lymphadenectomy)—excision of primary cancer, omentum, and first tiers of lymph nodes (N1) which drain the affected area of the stomach.

D2 resection (systemic lymphadenectomy)—excision of primary cancer, omentum, and first two tiers of lymph nodes (N1 and N2).

Extended lymphadenectomy—excision of lymph nodes beyond the second tier (e.g. hepatoduodenal ligament lymph nodes).

Box 30.8 Lymph node dissection—selection

Extent of lymph node dissection—remains controversial. In summary:
- Multicentre trials have shown no clear-cut significant survival benefits for D2 over D1 resection for curable gastric cancer.
- The International Gastric Cancer Association consensus recommends
- D2 resection for all resectable gastric cancers, although mortality seems to be higher.
- Many US centres recommend removal of >15 lymph nodes to achieve adequate dissection.
- Surgeon experience, age and fitness of patient, stage of cancer, and workload of cancer centre should all be taken into consideration.

and 30-d mortality rate. Laparoscopic surgery was found in a meta-analysis of 1,611 cases to be inferior to open surgery in terms of lymph node retrieval (mean difference 4.4 nodes, $p<0.001$).
  • *Safety*—laparoscopic surgery has a lower complication rate (OR=0.54) compared to open surgery.
• *Outcome measures.*
  • *Curative resection (R0)*—achieved when all evidence of cancer is removed.
  • *Absolute curative resection*—achieved if at least one tier of nodes beyond those affected is removed.

Recommendation for chemoradiotherapy

• Perioperative combination chemotherapy conveys a significant survival benefit and is a standard of care [A].
  • *Adjuvant chemotherapy*—increases survival (just marginal, OR=0.80) when compared with surgery alone in non-Western population. Insufficient evidence to recommend for all patients. Age, comorbidities, and expected beneficial effects should be considered in individual cases.
  • *Neo-adjuvant chemotherapy*—improves 5y survival rate (36% in 'perioperative chemotherapy' groups vs 23% in 'surgery alone' group), and should be considered in selected cases after MDT discussion.
  • *Adjuvant chemoradiotherapy*—improves survival and is a standard of care in USA; should be considered in high-risk cases for recurrence who have not received neoadjuvant therapy [A].
  • *Intraperitoneal chemotherapy*—is investigational [B].

Further reading

Allum WH, Blazeby JM, Griffin SM, Cunningham d, Jankowski JA, Wong R, On behalf of the Association of Upper Gastrointestinal Surgeons of Great Britain and Ireland, the British Society of Gastroenterology and the British Association of Surgical Oncology (2011). Guidelines for the management of oesophageal and gastric cancer. Gut 2011;60:1449-1472

Gastric Cancer: ESMO clinical practice guidelines. E. C. Smyth, M. Verheij, W. Allum, D. Cunningham, A. Cervantes and D. Arnold on behalf of the ESMO Guidelines Committee Oncology 27 (Supplement 5): v38–v49, 2016 doi:10.1093/annonc/mdw350

Japanese gastric cancer treatment guidelines 2014 (ver. 4)

Gastric Cancer (2017) 20:1–19 DOI 10.1007/s10120-016-0622-4 Cancer Research UK. Available from: http://www.cancerresearchuk.org/.

BMJ Clinical Evidence. Stomach cancer, 2011. URL: http://clinicalevidence.bmj.com/x/systematic-review/0404/guidelines.html. Accessed: February 2015

Ngoan LT, Mizoue T, Fujino Y, Tokui N, Yoshimura T (2002). Dietary factors and stomach cancer mortality. Br J Cancer 87:37–42.

Joossens JV, Hill MJ, Elliott P et al. (1996). Dietary salt, nitrate and stomach cancer mortality in 24 countries. European Cancer Prevention (ECP) and the INTERSALT Cooperative Research Group. Int J Epidemiol 25, 494–504.

Forman D, Newell DG, Fullerton F (1991). Association between infection with Helicobacter pylori and risk of gastric cancer: evidence from a prospective investigation. BMJ 302, 1302–5.

Hsing AW, Hansson LE, McLaughlin JK et al. (1993). Pernicious anaemia and subsequent cancer. A population-based cohort study. Cancer 71, 745–50.

Hansson LE, Nyren O, Hsing AW et al. (1996). The risk of stomach cancer in patients with gastric or duodenal ulcer disease. N Engl J Med 335, 242–9.

Tersmette AC, Offerhaus GJ, Tersmette KW et al. (1990). Meta-analysis of the risk of gastric stump cancer: detection of high risk patient subsets for stomach cancer after remote partial gastrectomy for benign conditions. Cancer Res 50, 6486–9.

Nakamura T, Nakano G (1985). Histopathological classification and malignant change in gastric polyps. J Clin Pathol 38, 754–64,

Drewitz DJ, Sampliner RE, Garewal HS (1997). The incidence of adenocarcinoma in Barrett's oesophagus: a prospective study of 170 patients followed 4.8 years. Am J Gastroenterol 92, 212–5.

Arents NL, Thijs JC, Kleibeuker JH (2002). A rational approach to uninvestigated dyspepsia in primary care: review of the literature. Postgrad Med J 78:707–16.

Dicken BJ, Bigam DL, Cass C, Mackey JR, Joy AA, Hamilton SM (2005). Gastric adenocarcinoma: review and considerations for future directions. Ann Surg 241:27–39.

Stephens MR, Lewis WG, White S et al. (2005). Prognostic significance of alarm symptoms in patients with gastric cancer. Br J Surg 92, 840–6.

Barr et al. Carcinoma of the stomach. In: Oxford Textbook of Surgery, 2nd ed. Oxford University Press, Oxford.

Pieslor PC, Hefter LG (1986). Umbilical metastasis from prostatic carcinoma—Sister Joseph nodule. Urology 27, 558–9.

Morgenstern L (1979). The Virchow–Troisier node: a historical note. Am J Surg 138, 703.

Gilliland R, Gill PJ (1992). Incidence and prognosis of Krukenberg tumour in Northern Ireland. Br J Surg 79, 1364–6.

Winne Burchard BE (1965). Blumer's shelf tumour with primary carcinoma of the lung. A case report. J Int Coll Surg 44, 477–81.

Fuchs CS, Mayer RJ (1995). Gastric carcinoma. N Engl J Med 333, 32–41.

Mulholland M (2006). Gastric neoplasms. In: Greenfield's surgery: scientific principles and practice, 2nd ed, Lippincott Williams & Wilkins, Philadelphia.

Graham DY, Schwartz JT, Cain GD, Gyorkey F (1982). Prospective evaluation of biopsy number in the diagnosis of oesophageal and gastric carcinoma. Gastroenterology 82, 228–31.

Karita M, Tada M (1994). Endoscopic and histologic diagnosis of submucosal tumours of the gastrointestinal tract using combined strip biopsy and bite biopsy. Gastrointest Endosc 40, 749–53.

Sussman SK, Halvorsen RA Jr, Illescas FF et al. (1988). Gastric adenocarcinoma: CT versus surgical staging. Radiology 167:335–40.

Pollack BJ, Chak A, Sivak MV Jr (1996). Endoscopic ultrasonography. Semin Oncol 23, 336–46.

Conlon KC, Karpeh MS Jr (1996). Laparoscopy and laparoscopic ultrasound in the staging of gastric cancer. Semin Oncol 23, 347–51.

Yoshida S, Saito D (1996). Gastric pre-malignancy and cancer screening in high-risk patients. Am J Gastroenterol 91, 839–43.

National Comprehensive Cancer Network (2007). Clinical practice guidelines in oncology: gastric cancer. Available from: http://www.nccn.org

Japanese Research Society for Gastric Cancer (1995). Japanese classification of gastric cancer, 1st English ed, Kanehara & Co Ltd, Tokyo.

Cunningham D, Allum WH, Stenning SP et al. (2006). Perioperative chemotherapy versus surgery alone for respectable gastroesophageal cancer. N Engl J Med 355, 11–20.

The Royal College of Surgeons of England (2017). National audit of oesophago-gastric cancer report. Available from: http://content.digital.nhs.uk/og.

National Institute for Health and Clinical Excellence (2008). Laparoscopic gastrectomy of cancer. Available from: http://www.nice.org.uk/Guidance/IPG269.

Whiting JL, Sigurdsson A, Rowlands DC et al. (2002). The long term results of endoscopic surveillance of premalignant gastric lesions. Gut 50, 378-381

Chapter 31

Neuroendocrine tumours (NETs)*

Basic facts *296*
Recommended investigations *298*
Recommended treatment *300*
Further reading *302*

Key guidelines

- UKNETwork for neuroendocrine tumours (2012). Guidelines for the management of gastro-enteropancreatic neuroendocrine (including carcinoid) tumours.
- European Neuroendocrine Tumour Society – ENETS (2012).
- National Comprehensive Cancer Network – NCCN (2011). Practice guidelines: neuroendocrine tumours.

* The guidelines on this chapter have been sourced and summarized from different UK, Europe, and international government sources, professional organizations, and medical specialty societies. Leading guidelines have been listed in the further reading section at the end of this chapter.

Basic facts

- *Definition*—NETs originate in the enterochromaffin cells (part of neuroendocrine cell system scattered throughout the body). NETs consist of a heterogeneous group of tumours that share specific 'biological' features and classified into one entity. NETs can be benign or malignant, functional or non-functional, may occur in the pancreas, stomach, small or large bowel, and can be diagnosed based on the function (gastrinoma, insulinoma, etc.) or the mass effect.
- *Incidence*—rare. NETS affect 72–73 per 100,000 population per year. Females are more affected, especially in the fifth decade. NETs run in families; the estimated life risk of developing NETs in individuals with one affected first-degree relative is ~4× compared to the general population, rising to 12× in the presence of two affected first-degree relatives.
- *Pathobiology*—very slow growing malignant tumours with the potential risk of metastasizing to lymph nodes, liver, bone, lungs, and brain (Box 31.1).
- *Clinical presentation*—most NETs remain asymptomatic or present with non-specific symptoms due to the local or metabolic effects (Box 31.2).

Box 31.1 Pathobiology of NETs

Frequency of primary NETs—appendix (35% of total), ileum (15% of total), lung (15% of total), rectum (10% of total), and pancreas (5% of total).

Genetics—most occur sporadically as isolated tumours and few as part of complex familial endocrine cancer syndromes, including multiple endocrine neoplasia (MEN) type 1 and 2, and neurofibromatosis type 1 (NF1). MEN1 incidence varies from 30% in gastrinomas to almost 0% in gut carcinoids. Detailed family history is essential in every case [C]. Further testing should be considered for individuals with a positive family history for carcinoid, NETs, or second endocrine tumour [C].

Box 31.2 Clinical presentation of neuroendocrine tumours

Local symptoms—differ depending on the site and biology of the NET tumour. Gastropancreatic tumours may invoke intense mesenteric desmoplastic reaction (in the case of carcinoid), and lead to shortening and fibrosis of the mesentery, with resultant small bowel obstruction. Bronchial carcinoid tumours may present with bronchial obstruction (e.g. obstructive pneumonitis, atelectasis).

Carcinoid syndrome—results from the release of hormones (serotonin, tachykinins, and other vasoactive compounds) directly into the systemic circulation following tumour metastases to the liver. Presents with episodes of intermittent abdominal pain (70% of patients), diarrhoea (50%), flushing (30%), and sometimes episodes of lacrimation, rhinorrhoea, and palpitations

Other syndromes—depend on the type, location, and biology of the tumour.

- *Insulinoma*—dizziness, confusion, and weakness (relieved by eating food).
- *Gastrinoma*—Zollinger–Ellison syndrome with severe peptic ulceration and diarrhoea.
- *Glucagonoma*—weight loss, diarrhoea, diabetes mellitus, necrolytic migratory erythema, and stomatitis.
- *Others*—e.g. vasoactive intestinal peptide (VIP) hypersecretion in VIPomas (watery diarrhoea, dehydration, lethargy, etc), somatostatin hypersecretion in somatostatinomas (triad of mild diabetes mellitus, steatorrhoea, and gallstones).

Recommended investigations

- *General approach*—the diagnosis requires a high index of suspicion and judicious combination of clinical, hormonal, radiological, and other imaging findings. Histopathologic confirmation defines the management plan.

Baseline tests—should include chromogranin A (CgA) test and 5-hydroxyindoleacetic acid (5-HIAA) test in the case of carcinoid (of no value in pancreatic NET) [C].
  - *Plasma CgA*—large protein produced by all neural crest-derived cells, and in very significant quantities by NET cells. CgA role in accurate monitoring of progression remains unclear.
  - *Urine 5-HIAA*—remarkably raised in certain NETs syndrome (70% in midgut tumours, sometimes in foregut tumours, and never in hindgut tumours).
- *Specific tests*—should be ordered as required, see Box 31.3.
- *Imaging tests*—should be based on clinical suspicion and be multi-modality. Imaging tests include USS, CT, endoscopy, MRI, somatostatin receptor scintigraphy (SSRS), EUS, gallium 68-PET (best for secondaries), and other selected imaging modalities (e.g. 5H-tryptamine imaging).
- *Searching for the primary and/or associated lesion*—is required [C] and might be very challenging, which may require a triple phase CT scan of the thorax and abdomen.
- *SSRS scan*—detects somatostatin receptors subtypes 2 and 5. SSRS scan has a central role in the assessment and localization of the primary in NETs as well as in looking for secondaries. Reported sensitivity achieves ~90%.
- *PET scan*—should be considered as well to increase sensitivity.
- *Intra-arterial calcium infusion*—followed by digital subtraction angiography (for gastrinomas) or hepatic venous sampling (for insulinoma); has high sensitivity (90% sensitivity).
- *Pathologic confirmation is required before commencing on treatment*—pathological characterization and classification of NETs should be based on the WHO 2010 classification, the Union for International Cancer Control (UICC) TNM (7th edition), and the European Neuroendocrine Tumour Society (ENETS) site-specific T-staging system. [D]
- All patients with midgut NETs, with or without hepatic metastasis, and all patients with the carcinoid syndrome, should be screened, and treated where necessary, for carcinoid heart disease (CHD). This may include N-terminal pro-brain natriuretic peptide (NT-proBNP) and echocardiography. [B]

Box 31.3 Other baseline tests

Should be considered depending on the clinical and histochemical features of the suspected tumour:

• Thyroid function tests (TFTs), parathyroid hormone (PTH), A-fetoprotein, carcinoembryonic antigen (CEA), B-human chorionic gonadotrophin (B-HCG), calcium, calcitonin, prolactin [D].

Recommended treatment

Main objective—should be curative (most, if not all, insulinomas are cured) where possible. Maintaining a good quality and symptom-free life for as long as possible may be considered occasionally to be a more realistic goal.

Surgical resection

- *Perioperative preparation*—is an essential step to correct abnormal physiologic disturbances relating to NET secretory behaviour and preventing carcinoid crises. If a functioning carcinoid tumour was found preoperatively, octreotide should be administered by constant IV infusion at a dose of 50μg/h for 12h prior to and at least 48h after surgery. Insulinomas require preoperative glucose infusion and sliding scale (glucose infusion should not be required once the insulinoma has been resected). Gastrinomas require PPIs and IV octreotide.
- *Surgical options*—depends on the site, type, and biologic features of the tumour. In general terms:
  - *Stomach NET*—can be managed by watchful monitoring, limited endoscopic resection, or major resection with regional lymph node clearance. Selection of the best procedure depends on the type, extent, and potential metastatic profile of the individual tumour.
  - *Small bowel NET*—should a NET be confirmed histologically post-laparotomy, then re-operation to achieve complete mesenteric lymphadenectomy should be considered.
  - *Appendix NET*—usually removed during emergency appendicec-tomy and the diagnosis is made post-operatively. If the size is <1cm and the tumour was completely removed, no further treatment or follow-up would be required. If the tumour size is >2cm, or there is serosal involvement, vascular invasion, or appendix base involve-ment, radical right hemicolectomy is indicated and 5y follow-up is recommended.
  - *Colorectal NET*—requires complete resection using the same cancer-type standards (see ➲ Chapter 38, pp.358–368).
  - *Pancreatic NETs*—localized enucleation of well-defined insulinomas is sometimes possible, but more radical resections may be necessary.
- Liver metastasis is not absolute contraindication to resection [D].
- Treatment choices for non-resectable disease include somatostatin analogues, targeted radionuclide therapy, biotherapy, loco-regional treatments including ablation and (chemo) embolization and chemotherapy [C].
- *Other comments*—somatostatin analogues are the mainstay of treat-ment for those hormone-secreting tumours. The actual tumour may stabilize or occasionally shrink. PPIs for gastrinomas, diazoxide for some insulinomas, and ondansetron benefits some patients. Interferon-A is suitable for symptomatic carcinoid patients with about 50% symptomatic improvement and 10–15% reduction in size. Limited benefits are seen with platinum-based chemotherapy and patients so treated should be entered into trials. Radionucleotide therapies as well as hepatic artery embolization and tissue ablation technologies are being used in some centres (see Fig. 31.1).

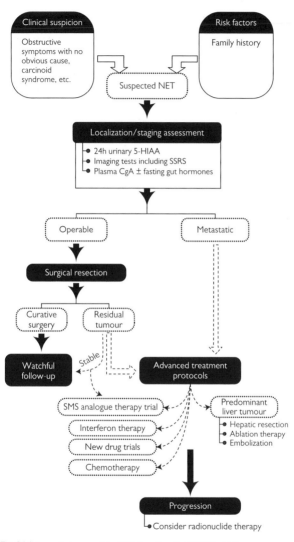

Fig. 31.1 Suggested approach to NETs, based on the UKNET guidelines.

Further reading

Ramage JK, Davies AH, Ardill J et al.; UKNETwork for neuroendocrine tumours (2012). Guidelines for the management of gastro-enteropancreatic neuroendocrine (including carcinoid) tumours. Gut 54 (Suppl 4), iv1–16.

European Neuroendocrine Tumour Society (2012). Available from: https://www.enets.org.

National Comprehensive Cancer Network (2011). Practice guidelines: neuroendocrine tumours. Available from: https://www.nccn.org/professionals/physician_gls/default.aspx.

Wareing TH, Sawyers JL (1983). Carcinoids and the carcinoid syndrome. Am J Surg 145, 769–72.

Kvols LK (1994). Metastatic carcinoid tumours and the malignant carcinoid syndrome. Ann N Y Acad Sci 733, 464–70.

Soga J, Yakuwa Y, Osaka M (1999). Carcinoid syndrome: a statistical evaluation of 748 reported cases. J Exp Clin Cancer Res 18, 133–41.

Hemminki K, Li X (2001). Familial carcinoid tumours and subsequent cancers: a nationwide epidemiologic study from Sweden. Int J Cancer 94, 444–8.

Surgery for obesity*

Basic facts *304*
Recommended treatment *306*
Further reading *310*

Key guidelines

- NICE (2014). Obesity: identification, assessment and management.
- World Health Organization (2000). Obesity: preventing and managing the global epidemic.
- National Obesity Forum (2010). Guidelines on management of adult obesity and overweight in primary care.
- European clinical practice guidelines (2015). Management of obesity in adults.
- Scottish Intercollegiate Guidelines Network (2010). Management of obesity.
- American Society for Gastrointestinal Endoscopy (2015). The role of endoscopy in the bariatric surgery patient.

---

* The guidelines on this chapter have been sourced and summarized from different UK, Europe, and international government sources, professional organizations, and medical specialty societies. Leading guidelines have been listed in the further reading section at the end of this chapter.

Basic facts

- *Definition*—obesity is a condition of excess adipose tissue mass that poses significant effect on the person's health.
- *Incidence*—serious 'global epidemic'. Trebled in the past 20y in the UK, shortening the lives of its sufferers by up to 9y. About 22% of men and women are clinically obese (BMI >30kg/m^2), and 43% of men and 34% of women are overweight (BMI 25–29.9kg/m^2).
- In 2011, about 3 in 10 children aged 2–15 years were overweight or obese. The estimated annual cost of care in England is £7.4 billion.
- *Comorbidities*—obesity increases risk of type 2 diabetes, contributes 35% of ischaemic heart disease cases, and 55% of hypertension cases among the adult population in Europe (Box 32.1).
- *Classification*—see Table 32.1
  - *BMI*—equals the weight divided by square of the height (weight/height2, i.e. kg/m^2). BMI directly correlates with total body fat content (reliable proxy).
  - *Other measures*—waist circumference and ratio of waist-to-hip circumference can identify people (esp. with BMI <35) at increased risk for cardiovascular event due to excess harmful fat as compared to people with increased muscular compartment without real obesity (Table 32.2). Bioimpedance is not a suitable alternative to BMI.
- *Pathogenesis*—complex and multifactorial.
  - From one aspect, obesity develops simply as a result of 'energy imbalance' due to persistent increased energy intake and/or decreased physical activity.
  - On the other hand, the regulation of energy balance and fat stores requires complex interactions between biological (genetic and epigenetic), social, behavioural, and environmental factors. This makes the process remarkably difficult to accurately quantify all implicated factors involved.
  - In general terms, there is no doubt that environmental factors (food intake and energy expenditure) play a key role in the development of obesity.
- *Clinical presentation*—related to the associated comorbidities (Box 32.1).

Box 32.1 Comorbidities associated with obesity

Common (RR ×3).

- Metabolic—high insulin resistance, type 2 diabetes*, dyslipidaemia, fatty liver*, gallstones*, hypertension*.
- Mechanical—pulmonary complaints, gastro-oesophageal reflux disease, sleep apnoea and daytime sleepiness, difficult mobility and osteoarthritis, social isolation and depression.

Fairly common (RR ×2–3).

- Metabolic—coronary artery disease, stroke, gout.
- Mechanical—hernia, respiratory difficulties, psychosocial disturbances, low self-esteem, and body image disturbances.

Slightly increased risk (RR ×1–2).

- Metabolic—polycystic ovaries, cancer (commonly breast, endometrial, endocrine, and colon), impaired fertility, cataract.
- Mechanical—varicose veins, backache, stress incontinence.

*Direct link

Recommended treatment

General approach

- Effective management requires a motivated and well-informed multidisciplinary team. All relevant factors should be identified.
  - Possible manageable aetiology—should be sought.
  - Degree of overweight and obesity—should be estimated (Table 32.1 and 32.2).
  - Comorbidities—should be assessed and managed as appropriate.
  - Willingness and motivation to change—should be validated.

Initial selection to appropriate management plan

Should be based on BMI, waist circumference, and the presence of comorbidities (Box 32.2). Recommended initial treatment should be formulated accordingly.

Lifestyle interventions

Include healthy eating and increased physical activity.

- *Dietary changes.*
  - Reduced total energy intake—diet should contain 600kcal (carbohydrate and/or fat) less than the person's usual needs to stay at the same weight.
  - Low-calorie diets (1,000–1,600kcal/d)—less likely to be nutritionally complete, but may be considered for treatment.
  - Very-low-calorie diets (<1,000kcal/d)—can be used continuously for a maximum of 12wk, or intermittently with a low-calorie diet under close medical supervision.
- *Physical activity.*
  - Moderate-intensity physical activity—for a minimum of 30min/d for at least 5d/wk.
  - Additional one session or more—with a duration of 10min or more.
  - Regular exercises for 45–60min—may be required to prevent obesity.

Pharmaceutical management

- *General concepts*—drugs should be added to the healthy lifestyle advice (including diet and exercises) and should not be used as the sole element of treatment. Regular monitoring is essential. Stop the drug treatment if the patient regained weight whilst receiving the medications
- *Formulas*—orlistat, sibutramine, and rimonabant (currently withdrawn). No evidence exists to favour one over the others.
  - Orlistat is recommended for patients on high-fat intake
  - Sibutramine or rimonabant are recommended for patients unable to control their eating habits. Thyroid hormones, diuretics, or amphetamines have no role in the treatment of obesity.

Surgical management (bariatric surgery)

- *Main objectives of preoperative selection*—is to ensure that surgery is being recommended for patients who are expected to get most benefits, lose most weight, and remain safe over the perioperative period (see Fig. 32.1).
- *Expected outcome*—in selected patients, bariatric surgery has a better long-term weight loss, improved comorbidities, and quality of life as well as a significant decrease in the overall mortality.

Table 32.1 Obesity classification

BMI (kg/m²)	Description	Risk of comorbidities
<18.5	Underweight	Low
18.5–24.9	Healthy weight	Average
25–29.9	Pre-obese (overweight)	Mildly increased
30–34.9	Obese class I (moderately obese)	Moderate
35–39.9	Obese class II (severely obese)	Severe
>40	Obese class II (morbidly obese)	Very severe

Table 32.2 Estimating risk of obesity

	Waist circumference		
BMI classification	<94cm	94–102cm	>102cm
Overweight	No increased risk	Moderately increased risk	High risk
Obese	Moderately increased risk	High risk	Very high risk

Box 32.2 Recommended initial treatment for obesity

Overweight (BMI <30).
- Provide advice on healthy diet and lifestyle.
- Special advice on lifestyle changes, including diet and exercises ('L advice') should be provided if the waist circumference is high.
- Drug treatment ('D advice') should be considered in the presence of comorbidities.

Mild obesity (BMI <35).
- Always provide 'L advice'.
- Consider 'D advice' if comorbidities exists.

Moderate obesity (BMI <40).
- Always provide 'L advice'.
- Always consider 'D advice'.
- Consider surgery ('S advice') if comorbidities exists.

Severe obesity (BMI ≥40).
- Always provide 'L advice'.
- Always consider 'D advice'.
- Always consider 'S advice'.

L = Lifestyle changes; D = drugs; S = surgery

4 Most Common Weight Loss Surgery
Procedures in the United States

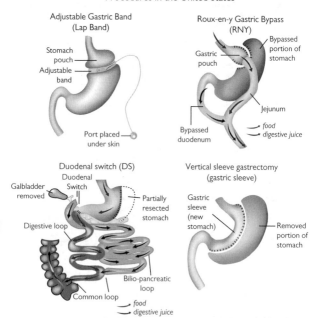

Fig. 32.1 Surgical management (bariatric surgery). Reprinted with permission of American Society for Metabolic and Bariatric Surgery, © 2009, all rights reserved

Indications
- First-line option (before lifestyle interventions or drug treatment) in adults with BMI ≥50kg/m² and acceptable operative risk [C*].
- Second-line option in patients with BMI ≥40 or 35–39.9kg/m² who have other obesity-related significant diseases (e.g. type 2 diabetes, cardiorespiratory disease, severe joint disease, and obesity-related depression), which put them at a significantly high risk for increased morbidity or premature mortality [C*].
- Patients should be well-motivated, psychologically fairly stable (stable home life, able to utilize adaptive coping skills, good social support), well-informed of disease management plans and the need for long-term follow-up, and in acceptance of operative risks.

Types
- Vertical banded gastroplasty (VBG).
  - *Technique*—the stomach size and function are restricted by using vertical staples and an annular band to create a small 15–20mL pouch with a restricted outlet stoma of 4.75–5.0cm. The pouch limits

the amount of food patients can eat at any one time and slows the passage of food to the rest of the stomach and small bowel.
  - *Efficiency*—can result in a mean weight loss of 32.2kg at 12mo follow-up (2,080 patients; 21 RCTs), and 32.0kg at and beyond 36mo (1,877 patients; 18 RCTs). The 30d mortality rate is ~0.2–0.3%, morbidity rate is 24%, and re-operation rate is 11%.
- Laparoscopic-adjusted vertical banded gastroplasty (LA-VBG).
  - *Technique*—same principle performed laparoscopically.
  - *Efficiency*—similar outcome to open surgery in reducing weight loss at 12mo. The operating time is significantly longer with the laparoscopic approach (2.10h with laparoscopic vs 1.45h with open), and no significant effect on average hospital stay (4d for both techniques). Complication rate is about the same at 12mo. The benefits of laparoscopic surgery still apply.
- Laparoscopic adjustable gastric banding (LAGB).
  - *Technique*—a tight adjustable prosthetic band is placed around the stomach entrance. The band is composed of a soft, locking silicone ring connected to an infusion port placed in the subcutaneous tissue. Injection of saline into the port reduces the band diameter, with resultant increased degree of restriction.
  - *Efficiency*—LAGB has replaced most other bariatric procedures due to its simplicity and relatively low complication rate. LAGB can result in a mean weight loss of 40–55% of excess weight at 12-mo follow-up, and 45–60% of excess weight at and beyond 48mo follow-up.
- Gastric bypass surgery (GBS).
  - *Technique*—the stomach is divided into an upper small pouch (15–30mL) and a lower remnant pouch. Appropriate bypass procedures are then used to ensure adequate drainage of pouches. The procedure restricts the volume of food which can be eaten and reduces weight.
  - *Efficiency*—can result in a mean weight loss of 43.5kg at 12mo follow-up (2,937 patients; 32 RCTs), and 41.5kg at and beyond 36mo follow-up (1,281 patients; 21 RCTs). Gastric bypass seems to be more effective at reducing weight compared to gastric banding procedure (18mo follow-up). There is no evidence of this beneficial effect beyond 1–3y follow-up.
  - *Laparoscopic approach*—has a similar effect on weight loss compared to open procedure, but gastric bypass has more side effects, including nutritional and electrolyte abnormalities, gastrointestinal symptoms, surgical complications, and a small risk of perioperative death.
- Biliopancreatic diversion.
  - *Technique*—complex operation. Rare in use due to side-effects. The stomach is resected to create a smaller volume and connected to the ileum to bypass the duodenum and jejunum.
  - *Efficiency*—can result in a mean weight loss of 51.9kg at 12mo follow-up (two systematic reviews, but no comparing RCTs), and 53.1kg at and beyond 36mo follow-up. The estimated 30d mortality rate is 0.9 and adverse events are fairly common, including surgical complications (6%), re-operations (4%), and gastrointestinal symptoms (38%).

Further reading

National Institute for Health and Clinical Excellence (2014). Obesity: identification, assessment and management of overweight and obesity in children, young people and adults Available from: https://www.nice.org.uk/guidance/cg189

World Health Organization. Obesity: preventing and managing the global epidemic. Report of a WHO consultation on obesity, Geneva, 1999 Available from : http://www.who.int/nutrition/publications/obesity/WHO_TRS_894/en/.

National Obesity Forum. Guidelines on management of adult obesity and overweight in primary care. Available from: http://www.nationalobesityforum.org.uk/images/stories/W_M_guidelines/NOF%20Adult%20Guidelines%20temporary%20revision%20June%202%202010.pdf http://nationalobesityforum.org.uk/images/stories/W_M_guidelines/NOF_Adult_Guildelines_Feb_06.pdf; National Obesity Forum. Pharmacotherapy guidelines for obesity management in adults. Available from: http://nationalobesityforum.org.uk/images/stories/W_M_guidelines/NOF_Pharma_Guidelines%284%29.pdf; (iii) An approach to weight management in children and adolescents (2–18 years) in primary care. Available from: http://www.icid.salisbury.nhs.uk/ClinicalManagement/ChildHealth/Documents/ade314857b384fb88e9fd0d752ddcdedAapproachotweightmanagementinchildrenazndadolescen.pdf

Tsigos C, Hainer V, Basdevant A et al. (2008). Management of obesity in adults: European clinical practice guidelines. Obes Facts 2008;1:106–116

Arterburn DE, DeLaet DE, Schauer DP (2008). Obesity in adults. BMJ Clin Evid 1, 604.

Scottish Intercollegiate Guidelines Network (2010). Management of obesity. Available from: http://www.sign.ac.uk/assets/sign115.pdf

CREST (2005). Guidelines for the management of obesity in secondary care. Available from: http://www.spitjudms.ro/_files/protocoale_terapeutice/gastro/obesity-guidelines-report.pdf

Clinical Knowledge Summaries (2007). Obesity—management. Available from: http://www.cks.library.nhs.uk/obesity.

Tsigosa C, Hainerb V, Basdevant A et al. (2008). Management of obesity in adults: European clinical practice guidelines. Obesity Facts 1, 106–16.

National Institutes of Health, National Heart, Lung, and Blood Institute (1998). Clinical guidelines on the identification, evaluation, and treatment of overweight and obesity in adults. The evidence report. Available from: http://www.nhlbi.nih.gov/guidelines/obesity/ob_gdlns.pdf .

Society of American Gastrointestinal Endoscopic Surgeons (2003). Guideline for clinical application of laparoscopic bariatric surgery. Available from: http://www.sages.org/publications/guidelines/guidelines-for-clinical-application-of-laparoscopic-bariatric-surgery/

American Society of Plastic Surgeons (2004). Practice advisory on liposuction. Available from: http://www.ncbi.nlm.nih.gov/pubmed/15060366

Maggard MA, Shugarman LR, Suttorp M et al. (2005). Meta-analysis: surgical treatment of obesity. Ann Intern Med 142, 547–59.

European Guidelines for Obesity Management in Adults (2015) available from: http://easo.org/education-portal/guidelines

The role of endoscopy in the bariatric surgery patient.Gastrointest Endosc 2015;81:1063–1072 DOI: http://dx.doi.org/10.1016/j.gie.2014.09.044

Part 5

Small bowel and appendix

Acute appendicitis*

Basic facts *314*
Recommended investigations *316*
Recommended treatment *318*
Further reading *320*

Key guidelines

- NICE (2016). Managing suspected appendicitis.
- Cochrane Library of Systematic Reviews. (i) (2005). Antibiotics versus placebo for the prevention of post-operative infection after appendicectomy; (ii) (2010). Laparoscopic versus open surgery for suspected appendicitis. (iii) (2011). Appendectomy versus antibiotics for the treatment of acute appendicitis (iv) (2014). Laparoscopy for the management of acute lower abdominal pain in women of childbearing age. (v) (2015). Abdominal drainage to prevent intra-peritoneal abscess after open appendectomy for complicated appendicitis.
- American College of Emergency Physicians. (2010) Clinical policy: Critical Issues in the Evaluation and Management of Emergency Department Patients With Suspected Appendicitis.Society of American Gastrointestinal and Endoscopic Surgeons (2010). SAGES guideline for laparoscopic appendectomy
- American College of Radiology(ACR). (i) (2013). ACR appropriateness criteria® right lower quadrant pain – suspected appendicitis.
- NIDDK (2014). Appendicitis.

---

* The guidelines on this chapter have been sourced and summarized from different UK, Europe, and international government sources, professional organizations, and medical specialty societies. Leading guidelines have been listed in the further reading section at the end of this chapter

Basic facts

- *Incidence*—the most common surgical emergency in general surgery. General lifetime risk is ~8.5% in men and 6.5% in women. Affects ~35,000 patients every year in England. Male to female ratio is 1.4:1. Most common in second and third decades of life. Peak incidence is age 10–19.
- *Pathogenesis*—most likely related to obstruction of appendix lumen, mostly due to lymphoid follicular hyperplasia (initiated or exacerbated by viral or bacterial infection) in young patients, and to fibrosis, faecoliths (often due to constipation or fruit stones), or neoplasia (carcinoid or caecal carcinoma) in older population.
- *Natural history*—secreted mucus becomes entrapped by obstruction, resulting in raised intramural pressure and considerably distended appendix distal to obstruction. Small vessels and lymphatic flow becomes occluded, resulting in ischaemic, necrotic, and then (usually in 48h) perforated appendix. This leads to the formation of localized mass, abscess, or diffuse peritonitis.
- *Bacterial pathogens*—most common (especially in gangrene and perforation) are *Escherichia coli*, *Peptostreptococcus*, *Bacteroides fragilis*, and *Pseudomonas* spp.
- *Clinical presentation*.
  - *Initial presentation*—non-specific symptoms (indigestion, feeling unwell, epigastric or periumbilical pain) caused by the luminal obstruction and distension of the appendix, stimulating the visceral autonomic pain nerves. Visceral pain is usually constant, moderate in severity and poorly localized.
  - *Intermediate period*—venous congestion associated with the inflammatory process stimulates bowel peristalsis, resulting in crampy pain, anorexia (90% of cases), nausea and vomiting (70%), and occasional diarrhoea (10%).

Box 33.1 Signs of acute appendicitis

McBurney's point—two thirds of the distance between the umbilicus and anterior superior iliac spine. Often overlies the base of appendix and is usually not variable with the appendix location.

Rovsing's sign—tenderness elicited in the RIF on palpation or gentle finger percussion on left iliac fossa (LIF). Indicates a right-sided peritoneal irritation.

Obturator sign—pain elicited by internal rotation of the hip. Usually associated with pelvic appendix.

Iliopsoas sign—pain in the RIF elicited by extension of the right hip. Usually indicates a retrocaecal appendix.

Rectal examination—may reveal tenderness or an inflammatory mass on the right side of the pelvis. Most useful in non-specific cases. Only used if absolutely necessary in children, and after obtaining a proper consent.

Vaginal examination—may show positive cervical excitation. Indicates acute salpingitis.

- *Localized pain*—somatic pain nerves are stimulated once the overlying parietal peritoneum is involved. Symptoms localize to the right
  iliac fossa (RIF), and become sensitive to movement.
- *Signs*—initial findings are usually non-specific. Localized signs become
  prominent once the overlying parietal peritoneum is irritated
  (Boxes 33.1, 33.2, 33.3); a completely soft abdomen is unlikely to
  harbour acute appendicitis.

Box 33.2 Unusual presentation of acute appendicitis

Retrocaecal appendix—appendix located far away from the anterior parietal peritoneum. Localized tenderness is usually less remarkable. Patients
may complain of diarrhoea, urinary irritation, haematuria, and pyuria.

Pelvic appendix—may resemble acute gastroenteritis, causing diffuse
pain, urinary frequency, dysuria, or rectal symptoms (tenesmus and
diarrhoea). Digital rectal examination may raise suspicion of acute
appendicitis.

Acute appendicitis during pregnancy—special challenge (See also
Box 33.3).

Perforated appendicitis—suspected in any patient with unusually remarkable high fever (over 39.4°C) or high white cell count.

Box 33.3 Acute appendicitis in pregnancy

Incidence—occurs in 1 in 2,000 pregnancies at any trimester. Higher perforation rate at third trimester.

Challenges.
Displaced appendix—superiorly by the enlarging uterus around the
second and third trimesters. The abdominal wall lies away from the appendix being pushed by the gravid uterus.

Masked signs—skeletal muscles are lax and signs of peritoneal irritation
are usually vague.

Physiologic response—physiologic leukocytosis is normal in
pregnant women.

Diagnosis—depends on repeated physical examination, clinical suspicion, ultrasound scan, and possibly MRI. Retrocaecal appendix can produce flank pain similar to pyelonephritis.

Risks of perforated appendicitis.
Higher foetal death—up to 36% of perforated cases vs 1.5% for non-
perforated ones. Aggressive but safe approach is justified, and negative
laparotomy rates are much more common in pregnant than non-pregnant
patients (35% vs 15%).

Pregnancy-related complications (e.g. spontaneous abortion)—occur frequently when an appendectomy is performed in the first trimester (33%)
as compared to the second (14%) or third trimester (0%).

Recommended investigations

- *General approach*—clinical findings can be used to risk stratify patients and guide decisions regarding further testing and management (discharge, observation, surgery). A detailed clinical history and repeated physical examination are usually sufficient in making the diagnosis of acute appendicitis in most cases. In suspected situations, hospital admission for 12–24h observation (a wait-and-watch policy) is a safe and effective approach (Fig. 33.1). In situations where the diagnosis is unclear, the use of clinical scoring systems such as the Alvarado score have been demonstrated to be inferior to imaging in identifying patients with acute appendicitis.
- *Laboratory tests*—no single laboratory test or any combination of tests have been shown to be as effective and accurate as the careful examination and clinical acumen of an experienced surgeon. Nevertheless, laboratory tests are useful adjuncts to the surgeon's clinical impression, particularly in high-risk patients and those with equivocal clinical presentation.
  - *Urinalysis*—helpful in excluding urinary tract infections. Positive results, however, might be confusing as up to a third of acute appendicitis can result in microscopic haematuria and pyuria due to the proximity of the inflamed appendix to the bladder and ureter.
  - *Pregnancy test (urine or blood)*—mandatory in childbearing age to rule out pregnancy (normal or ectopic).
  - *White cell count (WCC) test*—leucocytosis is found in 70–92% of cases, with a left shift in 95% of cases. Up to a third of patients with acute appendicitis may have a normal WCC; this does not rule out appendicitis.
  - *Serum C-reactive protein (CRP) levels*—have sensitivity of 93%, specificity of 80%, and accuracy of 91%, and are recommended by many authors in all cases.
  - *Other tests and investigations*—should be arranged in equivocal cases based on the clinical suspicion and if such investigations will improve outcome.
- *Imaging*—should only be performed in equivocal cases. Imaging is neither cost-effective nor helpful when there is a high or a low probability of acute appendicitis. There is a lower threshold for imaging in women of childbearing age, and the elderly in whom the accuracy of clinical diagnosis is lower. The best radiological test for acute appendicitis is CT imaging.
  - *Plain abdominal radiograph (AXR)*—usually unhelpful. AXR may show appendicolith or localized right lower quadrant ileus.
  - *Abdominal CT scan*—can show thickened wall (>2mm) appendix, appendicolith (25% of cases), concentric thickening of inflamed appendiceal wall, fat stranding, phlegmon, abscess, or free fluid. Sensitivity and specificity are 91% and 90%, respectively. Sensitivity of CT scanning increases with the addition of IV, while the role of enteral contrast is less clear.
  - *Ultrasonography*—in experienced hands, can be useful in diagnosing acute appendicitis in equivocal cases and in detecting pelvic pathologies

in women. Ultrasound is considered first line imaging in children with suspected appendicitis due to the absence of ionizing radiation. Algorithms using ultrasound as a first line investigation in young patients and the use of CT only in the setting of equivocal ultrasonographic findings have been demonstrated to reduce radiation dose exposure without affecting negative appendectomy rates [ACR]. Acute appendicitis presents as a non-compressible tubular structure at the base of the caecum, thickened wall (>2mm) appendix, luminal distension (diameter >6mm), and free fluid in the pelvis in some cases. Sensitivity and specificity are 78% and 83% respectively.

- *Magnetic resonance imaging* (MRI)—has been identified to have a sensitivity of 97% and specificity of 95%. However, its use is limited by its greater cost and relatively lower access to imaging. The use of MRI is advocated as a second-line imaging modality after ultrasound (in equivocal cases) for patients who are pregnant to avoid radiation exposure offered by CT.

- *Diagnostic laparoscopy*—should be viewed as an invasive procedure requiring general anaesthesia. During 'diagnostic' laparoscopy, if no other pathology is identified, (e.g. Crohn's, Meckel's, tubo-ovarian pathology), the decision to remove the macroscopically 'normal' appendix should be considered on an individual basis with the knowledge that up to 40% of these cases can have microscopic abnormalities. Removal of the macroscopically 'normal' appendix rules out inflammation by pathologic examination and makes the diagnosis of acute appendicitis less likely if the patient complains of similar pain in the future.

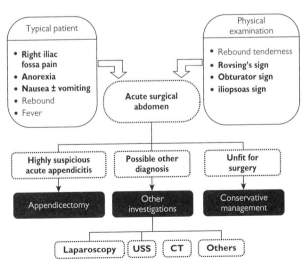

Fig. 33.1 Algorithm for approaching patients with suspected acute appendicitis.

Recommended treatment

- *Surgery plus perioperative systemic antibiotics*—is the default effective curative treatment, significantly reducing wound infection rate and intra-abdominal abscesses, shortening hospital stay, and enhancing the return to normal activities.
  - *Preoperative preparation*—includes adequate hydration, correction of electrolyte abnormalities, and commencement of systemic antibiotics.
  - *Choice of antibiotics (type, dose)*—remains to be standardized (see Chapter 19). A perforated appendicitis should be treated therapeutically against enteric Gram negative rods and anaerobes.
  - *Laparoscopic appendectomy in adults*—can reduce post-operative wound infections, pain, duration of hospital stay, and time off work when compared with open surgery. Early studies demonstrated an increased risk of intra-abdominal abscesses with laparoscopic appendectomy, though this has been disputed by later studies. Laparoscopic approach is more likely to benefit women of child-bearing age and obese patients requiring larger skin incisions during open appendectomy. The use of laparoscopy for acute appendicitis is regarded to be safe in all trimesters of pregnancy and in children.
- *Treatment with antibiotics alone*—although not the standard option, it has been shown by different RCTs to significantly reduce pain and morphine consumption. Most patients can be discharged from hospital within 48h with no reported mortality if surgery was used when and as appropriate (e.g. generalized peritonitis). The evidence, however, is very limited, and up to a third of those patients require readmission for appendectomy within 1y. Appendectomy should remain the standard treatment and antibiotics used in specific patients or situations where surgery is contraindicated.
- *Post-operative complications*—include wound infection (75–33%), intra-abdominal abscess formation (72% of cases), and possible effect on female fertility in cases of perforated appendix in childhood and increased risk of ectopic pregnancies in the future.

Further reading

Andersen BR, Kallehave FL, Andersen HK (2005). Antibiotics versus placebo for the prevention of post-operative infection after appendicectomy. Cochrane Database Syst Rev Issue 3, CD001439;

Sauerland S, Lefering R, Neugebauer EA (2010) Laparoscopic versus open surgery for suspected appendicitis. Cochrane Database Syst Rev Issue 10, CD001546.

Wilms IMHA, de Hoog DENM, de Visser DC, Janzing HMJ (2011) Appendectomy versus antibiotic treatment for acute appendicitis. Cochrane Database Syst Rev, Issue 11, CD008359.

Gaitán HG, Reveiz I, Farquhar C, Elias VM. Laparoscopy for the management of acute lower abdominal pain in women of childbearing age (2014). Cochrane Database Syst Rev, Issue 5, CD007683.

Cheng Y, Zhou S, Zhou R, Lu J, Wu S, Xiong X, Ye H, Lin Y, Wu T, Cheng N. (2015) Abdominal drainage to prevent intraperitoneal abscess after open appendectomy for complicated appendicitis. Cochrane Database Syst Rev, Issue 2, CD010168

Howell JM, Eddy OL, Lukens TW, Thiessen ME, Weingart SD, Decker WWI American College of Emergency Physicians. Clinical policy: Critical issues in the evaluation and management of emergency department patients with suspected appendicitis. Ann Emerg Med. 2010 Jan155(1):71–116

Korndorffer JR Jr, Fellinger E, Reed W. SAGES guideline for laparoscopic appendectomy. Surg Endosc, 2010 Apr;24(4):757-61

Smith MP, Katz DS, Rosen MP, Lalani T, Carucci LR, Cash BD, Kin DH, Piorkowski RJ, Small WC, Spottswood SEC, Tulchinsky M, Yaghmai V, Yee J, Expert Panel on Gastrointesinal Imaging. ACR Appropriateness Criteria® right lower quadrant pain—suspected appendicitis. [online publication]. Reston (VA): American College of Radiology (ACR); 2013. 10

Humes D, Speake W, Simpson J (2007). Appendicitis. BMJ Clin Evid 6, 408.

Addiss DG, Shaffer N, Fowler BS, Tauxe RV (1990). The epidemiology of appendicitis and appendicectomy in the United States. Am J Epidemiol 132, 910–25.

Hardin DM Jr (1999). Acute appendicitis: review and update. Am Fam Physician 60, 2027–34.

Guidry SP, Poole GV (1994). The anatomy of appendicitis. Am Surg 60, 68–71.

Lau WY, Teoh–Chan CH, Fan ST, Yam WC, Lau KF, Wong SH (1984). The bacteriology and septic complication of patients with appendicitis. Ann Surg 200, 576–81.

Morris PJ, Wood WC (2000). Chapter 27. In: Oxford Textbook of Surgery, 2nd ed. Oxford University Press, Oxford.

Mulholland MW (2005). Chapter 54. In: Greenfield's surgery: scientific principles and practice, 2nd ed, Lippincott–Raven Publishers.

Andersen B, Nielsen TF (1999). Appendicitis in pregnancy: diagnosis, management and complications. Acta Obstet Gynecol Scand 78, 758–62.

Longmore M, Wilkinson IB, Turmezei T, Cheung CK (2007). Oxford Handbook of Clinical Medicine, 7th ed. Oxford University Press, Oxford.

Jeffrey RB Jr, Laing FC, Townsend RR (1988). Acute appendicitis: sonographic criteria based on 250 cases. Radiology 167, 327–9.

Sivit CJ, Applegate KE, Stallion A et al. (2000). Imaging evaluation of suspected appendicitis in a paediatric population: effectiveness of sonography versus CT. AJR Am J Roentgenol 175, 977–80.

Eriksson S, Granstrom L, Carlstrom A (1994). The diagnostic value of repetitive preoperative analyses of C-reactive protein and total leucocyte count in patients with suspected acute appendicitis. Scand J Gastroenterol 29, 1145–9.

Connor TJ, Garcha IS, Ramshaw BJ et al. (1995). Diagnostic laparoscopy for suspected appendicitis. Am Surg 61, 187–9.

Grunewald B, Keating J (1993). Should the 'normal' appendix be removed at operation for appendicitis? J R Coll Surg Edinb 38, 158–60.

Kukreja N, Bhan C, Schizas A (2007). An audit of training in laparoscopic appendicectomy in the South Thames Region. Bulletin of the Royal College of Surgeons of England 89, 102–4.

NIDDK (2014) Guidlelines: Appendicitis. Available form: https://www.niddk.nih.gov/health-information/digestive-diseases/appendicitis

Part 6

Colorectal

Constipation in adults*

Basic facts *324*
Recommended investigations *326*
Recommended treatment *328*
Further reading *332*

Key guidelines
- CKS. NICE (2017). Constipation.
- British National Formulary 69 (2015). Constipation.

---

* The guidelines on this chapter have been sourced and summarized from different UK, Europe, and international government sources, professional organizations, and medical specialty societies. Leading guidelines have been listed in the further reading section at the end of this chapter.

Basic facts

- *Definition*—in simple patient terms, constipation is the passage of hard stool, the infrequent passage of stools, or the need for straining on defecation. The definition and diagnostic criteria (Rome III) have been recommended by the international working committee on functional constipation (Box 34.1).
- *Prevalence*—difficult to estimate (many do not seek medical advice). The average prevalence in Europe is 15.3%, ranging from 0.7% in paediatric population in Italy to 81% in elderly hospitalized male population.
- *Pathogenesis*—see Boxes 34.2 and 34.3.

Box 34.1 Rome III criteria for constipation*

Diagnostic requirements—the presence of two or more main complaints over the last year for a period of 12wk or more (not necessarily consecutive).

Main complaints.
- *Lumpy or hard stool*—for >25% of bowel movements.
- Decreased bowel movements—to <3 per wk.
- *Straining*—during more than 25% of bowel movements.
- *Sensation of anorectal blockage*—for >25% of bowel movements.
- *Sensation of incomplete evacuation*—for >25% of bowel movements.
- *The need for manual evacuation (digital or other techniques)*—for >25% of bowel movements.
- *The absence of*—loose stools or irritable bowel syndrome (diagnosed by full criteria).

* The Rome process is an international effort to define and categorize the functional gastrointestinal disorders.

Reproduced with permission from The Rome Foundation, Rome III criteria for constipation. http://www.romecriteria.org/assets/pdf/19_RomeIII_apA_885-898.pdf

Box 34.2 Causes of constipation

Physiologic changes.
- Pregnancy, irritable bowel syndrome.

Medications
- See Table 34.1

Underlying medical disorder.
- Neurologic disorder.
- Multiple sclerosis, spinal cord injury, Parkinson's disease, myotonic dystrophy.
- Peripheral neuropathy, diabetes mellitus, pseudo-obstruction, Hirschprung's disease, autonomic neuropathy.

Metabolic disorder.
- Hypokalaemia, hypercalcaemia, hypothyroidism, panhypopituitarism, anorexia nervosa.

Idiopathic.
- *Normal transit constipation*—about 60% of cases. Stools transverse the colon at normal speed and evacuate at similar frequency to average population, but the patient believes he/she is constipated.
- *Defecatory disorders*—about 25% of idiopathic cases. The rectum fails to effectively empty from stool. More common in:
  - Fear of defecation—due to pain associated with anal fissures, complicated haemorrhoids, or large hard stool.
  - Structural abnormalities—rectocoele, rectal intussusception, and excessive perineal descent.
  - Lack of coordination—among abdominal, rectoanal, and pelvic floor muscles during defecation.
- *Slow transit constipation*—occurs less frequently (13%) and is associated with delayed emptying of the colon, especially the proximal end.

Box 34.3 Medications causing constipation

Common surgical acute medications—analgesics, opiates, antispasmodics, antihistamines, 5HT3 antagonists.

Chronic disease medications—antidepressants, antipsychotics, antihypertensives, calcium channel blockers.

Supplements—iron supplements, antacids, sucralfate.

Recommended investigations

- See Fig. 34.1.
- *General approach*—the main reason for investigation is to exclude 'serious' disease. Accurate history and physical examination are essential [C].
    - *Clinical history*—patients will often complain about the urge to defecate, and this can be associated with the feeling of rectal fullness and crampy lower abdominal pain. The history should include the pattern of bowel movement (stool features, frequency, usual timing for defecation), general measures used to aid defecation (mobility and daily access to toilets, need for carer to go to toilet, high attention to privacy, laxatives taken and how efficient, dietary habits), nature and duration of constipation (onset, duration, pattern), presence of secondary causes (specific drugs, systemic disorders), presence

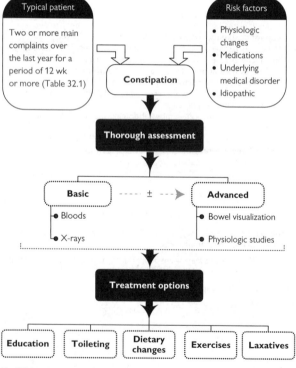

Fig. 34.1 Approaching patients with constipation.

of ALARM symptoms (e.g. weight loss, rectal bleeding, episodes of diarrhoea, and anaemia).
* *Physical examination*—may reveal malodorous breath, anal fissures, haemorrhoids (more likely effect rather than cause), and solid faeces on digital rectal examination. Some of these findings may be causative and some consequential upon the constipation.
* A change of bowel habit to constipation is not a high-risk symptom for colorectal cancer.

Diagnostic tests

* Not required when ALARM features are absent and the patient is under the age of 45 [C].
* *AXR*—may reveal faecal loading in the colon, and/or features of megacolon. Useful for regular monitoring of the bowel during treatment.
* *Bowel visualization*—indicated in patients with ALARM symptoms. Colonoscopy can reliably exclude underlying organic pathology (cancer, stricture, extrinsic compression). CT colonography and barium enema also have a place. Flexible sigmoidoscopy is the first-line investigation in younger patients [C].
* *Physiologic studies*—indicated in selected patients according to their response (or lack of response) to treatment in the absence of any justifying reason.
* *Colonic transit studies*—useful in evaluating patients whose major complaint is infrequent defecation.
  * *Technique*—patients need to swallow radio-opaque markers and undergo regular abdominal radiographs to monitor the passage throughout the colon.
  * *Outcome*—colonic inertia is diagnosed if the transit is delayed in the right colon. Outlet delay is diagnosed when the markers reach and accumulate in the rectum.
* *Defecography*—useful in diagnosing defecatory disorders.
* *Motility studies*—useful in some patients with severe constipation.
* *Wireless motility capsule*—has similar accuracy when compared to radiopaque marker tests.

Recommended treatment

- See Fig. 34.1.
- *General approach*—effective management requires a thorough approach that extends well beyond the simple use of laxatives. Attention to simple details is essential (associated pain, dietary habits, fluid intake, mobility, toileting).
- *Patient education*—includes appropriate reassurance, proper explanation of normal bowel habits, encouragement to reduce excessive use of laxatives, and advice on good toileting practice (consistent toileting each day, use of patient's own triggering factor like meal or morning call) [C].
- *Toileting education/support*—visual and auditory privacy should be safeguarded. Squat position is recommended for a good and effective defecation and should be achieved or, in the case of bedbound patients, simulated by left-side lying position [C].
- *Dietary changes*—high-fibre diet and adequate fluid intake should be encouraged [C]. Fibre intake should be increased to 25–30g/d with increased fluid intake (1.5–2L/d).
  - *Efficiency*—stool frequency is expected to increase significantly from a mean baseline of 1.8/wk to 4.2/wk with an improvement in stool consistency.
  - *Side-effects*—may be associated in the first week with some gastro-intestinal disturbance (flatulence and abdominal bloating), but disappears usually by the third week.
- *Preparations*—unprocessed wheat and oat bran, taken with food or fruit juice, is the most effective bulk-forming preparation. Table 34.1 shows some examples of dietary fibre contents.
- *Daily exercises*—effective in reducing the prevalence of constipation when compared with a sedentary lifestyle in adults (OR ×0.70) and should be encouraged [D].
  - *Walking*—highly recommended for mobile individuals, 15–20min once or twice a day, 3–5 times a week [D].
  - *Patients unable to walk or bedbound*—should be offered specific exercises such as pelvic tilt, low trunk rotation, and single leg lifts [D].
- Bulk-forming laxatives.
  - *Mechanism of action*—increase the volume of faecal mass which stimulates peristalsis.
  - *Efficiency*—increase the average mean frequency of bowel movements by 1.4 per wk.
  - *Preparations*—ispaghula (Fybogel→1 sachet or two level 5mL spoonfuls in water twice daily, preferably after meals), sterculia (Normacol→1–2 heaped 5mL spoonfuls, or the contents of 1–2 sachets, washed down without chewing with plenty of liquid once or twice daily after meals), and methylcellulose.
- Osmotic laxatives.
  - *Mechanism of action*—increase the water content within the large bowel by attracting fluid from the body into bowel lumen or by retaining water in colon, lowering the pH, and increasing colonic peristalsis.
  - *Macrogols (polyethylene glycols*—Movicol®).

Table 34.1 Estimated food fibre contents

Food	Each serving	Fibre content
Fruit		
Apple (with skin)	Medium size	✿✿✿✿
Apricots (dried)	1 cup	✿✿✿✿✿✿✿✿✿✿
Dates	1 cup (chopped)	✿✿✿✿✿✿✿✿✿✿✿✿
Grapes	10	✿✿✿
Orange	1	✿✿✿
Peach (with skin)	1	✿✿✿
Pear (with skin)	1	✿✿✿✿✿
Pineapple	1 cup (diced)	✿✿✿
Raspberries	1 cup	✿✿✿✿✿✿
Strawberries	1 cup	✿✿✿
Juice		
Apple	1 cup	✿
Grape	1 cup	✿✿
Orange	1 cup	✿
Cooked vegetables		
Bean (string, green)	1 cup	✿✿✿✿
Broccoli	1 stalk	✿✿✿✿✿
Brussels sprout	7–8	✿✿✿✿✿
Carrot	1 cup	✿✿✿✿✿
Cauliflower	1 cup	✿✿✿
Corn (canned)	1 cup	✿✿✿✿✿
Parsnip	1 cup (cooked)	✿✿✿✿✿✿
Peas	1 cup (cooked)	✿✿✿✿✿✿
Potato (without skin)	1 boiled	✿✿
Spinach	1 cup (raw)	✿✿✿✿✿
Tomato	1	✿✿
Legumes		
Baked beans, tomato sauce	1 cup	✿✿✿✿✿✿✿✿✿✿✿✿✿✿✿✿✿✿✿✿
Dried peas (cooked)	½ cup	✿✿✿✿✿
Bread, pasta, flour		
Bran muffin	1	✿✿✿✿✿✿
Mixed grains	-	✿✿✿✿
Oatmeal	1 cup	✿✿✿✿✿
White bread	1 slice	✿
Whole-wheat bread	1 slice	✿✿

✿ = about 1g/serving

- *Efficiency*—effective and reliable in treating chronic constipation and faecal impaction [A]. Can increase the number of bowel movements to 4.5 per wk (compared to 2.7 in placebo) at 2wk of use, and can achieve a return to normal bowel habits (three or more bowel movements per wk, no straining at defecation) in up to 70% of patients (compared to 30% in placebo) at 20wk of use.
- *Harm*—can cause abdominal pain and diarrhoea. Not significantly different from placebo in the overall frequency of adverse effects.
- *Dose*—Movicol® is given as 1–3 sachets daily in divided doses usually for up to 2wk for chronic constipation; as eight sachets daily dissolved in 1 litre of water and drunk within 6h, usually for maximum of 3d for faecal impaction.
- *Lactulose*.
  - *Efficiency*—effective and reliable in treating chronic constipation and faecal impaction [B].
  - *Benefits*—(30mL, 4 times/d) can significantly reduce the cramping, flatulence, tenesmus, and bloating sensation associated with the constipation. Lactulose does not increase the number of weekly bowel movements significantly (0.9 per week), but does achieve a good overall patient satisfaction at 1mo (satisfaction scores 5.2 on a score of 10 where 10 is 'excellent').
  - *Harm*—no serious side-effects.
  - *Dose*—initially 15mL twice daily, adjusted according to patient's needs.
  - *Other laxatives*—many available but little evidence to support one over the others. Few comparative clinical trials have been carried out, although a 2010 Cochrane review of studies in adults and children concluded that polyethylene glycol was superior to lactulose for outcomes such as stool frequency per week, form of stool, relief of abdominal pain, and the need for additional laxatives.
- *Stimulant laxatives*—act on the intestinal mucosa or nerve plexus and alter water and electrolyte secretion.
  - *Common preparations*—bisacodyl and senna.
  - *Harm*—often cause abdominal cramp and should be avoided in intestinal obstruction. Excessive use can cause diarrhoea and related effects such as hypokalaemia.
  - *Glycerol suppositories*—mild rectal stimulant.
  - *Arachis oil enemas*—contains ground nut oil and peanut oil. Act by lubricating and softening impacted faeces, and promoting bowel movement.
  - Prucalopride should only be considered in women who have tried at least two different types of laxatives from different classes (at the highest tolerated recommended doses) for at least 6mo, but have not had relief from constipation, and in whom invasive treatment is being considered. Prucalopride has not been tested in enough men to show that it works for them.
  - Lubiprostone is recommended as a possible treatment for people with chronic idiopathic constipation who have previously been treated with two different types of laxatives at the highest possible

recommended dose, for at least 6mo, but these haven't worked well enough, and when invasive treatment is being considered.

- *Surgery for constipation*—indicated occasionally to correct specific anatomical deformities (e.g. rectocoele) or for the very occasional longstanding debilitating symptoms refractory to conservative management. Total abdominal colectomy with anastomosis or ileostomy maybe indicated.

Further reading

CKS. NICE GUIDELINES (2017). Constipation. Available from: https://cks.nice.org.uk/constipation#!scenario

Brandt L, Schoenfeld P, Prather C, Quigley E, Schiller L, Talley N; American College of Gastroenterology Functional Gastrointestinal Disorders Task Force. (2005). An evidence-based approach to the management of chronic constipation in North America. Am J Gastroenterol 100, S1–21.

Peppas G, Alexiou VG, Mourtzoukou E, Falagas ME (2008). Epidemiology of constipation in Europe and Oceania: a systematic review. BMC Gastroenterol 8, 5.

British National Formulary 69 (2015). Constipation. Available from:https://bnf.nice.org.uk/treatment-summary/constipation.html .

Frizelle F, Barclay M (2007). Constipation in adults. BMJ Clin Evid 12, 413.

Registered Nurses' Association of Ontario (2005). Prevention of constipation in the older adult population. Available from: http://rnao.ca/bpg/guidelines/prevention-constipation-older-adult-population .

Hsieh C (2005). Treatment of constipation in older adults. Am Fam Physician 72, 2277–84.

Fallon M, O'Neill B (1997). ABC of palliative care. Constipation and diarrhoea. BMJ 315, 1293–6.

Locke GR 3rd, Pemberton JH, Phillips SF (2000). American Gastroenterological Association medical position statement: guidelines on constipation. Gastroenterology 119, 1761–6.

Ramkumar D, Rao SS (2005). Efficacy and safety of traditional medical therapies for chronic constipation: a systematic review. Am J Gastroenterol 100, 936–71.

Longstreth GF, Thompson WG, Chey WD, Houghton LA, Mearin F, Spiller RC (2006). Functional bowel disorders. Gastroenterology 130, 1480–91.

The Association of Coloproctology of Great Britain and Ireland (2007). Guidelines for the management of colorectal cancer. Available from: https://www.acpgbi.org.uk/content/uploads/2007-CC-Management-Guidelines.pdf.

Bandolier (1997). Constipation. Agency for Healthcare Research and Quality (AHRQ). Wireless motility capsule versus other diagnostic technologies for evaluating gastroparesis and constipation: A comparative effectiveness review (No. 110)

Chapter 35

Diverticular disease[*]

Basic facts *334*
Recommended investigations *336*
Recommended treatment *338*
Further reading *340*

Key guidelines

- NICE (2013). Diverticular disease and diverticulitis.
- World Gastroenterology Organization (2007). Diverticular disease.
- RCS and Assoc. of Coloproctolgy (2014). Colonic diverticular disease.

[*] The guidelines on this chapter have been sourced and summarized from different UK, Europe, and international government sources, professional organizations, and medical specialty societies. Leading guidelines have been listed in the further reading section at the end of this chapter.

Basic facts

- *Definitions*—diverticula of the colon are small, blind, narrow-necked pouches formed by mucosal herniation through the muscle layer of the bowel wall (Box 35.1).
- *Prevalence*—difficult to estimate. Ranges from ~10% at <40y to 70% at age 80. More common in Western countries and has been increasing over the years. Evidence to correlate diverticular disease with specific risk factors are insufficient to draw solid conclusions (Box 35.2). The sigmoid colon is mostly affected.
- *Pathogenesis*—results from the formation of false or pulsion diverticulum where the bowel mucosa and submucosa protrude through weakest areas of the muscular layer (where the vasa recta pass through) and form several outpouchings covered only by serosa.
- *Acute diverticulitis*—results from the inflammation of the diverticula, caused by stasis or obstruction with subsequent bacterial overgrowth and local tissue ischaemia. This results in a micro- or macroscopic perforation of the wall and confined or complicated pericolic infection.
- *Diverticular bleeding*—occurs when the vasa recta is exposed to injury and ruptures into the lumen.
- *Clinical presentation*.
  - *Uncomplicated diverticular disease*—may be associated with non-specific lower abdominal pain, bloating, and constipation.
  - About 10–25% of asymptomatic cases will develop symptoms with time. Diverticular colitis is now a recognized entity.
  - *Diverticulitis*—most cases (75–95%) are simple (Box 35.3). Hinchey classification scheme can be used for staging purposes.
- *Diverticular bleeding*—painless maroon or bright red rectal bleeding, usually self-limiting. Rare to coexist with acute diverticulitis. Frequent or small PR bleeding is unlikely to be caused by diverticulosis and requires further investigations.

Box 35.1 Definitions

Diverticula—small, blind, narrow-necked pouches formed by mucosal herniation through the muscle layer of the bowel wall.

Diverticulosis—incidental finding of asymptomatic diverticula in the colon.

Diverticular disease—a term used when diverticula cause symptoms.

Diverticulitis—a term used when diverticula are associated with inflammation

Box 35.2 Risk Factors

- *Low fibre intake*—inversely correlates to the incidence of diverticular disease. RR is 0.58 for highest vs lowest fibre intake (a 47,000 men study).
- *Western diet*—high fat, red meat, and low fibre. RR × 2.35–3.32.
- *Smoking, caffeine, or alcohol*—no specific correlation exists. Current smoking increases risk of perforation (OR ×1.89).
- *Physical activity*—lack of physical activity increases the risk of developing symptomatic diverticular disease (RR ×0.63 for highest vs lowest extremes) after adjustment for age and dietary habits. The effect of moderate exercise remains unclear.
- *Obesity* – increases the risk slightly (OR ×1.89).

Box 35.3 Hinchey classification of complicated diverticulitis

Paracolic abscess (stage 1)—small, confined paracolic or mesenteric abscesses.

Presentation—LIF pain (70% of cases), few days' history; previous similar episode (>50% of cases); nausea and vomiting (20–60%), constipation (50%), diarrhoea (25–35%), and urinary symptoms (10–15%). Right colon diverticulitis occurs in 1.5% of cases, mimicking appendicitis.

Pelvic abscess (stage 2)—abscesses are larger, but often confined to the pelvis. Mortality rate is <5%.

Perforated purulent diverticulitis (stage 3)—ruptured peridiverticular abscess, causing purulent peritonitis. Mortality rate is 15%.

Perforated faecal diverticulitis (stage 4)—rupture into the free peritoneal cavity, causing faecal contamination. Mortality rate is 45%.

This article was published in Advances in Surgery, Volume 12, Hinchey, E.J., Schaal, P.G. and Richard, G.K, Treatment of perforated diverticular disease of the colon, pp. 85–109, Copyright Elsevier 1978

Recommended investigations

- See Fig. 35.1
- *Uncomplicated diverticular disease*—symptomatic patients require investigation to exclude coexistent lesions such as polyps or carcinoma (see Chapter 38, pp.358–368), and confirm the presence of diverticular disease.
  - *Recommended investigations*—colon visualization includes full colonoscopy, flexible sigmoidoscopy with double contrast barium enema, or CT colonography.
- *Acute diverticulitis.*
  - *Abdominal and pelvis CT scan*—the first-line investigation of choice when indicated [A]. Oral, IV, and rectal contrasts are useful to enhance accuracy.
  - *Accuracy*—very high. Sensitivity, specificity, positive and negative predictive values (with contrast) are all well over 97%.
  - *Findings*—colonic diverticula (84% of cases), increased soft tissue density within the pericolic fat (98% of cases), thickening of bowel wall (70%), and soft tissue masses (pericolic fluid collections, abscess, or phlegmon) in 35% of cases.
  - *Other investigations*—include single contrast enema (preferably water-soluble), compression ultrasound scan, cystography, and possible limited and gentle flexible sigmoidoscopy in selected cases where the risk of perforation is minimal [B].
- *Diverticular bleeding.*
  - General approach—following active resuscitation, investigation choices depend on available resources and expertise.
  - *Early colonoscopy (for diagnosis and treatment)*—the first-line investigation of choice when experience and facilities are available [A].
    - —*Efficiency*—in dedicated centres, early colonoscopy can reduce the length of hospital stay (from 5 to 2d).
    - —*Preparation*—stop aspirin, warfarin, and NSAIDs if possible [C]. Consider upper GI endoscopy for severe bleeding as possible upper GI source, or if negative colonoscopy [A]. Bowel preparation using polyethylene glycol-based solutions when colonoscopy is indicated can improve visualization, therapeutic yield, and patient safety, providing the patient is fit enough.
- *Other investigations*—angiography and/or tagged red blood cell scanning can be used with high identification rate (75%) in active persistent bleeding (0.1mL/min for tagged red blood cell scanning and 1mL/min for angiography) or in cases of non-diagnostic endoscopic findings.
- *Control of bleeding*—by superselective arterial embolization can be achieved in 45–90% of cases, and may be required for diagnostic and therapeutic purposes in severe unstable cases (e.g. >6 units of blood transfusion in 24h). Colonoscopy with thermal, laser, injection, or clip modalities may be possible. Preoperative localization of bleeding site should always be attempted to allow for limited segmental colonic resection rather than 'blind' colectomy, with resultant high morbidity and mortality.

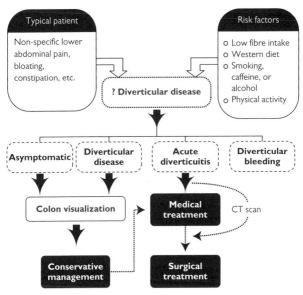

Fig. 35.1 Approaching patients with diverticular disease.

Recommended treatment

- See Fig. 35.1.
- Good quality randomized trials are few.
- The use of antibiotics in uncomplicated disease has been called into question. Use of antibiotics for uncomplicated acute diverticulitis has been the subject of a Cochrane review and three randomized clinical trials (RCTs). The AVOD trial from northern Europe randomized 669 patients with CT-confirmed acute uncomplicated diverticulitis into those treated with antibiotics and those without. No statistical difference in complication rates, emergency surgery, or recurrence. It should be recognized that this only applies to patients who have no overt signs of sepsis or underlying immunosuppression, or significant co-morbidities. The most recent Cochrane review has recommended that further RCTs are required to confirm these findings.
- *Asymptomatic incidental diverticulosis*—no further investigations are required. Encourage a healthy diet and an active lifestyle. Despite usual practice, there is little evidence to support the use of added fibre (bran or ispaghula husk) or laxatives (lactulose, methylcellulose) to prevent complications in diverticulosis (no significant difference from placebo in long-term follow-up).
- *Symptomatic uncomplicated diverticular disease*—following appropriate investigations, a healthy diet and an active lifestyle are advised. Simple analgesia may be required (paracetamol is better than NSAIDs or opioid).
  - *Added fibre or laxatives*—evidence to support the efficiency of this practice compared to placebo and is recommended by NICE.
  - *Dietary fibre supplements + antibiotics (US practice: Rifaximin 400mg bd for 12mo)*—may relieve symptoms at 12mo more than fibre alone (70% with rifaximin vs 40% with placebo alone), but may cause side effects (nausea, headache, and weakness). This is currently not the recommended practice in the UK. The place of mesalazine, pre- and probiotics is not clear. More evidence is required to draw solid recommendations.
  - *Elective open or laparoscopic surgery*—no evidence to recommend preventive surgery in uncomplicated diverticular disease.
- *Diverticulitis*—treatment options depend on the severity of the case and the individual patient circumstances (Box 35.4).
  - *Recurrent attacks*—a later second attack of diverticulitis occurs in 10–35% of cases, and a further third of patients will have a third attack. Recurrent diverticulitis is more likely in patients who already had recurrent attacks (the risk doubles in each subsequent hospital admission), young patients (<50y), and patients with other coexisting conditions (e.g. obesity). Recommendation for elective surgery should be tailored according to the individual patient risk–benefit assessment [B]. Patients willing to avoid a second severe attack of diverticulitis or recurrent attacks, who have acceptable operative risk and understands the implication of surgery, should be offered sig-moid resection. This can be performed 6wk after the acute attack.
- *Diverticular bleeding*—see Oxford Handbook of Clinical Surgery 4e Ch. 11.

Box 35.4 Treatment of diverticulitis

Primary or secondary care
- *Treat as outpatient*—for uncomplicated mild cases where patient can tolerate oral fluid and be followed up. Patients not improving after 48h of treatments require hospitalization.
- *Treat as inpatient*—if patient is unable to tolerate oral fluid and in more severe cases (fever, peritoneal irritation), elderly patients, and immunosuppressed patients [B].

Medical treatment
- *Oral intake*—clear fluid (or NBM with IV hydration) is commonly recommended initially for 2–3d. Solid food can be gradually introduced thereafter.
- *Broad spectrum antibiotics*—to cover both aerobic and anaerobic bacteria [B].
  - *Recommended antibiotics*—co-amoxiclav (500mg/125mg tablets tds) or ciprofloxacin (500mg bd) and metronidazole (400mg tds) for penicillin allergics.
  - *Duration*—minimum 7d.
- *Analgesia*—paracetamol is safe and effective. NSAIDs and long-term opioids should be used with caution as they have been identified as risk factors for diverticular perforation. If required, give Pethidine whilst awaiting admission.
- *Treatment outcome*—most cases (75–100%) respond to conservative management within 48–72h. Severe unresolving cases should be approached as complicated cases (see above) and treated accordingly. Other causes should be considered.
- *Follow-up*—confirmation of diagnosis is recommended following resolution of the acute attack [D], usually within 4–6wk.
- *Percutaneous drainage of abscess*—the recommended best treatment for large (>2–4cm) diverticular abscesses [B]. This approach reduces the need for emergency surgery and improves overall patient outcome.
- *Emergency surgery*—required for severe unresponsive cases or for patients with significant complications (peritonitis, bowel obstruction) [B]. Options include Hartmann's procedure (sigmoid colectomy with end colostomy) and sigmoid colectomy with primary anastomosis (± proximal colonic washout and diverting ileostomy).
- *Laparoscopic lavage* has also been used as an alternative in Hinchey stage 3 disease.
- *Elective surgery*—the role of elective resection after an acute episode of diverticulitis should be assessed on a case by case basis taking into account the presence of complicated diverticular disease and a risk–benefit assessment of the patient.

Further reading

NICE (2013). Diverticular disease and diverticulitis. Available from: https://cks.nice.org.uk/diverticular-disease

Rafferty J, Shellito P, Hyman NH, Buie WD (2006). Practice parameters for sigmoid diverticulitis. Dis Colon Rectum 49, 939–44.

BMJ Clinical Evidence. Available from: http://clinicalevidence.bmj.com/x/systematic-review/0405/overview.html.

The Society for Surgery of the Alimentary Tract (1999). Surgical treatment of diverticulitis. Available from: J Gastrointest Surg. 1999 Mar-Apr;3(2):212-3.

World Gastroenterology Organization (2007). Diverticular disease. Available from: http://www.worldgastroenterology.org/guidelines/global-guidelines/diverticular-disease

Meyers MA, Alonso DR, Gray GF, Baer JW (1976). Pathogenesis of bleeding colonic diverticulosis, Gastroenterology 71, 577–83.

Painter NS, Truelove SC, Ardran GM, Tuckey M (1965). Segmentation and the localization of intraluminal pressures in the human colon, with special reference to the pathogenesis of colonic diverticula. Gastroenterology 49, 169–77.

Jacobs DO (2007). Clinical practice. Diverticulitis. N Engl J Med 357, 2057–66.

Painter NS, Burkitt DP (1971). Diverticular disease of the colon: a deficiency disease of Western civilization. Br Med J 2, 450–4.

Aldoori WH, Giovannucci EL, Rimm EB, Wing AL, Trichopoulos DV, Willett WC (1994). A prospective study of diet and the risk of symptomatic diverticular disease in men. Am J Clin Nutr 60, 757–64.

Aldoori WH, Giovannucci EL, Rimm EB, Wing AL, Trichopoulos DV, Willett WC (1995). A prospective study of alcohol, smoking, caffeine, and the risk of symptomatic diverticular disease in men. Ann Epidemiol 5, 221–8.

Aldoori WH, Giovannucci EL, Rimm EB et al. (1995). Prospective study of physical activity and the risk of symptomatic diverticular disease in men. Gut 36, 276–82.

Konvolinka CW (1994). Acute diverticulitis under age forty. Am J Surg 167, 562–5.

Ngoi SS, Chia J, Goh MY, Sim E, Rauff A (1992). Surgical management of right colon diverticulitis. Dis Colon Rectum 35, 799–802.

Meyers MA, Alonso DR, Gray GF, Baer JW (1976). Pathogenesis of bleeding colonic diverticulosis. Gastroenterology 71, 577–83.

Janes SE, Meagher A, Frizelle FA (2006). Management of diverticulitis. BMJ 332, 271–5.

American Society for Gastrointestinal Endoscopy (2005). The role of endoscopy in the patient with lower GI bleeding. Available from http://www.asge.org/uploadedFiles/Publications_(public)/Practice_guidelines/2014_The%20role%20of%20endoscopy%20in%20the%20patient%20with%20lower%20GI%20bleeding.pdf.

Jensen DM, Machicado GA, Jutabha R, Kovacs TO (2000). Urgent colonoscopy for the diagnosis and treatment of severe diverticular haemorrhage. N Engl J Med 342, 78–82.

Sarin S, Boulos PB (1994). Long-term outcome of patients presenting with acute complications of diverticular disease. Ann R Coll Surg Engl 76, 117–20.

State LL, Syngal S (2003). Timing of colonoscopy: impact on length of hospital stay in patients with acute lower intestinal bleeding. Am J Gastroenterol 98, 317–22.

Chabok A, P"ahlman L, Hjern F, Haapaniemi S, Smedh K; AVOD Study Group. Randomized clinical trial of antibiotics in acute uncomplicated diverticulitis. Br J Surg 2012; 99: 532–539.

Shabanzadeh DM, Wille-Jørgensen P. Antibiotics for uncomplicated diverticulitis. Cochrane Database Syst Rev 2012; (11)CD009092.

Myers E, Hurley M, O'Sullivan GC, Kavanagh D, Wilson I, Winter DC. Laparoscopic peritoneal lavage for generalized peritonitis due to perforated diverticulitis. Br J Surg 2008; 95: 97–101.

Afshar S, Kurer MA. Laparoscopic peritoneal lavage for perforated sigmoid diverticulitis. Colorectal Dis 2012; 14: 135–142.

ACPGBI position statement on elective resection for diverticulitis. Fozard JB, Armitage NC, Schofield JB, Jones OM; Association of Coloproctology of Great Britain and Ireland. Colorectal Dis. 2011 Apr;13 Suppl 3:1-11

RCS Commissioning Guidelines (2014). Colonic Diverticular disease.

Anal fissures[*]

Basic facts *342*
Recommended treatment *344*
Further reading *348*

Key guidelines

- NICE Clinical Knowledge Summaries (2016). Anal fissure: management.
- American Society of Colon and Rectal Surgeons (2010). Practice parameters for the management of anal fissures (3rd revision).
- The management of anal fissure: ACPGBI position statement (2008).
- ACG Clinical Guideline: Management of Benign Anorectal Disorders 2014.

[*] The guidelines on this chapter have been sourced and summarized from different UK, Europe, and international government sources, professional organizations, and medical specialty societies. Leading guidelines have been listed in the further reading section at the end of this chapter.

Basic facts

- *Definition*—tear or split in the squamous lining of the anal canal distal to the dentate line (Box 36.1).
- *Incidence*—common condition. The lifetime incidence is 11.1%. Anal fissures affect both genders equally at any age. Anterior fissures are more common in females than males.
- *Pathogenesis*—no simple or unified theory to explain pathogenesis. Increased anal tone is common. Elevated internal sphincter pressure exacerbates local ischaemia, and impairs wound healing. Severe pain is thought to be ischaemic in origin.
  - *Anatomic location*—about 90% of primary anal fissures occur posteriorly, possibly due to the distinctive distribution of blood flow into the anoderm, where blood supply is less than one half that in other parts of the anal canal.
  - *Secondary causes of anal fissures*—see Box 36.2.
- *Clinical presentation*—severe anal pain, spontaneously or during the passage of stool, lasting from a few minutes to a few hours, and accompanied commonly by rectal bleeding. Rectal bleeding presents with small amounts of bright red blood, on the toilet paper or the surface of the stool (typically separated from stool). Other symptoms may include perianal discharge; itching and skin irritation can be prominent. Multiple fissures occurring away from the midline and other aberrant-shaped fissures may hide some serious underlying disease, including Crohn's, sexually transmitted diseases, tuberculosis, or malignancies. See Box 36.3.

Box 36.1 Anal fissures—definitions

Acute anal fissures—fissures presenting for <6wk.

Chronic anal fissures—fissures oresenting for >6wk with morphological signs of chronicity.

Primary anal fissures—fissures associated with increased anal tone or posterior ischaemia, but no identifiable underlying cause can be found.

Secondary anal fissures—fissures associated with an identifiable underlying cause, not with increased anal tone or posterior ischaemia.

Box 36.2 Secondary causes of anal fissures

Severe constipation.

Inflammatory bowel disease —associated inflammatory process causes ulceration of mucosa.

Pregnancy (especially third trimester) and childbirth—commonly located anteriorly and often associated with low anal sphincter pressures.

Sexually transmitted disease—the infectious process may result in tissue breakdown.

Rectal cancer.

Box 36.3 Physical examination for anal fissures

Acute anal fissure.

- *Technique*—best performed by spreading the buttocks apart gently and looking carefully at the posterior midline. Inspection of the entire anal canal is essential.
- *Appearance*—fresh laceration in the anoderm, with sharply demarcated edges.
- *Other findings*—involuntary spasm of the anus may indicate the presence of anal fissure, perianal abscess.
- *Digital rectal examination and proctoscopy*—often too uncomfortable and best to avoid.

Chronic anal fissure.

Appearance—linear or pear-shaped split with raised edges and exposed white, horizontally oriented fibres (internal anal sphincter) at the base.

Secondary features—include external (sentinel) skin tags, hypertrophied anal papillae at the proximal end, and induration of the edges.

Recommended treatment

- An optimal strategy for the management has not been well established yet.
- *Conservative measures*—can eventually reach a healing rate of 35% without any other intervention and is the first treatment of choice [B] (Box 36.4).

Medical management

- *Indications*—persistent symptoms (>1wk) despite conservative management in the absence of contraindications (e.g. pregnancy, breastfeeding).
- *Objectives*—to reduce the internal sphincter spasm, decrease the pressure in the anal canal, and enhance blood flow to the anoderm with subsequent healing of the fissure.

Topical glyceryl trinitrate (GTN).

- First-line treatment for chronic anal fissures [A]. Marginally superior to placebo.
  - *Mechanism*—increases local blood flow in the anal canal and reduces pressure in the internal anal sphincter, which may further facilitate healing.
  - *Applications*—apply as a 0.2–0.6% topical ointment (a pea-sized amount) to the anal margin twice a day. This should be continued for 8 weeks or until complete healing of the anal mucosa.
  - *Risks and benefits*—see Box 36.5.

Topical diltiazem.

- Insufficient evidence to conclude whether this is superior to placebo, but widely used. Less headache side-effects than GTN.
  - Mechanism—calcium antagonist that inhibits calcium ion entry through voltage-sensitive areas of vascular smooth muscles, causing relaxation and dilatation.
  - Application—topical diltiazem 2% gel to the anal margin twice a day (not widely available or licensed).
  - Risks and benefits—see Box 36.5.

Botulinum toxin injection.

  - *Mechanism*—potent inhibitor of acetylcholine release from nerve endings. Historically been used in treating certain spastic disorders of skeletal muscles.
  - *Application*—inadequate consensus on dosage, precise site of administration, number of injections, or efficacy.
  - *Risk and benefits*—see Box 36.5.

Box 36.4 Conservative measures in managing anal fissures

Patient education—essential to achieve compliance.

Ensure soft and easily passed stool—advise patients on increasing fluid (1.5–2L/d) and fibre (18–30g/d) intake, add laxatives if necessary (osmotic laxatives for children, and bran or bulk-forming laxatives for adults), and manage constipation as appropriate (see ➾ Chapter 34, pp.324–332).

Warm sitz baths—using salted warm water for 10 or 15min after each bowel movement. This traditional measure, although shown previously to be safe and effective in reducing anal sphincter tone, is not anymore recommended by expert reviewers.

Pain relief and soothing.
- *Topical lubricants (petroleum jelly)*—instilled before opening the bowel.
- *Topical anaesthetic creams*—useful and effective [D]. Long-term use is not recommended.

Box 36.5 Medical treatment for anal fissures

Topical GTN.
- *Benefits*—healing rate is 50–70%, which is marginally but significantly better than the best supportive conservative treatment. The median time to heal is 6wk (range 4–8wk). The relapsing rate is 25–40% and may require further prescription of GTN.
- *Risks*—main side effect is headache, which occurs in 20–50% of patients and causes up to 20% of patients to stop therapy.
Topical diltiazem.
- *Benefits*—healing rate comparable to GTN ointment. Few studies showed better response rate in cases unresponsive to GTN. Similar indications to GTN if available and licensed [A].
- *Risks*—fewer side-effects than GTN. May cause headache (33%) or pruritus ani.

Botulinum toxin.
- *Benefits*—acceptable alternative to GTN in 'failed to respond' cases [B]. Short-term healing rate is >90%, but similar to GTN in the long term. The relapsing rate is 40% and may require further injections.
- *Risks*—invasive and expensive. The main side-effect is the occasional transient incontinence to flatus.

Surgical management

- *Objectives*—to reduce the internal sphincter tone and enhance blood flow to the anoderm with subsequent healing of the fissure.
- *Indications*—usually reserved as a backup treatment for refractory cases not responding to medical therapy, but is considered a completely acceptable first-line treatment (after failed conservative measures) for some patients following informed decision on risks and benefits [A].

Anal stretch

- Lord's or four finger dilatation (healing rate 75–90%) is no longer recommended due to the risk of anal sphincter injury and consequent risk of incontinence (0–25%).

Lateral sphincterotomy

- *Technique*—divide the internal anal sphincter linearly from the distal external end up to the dentate line or to a distance equal to that of the fissure, using closed or open technique.
- Sphincterotomy healing is better if performed on the right or left lateral positions (compared to posterior or anterior midline).
- No surgical repair of the fissure itself is required. Biopsy may be warranted for fissures with atypical appearance.
- *Benefits*—highest healing rate (>95%) at 8wk compared to GTN (OR ×6.6) or other modalities.
- *Risks*—some degree of flatus and faecal incontinence may occur quite often in the immediate post-operative period (25–40%), and therefore, it is imperative to err on the side of doing too little rather than too much. It is always possible to go back and do more.

Anal advancement flap

- This operation avoids disruption to the anal sphincter by using a triangular or square-shaped sliding graft skin flap. It was shown to be as effective as an internal anal sphincterotomy in fissure healing rates at 3mo, but further studies are required to draw solid conclusions.

Further reading

Clinical Knowledge Summaries (2016). Anal fissure: management. Available from: https://cks.nice.
org.uk/anal-fissure

Nelson R (2007). Anal fissure (chronic). BMJ Clin Evid 12, 407

Lindsey I, Jones OM, Cunningham C, Mortensen NJ (2004). Chronic anal fissure. Br J Surg 91, 270–9.

Haemorrhoid disease[*]

Basic facts 350
Recommended treatment 352
Further reading 356

Key guidelines

- NICE (2016). Haemorrhoids: management.
- American Society of Colon and Rectal Surgeons (2010). Practice parameters for the management of haemorrhoids.
- National Institute for Health and Clinical Excellence: (i) (2010). Haemorrhoidal artery ligation[IPG342] (ii) (2007). Stapled haemorrhoidopexy for the treatment of haemorrhoids [TA128].
- Cochrane database of systemic reviews: (i) (2010). Rubber band ligation versus excisional haemorrhoidectomy for haemorrhoids, (ii) (2010). Stapled versus conventional surgery for hemorrhoids, (iii) (2011). Conventional versus LigaSure hemorrhoidectomy for patients with symptomatic hemorrhoids.

[*] The guidelines on this chapter have been sourced and summarized from different UK, Europe, and international government sources, professional organizations, and medical specialty societies. Leading guidelines have been listed in the further reading section at the end of this chapter.

Basic facts

- *Definition*—chronic engorgement of the haemorrhoidal physiologic complex, causing enlargement and displacement of the vascular cushions within the anal canal, with resultant bleeding, prolapse, and pain.
- *Incidence*—common condition. Estimated prevalence in Europe and US is 74% of the population. Affects both genders equally (men report their complaint more commonly to GPs), peaking between 45 and 65y of age to decline thereafter.
- *Pathogenesis*—normal haemorrhoids are physiologic vascular and connective tissue structures in the anal canal, contributing to the anal continence mechanism by providing compressible spongy cushions that allow for complete closure of the anus. Risk factors include advancing age, prolonged sitting and straining, pregnancy and pelvic tumours, diarrhoea and chronic constipation. Different pathogenesis theories exist (Box 37.1).
- *Clinical presentation*—often presents with painless bleeding (bright red, on toilet paper, or drips into toilet bowel), prolapsing piles (reducible initially), mucus discharge, and pruritus. Pain is rarely significant in internal haemorrhoids (see below), but may be so prominent in thrombosed external piles to warrant hospitalization. Other causes of perianal pain should be investigated.
- *Classification*—see Box 37.2.

Box 37.1 Pathogenesis of haemorrhoids

Aging theory—advancing age or other aggravating conditions cause weakness in the connective tissue anchoring haemorrhoidal tissue to the underlying sphincter, with resultant sliding into the anal canal.

Straining theory—abnormally increased tone of internal anal sphincter causes solid faecal material to forcefully squeeze haemorrhoidal plexus against the firm internal sphincter, with resultant congested and enlarged haemorrhoids.

Abnormal cushions' theory—haemorrhoidal cushions with its erectile properties become abnormally swollen, accompanied by possible congenital weakness in venous plexus walls, causing enlarged haemorrhoids.

Box 37.2 Classification of haemorrhoids

Internal vs external.

- *Internal haemorrhoids*—arise from superior haemorrhoidal cushions above the dentate line. Located in the left lateral, right anterior, and right posterior positions. The overlying mucosa has visceral innervation.
- *External haemorrhoids*—arise from the inferior haemorrhoidal plexus beneath the dentate line. Overlying squamous epithelium contains somatic pain receptors.
    - *Skin tags*—residual excess skin (remnant external thrombosed piles) and not haemorrhoidal tissue.
    - *Acutely thrombosed piles*—present with severely tender, tense, and oedematous mass.

Internal haemorrhoid severity classification

- *First degree*—painless bleeding with no prolapse.
- *Second degree*—bleeding associated with prolapse (with Valsalva manoeuvres) and spontaneous reduction.
- *Third degree*—bleeding with associated prolapse which requires manual reduction.
- *Fourth degree*—chronically prolapsed and is irreducible.

Box 37.3 Conservative management of haemorrhoids

Topical agents.

- *Action*—reduce symptoms by applying local anaesthetic or anti-inflammatory effects. No effect on haemorrhoids cure rate.
- *Efficiency*—quite efficient as short-term first-line measures [C].
- *Options*—no clinical trials to support one product over the others. Options include simple analgesia, sitz bath, soothing (astringent) preparations, anaesthetic preparations, and topical corticosteroids.
- *Harm*—avoid using opioids (risk of constipation) or NSAIDs (in rectal bleeding). Long-term use of local steroids can produce perianal dermatitis [B].

High-fibre diet.

- *Method*—ensure adequate fluid and fibre dietary intake (see ➲ Chapter 32, pp.324–332), with bulk-forming agents if necessary [B].
- *Efficiency*—relief of constipation occurs usually in a few days and relief of haemorrhoidal symptoms in a few weeks. Fibre supplement for 6wk can reduce haemorrhoidal bleeding in 95% of patients (compared to 56% in placebo). NNT is 3 (need to treat three patients to achieve one significant response).

Behavioural modifications—include avoiding reading in toilet, excessive straining, and encourage to lose weight and to maintain good anal hygiene.

Recommended treatment

- See Fig. 37.1.
- *Natural history*—untreated haemorrhoids heal spontaneously (25%), progress into recurrent condition (66%), or develop complications (ulceration, maceration, thrombosis, sepsis, and anaemia). Most patients use over-the-counter preparations and only seek medical advice for relatively severe disease.

Conservative management

- The first-line treatment of choice [B].
- Successful for most patients with mildly symptomatic haemorrhoids.
- *Main objectives*—to relieve symptoms as quick as possible and maintain remission.
- *Options*—dietary modification with high fibre and improved fluid intake should be the primary intervention. Other conservative options include laxatives, topical agents, and behavioural modifications

Non-surgical management for patients who fail medical management

Injection sclerotherapy

- *Indications*—alternative therapy for first and second degree haemorrhoids [B].
- *Technique*—a total of 3mL of 5% phenol (an irritant chemical solution) is injected into the submucosa of each pile. Sclerosants induce intense inflammatory reaction, provoke fibrosis, destroy redundant haemorrhoidal tissue, and ultimately fix the haemorrhoidal cushion.
- *Benefits and risks*—see Box 37.4.

Other options

- *Bipolar, infrared, and laser coagulation*—bipolar current, infrared, or laser light is applied to induce coagulation and necrosis, with resultant fibrosis in the submucosal layer. May be as effective as RBL with few side-effects, but more frequent recurrences.
- *Cryosurgery*—special probes cooled with liquid nitrogen is used to induce freezing and necrosis, with resultant fixation of the haemorrhoidal cushion. Has higher rate of complication and decreased patient satisfaction.
- *Rubber band ligation (RBL)*.
  - *Indications*—common choice for first, second, and selected third grade haemorrhoids in conjunction with conservative management [B].
  - Most effective office-based management option compared to injection sclerotherapy and infra-red coagulation. Long-term outcomes inferior to surgical excisional haemorrhoidectomy.
  - *Technique*—using anoscope to identify diseased haemorrhoids, a special machine with suction is used to place a special rubber ring on the base of the selected haemorrhoid.
  - *Benefits and risks*—see Box 37.5. All patients should be formally consented before using this procedure due to the serious, but rare, possible side-effects.

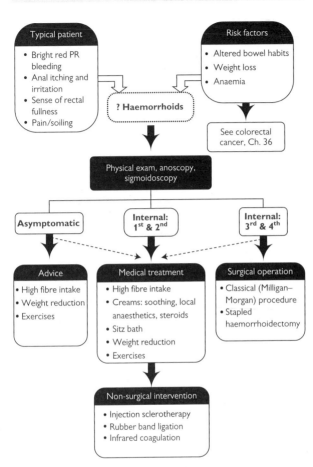

Fig. 37.1 Approaching patients with haemorrhoids.

Box 37.4 Injection sclerotherapy—benefits and risks

Efficacy—effective in treating haemorrhoidal bleeding or prolapse in ~60–90% of cases at 1y follow-up. About 30% of patients require repeated therapy over this period. A 4y recurrence of bleeding and/or prolapse occurs in 81% and 36% of patients, respectively.

Harm—uncommon, but serious side-effects include septic complications and chemical prostatitis (therefore, injecting anteriorly should not be performed).

Box 37.5 Rubber band ligation–benefits and risks

Efficacy—effective in treating haemorrhoidal bleeding or prolapse in ~75–95% of cases at 1y follow-up. About 10% of patients require repeated therapy over this period. A 4y recurrence of bleeding and/or prolapse occurs in 61% and 12% of patients, respectively.

Harm.
- *Pain*—occurs in ~13% of patients.
- *Anal stenosis*—requires anal dilatation, occurs rarely.

- *Stapled haemorrhoidopexy.*
  - *Indications*—effective in prolapsing internal haemorrhoids, but not in large external haemorrhoids.
  - Immediate postoperative pain has been demonstrated to be significantly less compared to surgical excisional haemorrhoidectomy thereby enabling earlier return to work. However, no difference in pain is identified after 21d.
  - Stapled haemorrhoidopexy is associated with a higher risk of long-term recurrence and prolapsing haemorrhoids compared to excisional haemorrhoidectomy.
- *Haemorrhoidal artery ligation.*
  - This procedure involves the selective ligation of the haemorrhoidal arteries which can be assisted by the use of a Doppler probe. An adjunctive mucosal plication can be performed for large prolapsing haemorrhoids. Often done under a general anaesthetic.
  - Long-term outcomes following haemorrhoidal artery ligation is currently lacking. A systemic review in 2013 suggested its use in grade II and III haemorrhoids, with a wide heterogeneity in outcomes from studies in the literature.
- *Surgical excisional haemorrhoidectomy.*
  - *Indications*—usually reserved for refractory cases to above procedures, patients who are unable to tolerate minor procedures, large external haemorrhoids, and combined internal and external haemorrhoids with significant prolapse [B].
  - *Ligasure haemorrhoidectomy*—appears to be better tolerated compared to conventional haemorrhoidectomy with less postoperative pain, with no impact on recurrence or complications.
  - *Options*—see Box 37.6.
- *Complications.*
  - *Urinary retention*—can be up to 30% of patients. Some patients require urinary catheterization.
  - *Urinary tract infection*—about 5% of cases, possibly secondary to urinary retention.
  - *Delayed haemorrhage*—in 1–2% within 7–16d. Possibly results from sloughing of primary clot.
  - *Faecal impaction*—associated with post-operative pain and opiate use.

Box 37.6 Surgical options

Closed haemorrhoidectomy.

- *Technique*—a narrow incision is made around the external haemorrhoidal tissue and extended across the dentate line to the superior base of the haemorrhoidal column; the defect is closed with a continuous suture.
- *Efficiency*—effective in relieving symptoms (>95%). Recurrence rate at 1y ranges from 4% for small haemorrhoids to 22% for large ones.
- *Harm*—associated with more post-operative complications than stapled haemorrhoidopexy.

Open haemorrhoidectomy

- *Technique*—the excision and ligation are left open without mucosal closure.
- *Efficiency*—effective in relieving symptoms (>95%) in first to fourth degree haemorrhoids. Recurrence rate at 1y is 3.8% for small haemorrhoids and 15.4% for large ones.
- *Harm*—similar to closed procedure.

Stapled haemorrhoidopexy

- *Technique*—a special device is used to excise a circumferential column of mucosa and submucosa from the upper anal canal. This brings protruding haemorrhoids back and fixes the lining in position.
- *Efficiency*—effective where the operative treatment of haemorrhoids is indicated. Have shorter length of hospital stay (1d), less post-operative pain, but no significant difference in recurrence rates from traditional methods.
- *Harm*—this procedure should only be performed by a fully trained colorectal surgeon.
- *Recommendations*—NICE recommends this procedure as an alternative option to traditional surgery where appropriate skills and clinical governance setting exist

---

- *Local infection*—is very uncommon. Submucosal abscess affects
- <1% of cases.
- *Pain*—nearly universal and may in part be due to spasm of the internal sphincter. Topical diltiazem ointment (2%) can be applied three times daily for 7d post-operatively.
- *Other complications*—include delayed healing, sphincter damage, and stricture formation.

Further reading

NICE (2016). Haemorrhoids: management. Available from: https://cks.nice.org.uk/haemorrhoids#!scenario

Rivadeneira DE, Steele SR, Ternent C, Chalasani S, Buie WD, Rafferty JL; Standards Practice Task Force of the American Society of Colon and Rectal Surgeons. Dis Colon Recum. 2011 Sep;54(9):1059-64

National Institute for Health and Clinical Excellence (i) (2010) Haemorrhoidal artery ligation [igp342] www.nice.org.uk/ipg342 (ii) (2007). (ii) (2007) Stapled haemorrhoidopexy for the treatment of haemorrhoids [ta128]. www.nice.org.uk/guidance/ta128

Cochrane database of systemic reviews: (i) Shanmugam V, Hakeem A, Campbell KL, Rabindranath KS, Steele RJC, Thaha MA, Loudon MA. Rubber band ligation versus excisional haemorrhoidectomy for haemorrhoids.(2005), Issue 1. CD005034. (ii) Lumb KJ, Colquhoun PH, Malthaner R, Jayaraman S. Stapled versus conventional surgery for hemorrhoids (2006), Issue 4 CD005393. (iii) Nienhuijs SW, de Hingh IHJT. Conventional versus LigaSure hemorrhoidectomy for patients with symptomatic hemorrhoids.(2009), Issue 1. CD006761

Reese GE, von Roon AC, Tekkis PP (2009). Haemorrhoids. BMJ Clin Evid 1, 415.

Studd P (2005). Haemorrhoids: prevention and treatment. Nursing in Practice 25, 50–3.

Arabi Y, Alexander–Williams J, Keighley MR (1977). Anal pressures in haemorrhoids and anal fissure. Am J Surg 134, 608–10.

Thomson WH (1975). The nature of haemorrhoids. Br J Surg 62, 542–52

Kluiber RM, Wolff BG (1994). Evaluation of anaemia caused by haemorrhoidal bleeding. Dis Colon Rectum 37, 1006–7.

Jensen SL, Harling H, Arseth–hansen P, Tange G (1989). The natural history of symptomatic haemorrhoids. Int J Colorectal Dis 4, 41–4.

Johanson JF (2002). Evidence-based approach to the treatment of haemorrhoidal disease. Evidence-based Gastroenterology 3, 26–31.

Pucher PH, Sodergren MH, Lord AC, Darzi A, Ziprin P. Clinical outcome following Doppler-guided haemorrhoidal artery ligation: a systemic review. Colorectal Dis. 2013 Jun;15(6):e284-94

Chapter 38

Colorectal cancer

Basic facts *358*
Recommended investigations *362*
Recommended staging *363*
Recommended treatment *364*
Further reading *368*

Key guidelines
- NICE (2014). Colorectal cancer.
- Cancer research UK (2014). Bowel cancer.
- The Association of Coloproctology of Great Britain and Ireland (2017). Guidelines for the management of colorectal cancer.
- SIGN (2016) Diagnosis and management of colorectal cancer.

Basic facts

- *Incidence*—fourth most common cancer in the UK. Incidence has increased by 6% over last decade. The lifetime risk for developing CRC is 1 in 14 for men (19 for women). The male to female ratio is 1.2:1.
- *Pathogenesis*—the attributes of malignancy (genetic damage, invasiveness, lack of normal differentiation, increased rate of growth, ability for local invasion, and distant spread) are acquired in a stepwise fashion, a process known as tumour progression. This correlates at the genetic level with the accumulation of successive mutations. Most risk factors are related to environmental and genetic factors (Boxes 38.1 and 38.2).
- *Natural history*—most CRCs result from malignant changes in polyps (adenomas) that developed at least a decade earlier. CRC growth usually follows an exponential curve, with a doubling time of about 40mo for early cancer to 4mo or less for advanced cancer. Patients with hepatic metastases, diagnosed at the time of surgery, have a median survival period of only 4.5mo.
- *Cancer distribution*—caecum: 13%; ascending colon, hepatic flexure, transverse colon, and splenic flexure: 13%; descending and sigmoid colon: 20%; rectosigmoid and rectum: 36%; anus 2%; unspecified: 15%.
- *Clinical presentation*—see Box 38.3. Commonly presents with abdominal pain (45%), change in bowel habits (5%), rectal bleeding of short

---

Box 38.1 Risk factors

Age
- Major risk factor. Risk increases dramatically after the age of 40. Most cases (95%) occur after the age of 50.

Dietary factors
- Promotional or protective role.
- Risk increases (proven) with alcohol consumption, red and processed meat, and may decrease with dietary fibre, garlic, milk and calcium consumption.
- Smoking—RR 1.5–3.0 has been linked with increased polyp formation and bowel cancer risk.

Medications
- NSAIDs—the long-term (>10y) regular use of NSAIDs can significantly reduce the risk of bowel cancer, possibly due to the inhibition of cyclooxygenase-2, with resultant increased apoptosis and impairment of tumour cells.
- HRT—may reduce the risk of CRC by 20–50% with 5–10y of use.
- Oral contraceptives—may reduce the risk of CRC by 11–18%.

Medical conditions
- Type 2 diabetes mellitus—increases the risk of CRC by 30%. One possible reason is the hyperinsulinaemia status as insulin is an important growth factor for colonic mucosal cells and can stimulate colonic tumour cells.
- Inflammatory bowel disease.

Familial predisposition
- Has a strong link to colon cancer (Box 38.2).

duration or blood mixed with stool (40%), and/or iron deficiency anaemia (10%). Advanced cancer is the initial presentation in about one fifth of patients. Cancer can present initially with bowel obstruction or perforation causing peritonitis. Distant metastasis is found in 15–20% of cases at initial presentation.

- All high-risk patients (Box 38.4) should be referred urgently for further investigations [C].

Box 38.2 Familial predisposition in CRC—facts and figures

- *Estimated risk*—one member of the family who has had bowel cancer (4–10% of all presentations) doubles the risk to other members. The advice of regional genetic services is strongly recommended in patients with significant family history.

FAP surveillance
- *With negative mutations (minority)*—annual flexible sigmoidoscopy is indicated for age 13–30 and 3–5 yearly until 60.
- Patients identified as having FAP should be considered for proctocolectomy and offered an ileoanal pouch between the ages of 16 and 20 [B]. If stapled, the anastomosis and anorectal cuff must be checked subsequently on a yearly basis. Patients with FAP have a significant risk of upper GI cancer and should have 2-yearly OGDs, or more frequently if there is any duodenal polyposis [B].

HNPCC surveillance
- Should be biennial from the age of 25 or 5y younger than the incidence in the youngest family member.
- *Colonoscopy*—is the investigation of choice and should be continued to the age of 75 if the mutation abnormality is not identified [B].
- At present, there is insufficient data to recommend prophylactic colectomy in patients with known mutations, but total colectomy should be offered for patients who develop a curative colonic carcinoma, and continue with regular surveillance of remaining bowel.
- OGDs should be advised for patients in families with known gastric cancers from the age of 50 or 5y earlier than the youngest reported case in the family [C].
- *High–moderate risk*—three or more affected relatives, none aged <50y, should be offered 5-yearly colonoscopy (or 3-yearly if adenomas found) aged 55–75.
- *Moderate risk*—one first-degree relative aged <45 or two affected first-degree relatives should be offered a single colonoscopy at the age of 55 and continued surveillance if adenomas are found. Earlier guidance had suggested that consideration for surveillance should be at age 35–40; this was a relative recommendation, but took into consideration the anxiety of a patient having to wait until the age of 55.
- *Low risk*—patients should be reassured and advised to be involved in population screening (FOB test).
- *US guidelines*—differ. A family history of CRC or adenomas in a first-degree relative aged <60 or in two or more relatives of any age, then colonoscopy from age 40 or 10y before the youngest case in the immediate family every 5y.

Box 38.3 CRC by site

Right colon tumours
- Usually become fairly large before giving any obstructive symptoms or causing significant change in bowel habit. Right colon cancers usually ulcerate and cause chronic occult blood loss. Patients frequently present with iron deficiency anaemia and with related symptoms.

Transverse and left colon tumours
- Transverse colon/splenic flexure tumours are uncommon, but may present with change of bowel habit, anaemia, crampy abdominal pain or occasionally obstruction.

Descending colon and sigmoid cancers
- Commonly present with rectal bleeding, abdominal discomfort, change in bowel habit to looser and more frequent motions. Iron deficiency anaemia is uncommon as the initial presentation.

Rectal cancers
- These are defined as cancers where the distal margin lies at 15cm or less from the anal verge using a rigid sigmoidoscope. Tend to present with rectal bleeding and tenesmus as main symptoms.

Box 38.4 High-risk patients

All patients >40y old.
- With rectal bleeding associated with change in bowel habit (looseness or increased bowel frequency) for ≥6wk.

All patients >60y old.
- With change in bowel habits (looseness or increased bowel frequency) for ≥6wk and no PR bleeding.
- With rectal bleeding for ≥6wk and no anal complaints (pain, itching, or lumps) or change in bowel habits.

All patients (any age).
- With palpable right lower abdominal mass.
- With palpable rectal mass (intraluminal and not pelvic).
- With iron deficiency anaemia and Hb <11 (any male) or Hb <10 (any non-menstruating female).

Recommended investigations

- Colonoscopy should be offered to all patients without significant morbidity. Biopsies of any suspicious lesion should be taken if safe to do so. Flexible sigmoidoscopy and barium enema can be considered in patients with major co-morbidity.
- *CT colonography*—is an alternative to colonoscopy when available [A]. The SIGGAR trials show no difference between CT colonography and colonoscopy in sensitivity for CRC.
- *Histologic confirmation*—essential in rectal tumours, and optional in highly suspicious lesions on CT colonography in patients with iron deficiency anaemia and/or symptoms suggestive of cancer.
- *Screening*—cancer screening involves testing an asymptomatic person for cancer. The UK Bowel Cancer Screening programme aims to detect bowel cancer at an early stage or, by removing polyps, preventing bowel cancer from developing in the first place. Currently screening is offered to 60–69 year olds (up to 74 years on request) and uses guaiac-based faecal occult blood test (FOB) followed by colonoscopy if three FOBs positive. The faecal immunochemical test (FIT) is replacing the FOB test due to higher sensitivity. This will increase colonoscopy burden, however. Flexible sigmoidoscopy screening is also currently being implemented in the UK from the age of 55.

Recommended staging

- *Basic investigations*—chest, liver, and pelvis imaging is essential prior to any elective treatment of CRC [B].
- *Thoracic, abdominal, and pelvic CT scan*—should be performed on all patients with CRC [B].
- *Accuracy*—CT scan can demonstrate transmural invasion of tumour with 86% sensitivity, regional lymph nodal involvement with 70%, and distant metastases in 75–90% of cases.
- *Special cases*—complete staging is not necessary if no influence on management is expected. The 18-fluoro-2-deoxyglucose (18-FDG) PET-CT can be used to accurately detect hepatic and extra-hepatic disease. It is used to help difficult interpretation of CT scans.
- *Magnetic resonance imaging (MRI) rectum*—assesses local staging. It provides detailed information of the anticipated resection margin (ability to predict a clear margin 90%), local tumour and lymph node staging in all patients with rectal cancer unless it is contraindicated.
- *Magnetic resonance imaging (MRI) liver*—MRI of the liver is of value in characterizing any indeterminate lesion found on CT. In addition, MRI of the liver can identify liver metastases accurately and is of value in evaluating these lesions if resection or radiofrequency ablation is being considered
- *Decisions are taken in the context of MDT discussion*—essential requirement prior to commencing any definitive staging or treatment.
- *Breaking bad news*—should be done in a professional and effective way. The role of the cancer care nurse is essential [G].
- *TNM staging*—see Table 38.1.

Table 38.1 Classification of resectable rectal cancer

Risk of local recurrence	Characteristics of rectal tumours predicted by MRI
High	• A threatened (<1mm) or breached resection margin or • Low tumours encroaching onto the inter-sphincteric plane or with levator involvement
Moderate	• Any cT3b or greater, in which the potential surgical margin is not threatened or • Any suspicious lymph node not threatening the surgical resection margin or • The presence of extramural vascular invasion [A]
Low	• cT1 or cT2 or cT3a and • No lymph node involvement

Annals of Surgical Oncology, Diagnostic Accuracy of MRI for Assessment of T Category, Lymph Node Metastases, and Circumferential Resection Margin Involvement in Patients with Rectal Cancer: A Systematic Review and Meta-analysis, volume 19, 2012, pp.2212-23, Eisar Al-Sukhni MD, With permission of Springer

Recommended treatment

General principles

- Complete surgical resection of CRC in suitable patients with or without adjuvant/neo-adjuvant therapy represents the best opportunity for long-term survival.
- In general, 70% of CRC patients present with a resectable cancer.
- Complete curative resection is expected to be around 60% overall.
- *In metastatic disease*—chemotherapy alone, or chemotherapy combined with surgery can prolong survival or palliate symptoms.

Standards for surgical resection

- *Perioperative preparation*—see Box 38.5.
- *Extent of cancer resection*.
  - Laparoscopic resection of colon and rectal cancers is well established. Laparoscopic surgery has not shown non-inferiority when compared with open surgery in rectal cancer in pathological outcomes, and takes longer, but blood loss and hospital stay is lower.
  - *Robotic surgery*—early indications are that this is as safe and effective as laparoscopic surgery, with a possible benefit in males and the obese.
  - *Cancers in the right and transverse colon*—best treated using right or extended right hemicolectomy rather than segmental resection. Involved extracolonic organs should be carefully resected (partially or totally) to achieve clear margins as appropriate.
  - *Rectal cancer*—requires total mesorectal excision (TME) for all tumours in the lower two thirds. Rectal cancers in the upper third require a minimum of 5cm mesorectal excision below the lower margin of cancer while preserving the pelvic autonomic nerves [B]. The Trans Anal TME (TATME) is currently being evaluated for low rectal tumours.
  - *Abdominal perineal resection (APR)*—should be considered in operations expected to fail in achieving ≥1cm clearance from the lower limit of the tumour. The APR rate should not exceed 30% of all rectal cancer resections [G]. Hartmann's procedure (see below) is appropriate in some older patients with poor sphincter control. Locally advanced low rectal cancer should undergo extralevator AP excision (ELAPE) [C].
  - *Other issues*—the no-touch isolation technique (vascular control before manipulating the tumour) has no significant effect on outcome. Tumour perforation during surgical manipulation adversely affects the local recurrence rate independent from preoperative cancer stage.
- *Anastomosis*.
  - *Technique*—the lowest anastomotic leak rate can be achieved using interrupted sero-submucosal method [B]. Stapling techniques are used for low pelvic anastomoses [B].
  - *Rectal stump washout*—is highly recommended using cytocidal solution prior to anastomosis [G].
  - *Defunctioning stoma*—should be considered in low rectal anastomosis [B].

Box 38.5 Preoperative preparation in CRC

Preparation for possible stoma formation
- Should be done by a specialist stoma nurse, or in the case of an emergency, by an experienced surgeon who should mark the stoma site [C].

Blood cross-matching
- Recommended in rectal cancer operations and other extensive procedures. Right hemicolectomy requires 'group and save' only [C]. Blood transfusion has no significant effect on cancer recurrence and is indicated where necessary [C].

Bowel preparation
- Not recommended routinely before colonic operations [B]. There is a recommendation for bowel preparation for rectal cancer operations where a diverting ileostomy is to be used.

Thromboembolism prophylaxis
- Using mechanical and pharmaceutical measures is recommended (see ➲ Chapter 12, pp. 123–124) [A].

Antibiotic prophylaxis
- Recommended before any CRC surgery [A].
- The exact regime of antibiotics for best prophylaxis remains unclear. Post-operative surgical site infection rate should not exceed 10% [A].

Enhanced recovery programme (ERP)
- Has gained wide acceptance.
- The programme requires a dedicated team to ensure smooth preoperative planning, appropriate bowel preparation if indicated, avoidance of drains and nasogastric tubes early post-operative mobility, and special diet regime perioperatively (high-calorie drinks preoperatively and rapid diet-and-fluid build-up on day 1post-operatively)

- *Local excision of rectal cancers*—is appropriate for (pathologic staging) T1 tumours, <3cm in diameter, and with well or moderately well differentiated histology [B]. Benefits and risks of local recurrence should be fully discussed with patient.
- *Laparoscopic approach*—should be offered to patients and performed by properly trained surgeons [C]. These procedures are becoming the standard procedure in most units.
- *Emergency surgery for obstructing CRC*—should be preceded by CT scanning to exclude pseudo-obstruction, and is preferably performed during daytime by the colorectal team [C]. Immediate cancer re-section (segmental or subtotal colectomy) with proximal colostomy (Hartmann's) or primary anastomosis (with possible temporary defunctioning ileostomy) is an option [A], as is a defunctioning stoma as a bridge to later resection. Insertion of an expanding stent for palliation or bridging to definitive surgery is also recommended as an alternative. This has similar mortality to surgery, but lower risk of stoma [A].

- *Chemo/radiotherapy in rectal cancer.*
  - *Radiotherapy*—should be considered by the MDT for patients with moderate or high risk rectal cancer (see Table 38.1). Preoperative short-course radiotherapy (25Gy in 5 fractions in 1wk) is recommended in moderate risk rectal cancer, and surgical resection can be performed within 1wk of completion of radiation [A].
  - *Long-course chemoradiotherapy (45–50Gy in 25 fractions over 5wk)*—is used to downstage more locally advanced or low rectal tumours—classified as 'high risk'—and surgery is postponed for an interval (at least 8wk) after finishing the treatment. There is a full re-staging following neo-adjuvant treatment.
  - Complete clinical response after long course chemoradiotherapy is seen in around 16% of cases. A 'watch and wait' policy can be an alternative to radical surgery. The local relapse rate is 34%. Surveillance in patients opting for 'watch and wait 'should be intensive with imaging and endoscopy.
  - *Post-operative radiotherapy*—should be considered for patients who have not received preoperative radiotherapy and have histologic risk factors for local recurrence (e.g. tumour at circumferential resection margins).
- *Chemotherapy.*
  - Should be considered for patients with node-positive colon or rectal cancers. Choices to be jointly made with the patient taking into account contraindications and side-effects. Benefits and risks should also be extensively discussed with patients who have node-negative, but high- risk cancers, i.e. with adverse features (peritoneal involvement, vascular invasion, etc.) [A].
  - *Timing*—should start within 6wk of surgery, and standard treatments with 6mo of 5-fluorouracil (5-FU) and folinic acid (FA) have been updated with capecitabine as monotherapy or oxaliplatin in combination with 5-FU/FA. Where possible, patients should be entered into RCTs as this is a fast developing field with new agents and combinations becoming available.

Early rectal cancer

- There are significant dilemmas about local excision options (TEMS) with or without neo-adjuvant therapy vs radical resection.
- An early rectal cancer MDT should decide treatment.
- Discuss management of stage 1 rectal cancer with patient and relatives including uncertainties about risk/benefit of treatment options, and explaining the lack of good quality evidence.
- Offer patients entry into a trial.

Follow-up

- Remains controversial. Limited evidence exists for intensive follow-up following CRC resection.
- A minimum of 2 CTs of the chest abdomen and pelvis is recommended in the first 3 years.
- CEA estimations should be at least every 6 months in the first 3 years.
- Surveillance colonoscopy at 1 year, followed by 5 yearly colonoscopies, or as determined by findings.

Further reading

The Association of Coloproctology of Great Britain and Ireland (2017). Guidelines for the management of colorectal cancer. Available from www.acpgbi.org.uk/resources

The diagnosis and management of colorectal cancer December 2014 NICE clinical guideline 131 guidance.nice.org.uk/cg131

Scottish Intercollegiate Guidelines Network (2016). Management of colorectal cancer. Available from: http://www.sign.ac.uk/assets/sign126.pdf

Cancer Research UK (2014) About Bowel Cancer – A Quick Guide

Giovannucci E. An updated review of the epidemiological evidence that cigarette smoking increases risk of colorectal cancer. Cancer Epidemiol Biomarkers Prev 2001;10(7):725–31

Giovannucci E, Stampfer MJ, Colditz GA et al. (1998). Multivitamin use, folate, and colon cancer in women in the Nurses' Health Study. Ann Intern Med 129, 517–24.

Matsui T, Yao T, Yao K et al. (1996). Natural history of superficial depressed colorectal cancer: retrospective radiographic and histologic analysis. Radiology 201, 226–32.

Bengtsson G, Carlsson G, Hafström L, Jönsson PE (1981). Natural history of patients with untreated liver metastases from colorectal cancer. Am J Surg 141, 586–9.

Speights VO, Johnson MW, Stoltenberg PH, Rappaport ES, Helbert B, Riggs M (1991). Colorectal cancer: current trends in initial clinical manifestations. South Med J 84, 575–8.

Steinberg SM, Barkin JS, Kaplan RS, Stablein DM (1986). Prognostic indicators of colon tumours. The Gastrointestinal Tumour Study Group experience. Cancer 57, 1866–70.

Niederhuber JE (1993). Colon and rectum cancer: patterns of spread and implications for workup. Cancer 71 (12 Suppl), 4187–92.

Hundt W, Braunschweig R, Reiser M (1999). Evaluation of spiral CT in staging of colon and rectum carcinoma. Eur Radiol 9, 78–84.

Isbister WH, al-Sanea O (1996). The utility of preoperative abdominal computerized tomography scanning in colorectal surgery. J R Coll Surg Edinb 41, 232–4.

Selvachandran SN, Hodder RJ, Ballal MS, Jones P, Cade D (2002). Prediction of colorectal cancer by a patient consultation questionnaire and scoring system: a prospective study. Lancet 360, 278–83.

Renehan AG, Egger M, Saunders MP, O'Dwyer ST (2002). Impact on survival of intensive follow-up after curative resection for colorectal cancer: systematic review and meta-analysis of randomized trials. BMJ 324, 813.

Scholefield JH, Steele RJ, British Society for Gastroenterology, Association of Coloproctology for Great Britain and Ireland (2002). Guidelines for follow-up after resection of colorectal cancer. Gut 51 (Suppl 5), V3–5.

Anthony T, Simmang C, Hyman N et al. (2004). Practice parameters for the surveillance and follow-up of patients with colon and rectal cancer. Dis Colon Rectum 47, 807–17.

Dunlop MG, British Society for Gastroenterology, Association of Coloproctology for Great Britain and Ireland (2002). Guidance on gastrointestinal surveillance for hereditary non-polyposis colorectal cancer, familial adenomatous polyposis, juvenile polyposis, and Peutz–Jeghers syndrome. Gut 51 (Suppl 5), V21–7.

Dunlop MG, British Society for Gastroenterology, Association of Coloproctology for Great Britain and Ireland (2002). Guidance on large bowel surveillance for people with two first- degree relatives with colorectal cancer or one first-degree relative diagnosed with colorectal cancer under 45 years. Gut 51 (Suppl 5), V17–20.

Levin B, Lieberman DA, McFarland B (2008). Screening and surveillance for the early detection of colorectal cancer and adenomatous polyps, 2008: a joint guideline from the American Cancer Society, the US Multi-Society Task Force on Colorectal Cancer, and the American College of Radiology. Gastroenterology 134, 1570–95.

ASGBI Enhanced recovery protocol guidelines 2009

Cairns S, Scholefield JH, Steele RJ, Dunlop MG, Thomas HJ, Evans GD, Eaden JA, Rutter MD, Atkin WP, Saunders BP, Lucassen A, Jenkins P, Fairclough PD, Woodhouse CR; British Society of Gastroenterology; Association of Coloproctology for Great Britain and Ireland. Guidelines for colorectal cancer screening and surveillance in moderate and high risk groups (update from 2002). Gut 2010;59(5):666-89.

Primrose JN, Perera R, Gray A, et al: Effect of 3 to 5 years of scheduled CEA and CT follow-up to detect recurrence of colorectal cancer: The FACS randomized clinical trial. JAMA 311:263-270, 2014.

Al-Sukhni E, Milot L, Fruitman M, Beyene J, Victor JC, Schmocker S, Brown G, McLeod R, Kennedy E . Diagnostic accuracy of MRI for assessment of T category, lymph node metastasis, and circumferential resection margin involvement in patients with rectal cancer: a systematic review and meta-analysis. Ann Surg Oncol. 2012 Jul;19(7):2212-23. Epub 2012 Jan 20.

Health Improvement Scotland. SIGN 126, Diagnosis and management of colorectal cancer. http://www.sign.ac.uk/assets/sign126.pdf.

Part 7

Pancreas

Acute pancreatitis*

Basic facts 372
Recommended treatment 374
Further reading 378

Key guidelines

- International Association of Pancreatology; American Pancreatic Association evidence-based guidelines for the management of acute pancreatitis (2013).
- Working Party of the British Society of Gastroenterology, Association of Surgeons of Great Britain and Ireland, Pancreatic Society of Great Britain and Ireland, Association of Upper GI Surgeons of Great Britain and Ireland (2005). UK guidelines for the management of acute pancreatitis.
- ACG (2013). Management of acute pancreatitis.
- Classification of acute pancreatitis 2012: Revision of the Atlanta classification and definitions by international consensus.

---

* The guidelines on this chapter have been sourced and summarized from different UK, Europe, and international government sources, professional organizations, and medical specialty societies. Leading guidelines have been listed in the further reading section at the end of this chapter

Basic facts

- *Incidence*—30 persons per 100,000 population and appears to be rising.
- *Pathogenesis*—inflammatory process resulting from autodigestion of pancreatic substance by inappropriately activated pancreatic enzymes. Most common causes are obstructing gallstone and alcohol abuse (Box 39.1).
- *Clinical presentation*—typically presents with severe and persistent epigastric or upper abdominal pain radiating through to the back (40–70% of cases), often following the consumption of a large meal, and is associated with nausea, vomiting, and retching. Systemic signs may be prominent in severe cases (Box 39.2).
- *Scoring of severity*—should support the clinical assessment to formulate appropriate management plan [A].
- *Definitions*—severe acute pancreatitis (potentially lethal pancreatitis) is defined as the presence of persistent organ(s) failure and/or local pancreatic complications, (Atlanta).
- *Benefits of predictive scoring*—early prediction of severe cases allows appropriate admission to higher level of care (see Chapter 16, pp.144–150), aggressive fluid management, timely correction of metabolic abnormalities, and possible institution of severity reduction procedures.

Box 39.1 Acute pancreatitis—aetiology

Gallstone disease.

- Accounts for 35–40% of cases (only 3–7% of patients with gallstone develop acute pancreatitis).
- Small stones (<5mm) and male gender increases the risk of developing acute pancreatitis.
- Other obstructive lesions—periampullary tumours, ascariasis, and periampullary diverticula.
- *Alcohol*—accounts for 20–25% of cases (about 10% of chronic alcoholics develop attacks of acute pancreatitis).
- *Other toxic aetiologies*—scorpion venom and organophosphate poisoning.
- *Other causes*—include metabolic (serum triglycerides >11mmol/L*, hypercalcaemia), drug-induced (e.g. steroids, furosemide, thiazides, azathioprine, valproic acid), infection-related (e.g. mumps, CMV, HIV, *Salmonella, Aspergillus, Toxoplasma, Ascaris*), trauma-induced (blunt or penetrating, surgery, ERCP), congenital (pancreas divisum), vascular (ischaemia, vasculitis), genetic (CFTR), other miscellaneous reasons (pregnancy, renal transplantation, cardiac surgery), and idiopathic (only after vigorous search for underlying cause. Should not exceed 20–25% of cases [B]).

* In the absence of gallstones and/or history of significant history of alcohol use, a serum triglyceride should be obtained and considered the aetiology if > 1,000mg/dl. [ACG]

- *First 24h*—severity is best predicted by experienced clinical judgement (initial low accuracy, but equivalent to APACHE II prediction power by 48h), APACHE II score >8 (sensitivity and specificity 70%) (Box 39.3), and obesity [B].
- *At 48h*—severity is best assessed using Glasgow score ≥3 (Box 39.3), CRP >150mg/L, and persistent organ failure [B].
- Other scoring systems—have also been developed and used (APACHE III, APACHE IV, SAPS II, etc.).

Box 39.2 Acute pancreatitis—possible physical findings

- *Local features*—epigastric tenderness, flank discoloration (Grey–Turner's sign) or discolouration in the periumbilical region (Cullen's sign) (<1% of cases, non-diagnostic), epigastric mass (pancreatic pseudocyst).
- *Systemic features*—fever, multiorgan failure, jaundice (gallstone-related or alcoholic liver disease), subcutaneous nodular fat necrosis (panniculitis), thrombophlebitis in the legs, and polyarthritis.

Box 39.3 Severity scoring systems

APACHE II—score
- Check the following parameters:
  - General: age, presence of chronic organ insufficiency.
  - Vital signs: temperature, heart rate, respiratory rate.
  - Basic tests: WCC, Hct, Na, K, Cr.
  - ABG: PH, A-a Gradient, PO_2.
- Calculate APACHE II score using appropriate online tool:
  - https://www.mdcalc.com/apache-ii-score
  - www.medicalcriteria.com/sitei/apacheII.jpg

Glasgow scoring
- Modified Glasgow Criteria.
  - Age >55y.
  - LDH >600 U/L.
  - WCC >15 × 10^9/L.
  - Alb <32 g/L.
  - Urea >16 mmol/L.
  - PaO_2 <8 kPa.
  - Glucose (Blood) >10 mmol/L.
  - Ca <2 mmol/L.
- Score ≥ 3 within 48h is consistent with severe disease.

Recommended treatment

- See Fig. 39.1
- *Level of care*—all patients with severe acute pancreatitis should be treated in a level 2/3 care (HDU or ICU; see Chapter 16, pp.144–150).
- *General supportive treatment*—should follow the care of critically ill surgical patient principles (Box 39.4) (see also Chapter 16).
- *Pain management*—should be effective and multimodal (see ➜ Chapter 21, pp.192–198).
- *Prophylactic antibiotics*—remain of unproven benefits and specific recommendations cannot be made.
  - A Cochrane systematic review suggested that although there was a trend to survival advantage and reduced rate of pancreatic and non-pancreatic infected complications, it did not reach statistical significance. This is consistent with the American College of Gastroenterology Guideline recommendations of not using prophylactic routine antibiotics in patients with severe pancreatitis.
  - Selective gut decontamination is not recommended as there is no clear benefit and no statistically significant reduction in mortality.
- *Nutritional support*—not recommended for mild acute pancreatitis (no restriction on diet and fluid). UK guidelines have made no specific recommendations on nutritional support for severe acute pancreatitis. A more recent meta-analysis and systematic review are also inconsistent with the AGA recommendations of using nutritional support (preferably enteral [A]) to reduce the infection rate (RR ×0.46), length of hospital stay (4d) and possible mortality (RR ×0.26).
- *Treatment of gallstone-related pancreatitis.*
  - *Urgent therapeutic ERCP (within 72h)*—is recommended for all gallstone-related pancreatitis patients who have signs of obstructed bile duct or cholangitis [A]. ERCP is best performed within 72h of the onset of pain, and sphincterotomy should be performed on all those patients regardless of finding a stone [C].
  - *Early laparoscopic cholecystectomy (in the same hospital admission and no more than 2–4wk)*—should be recommended for all fit patients [B].
- *Treatment of complications.*
  - *Infected pancreatic necrosis*—requires fine needle aspiration (FNA) for culture and sensitivity if the necrosis is over 30% [B]. This should be performed in 1–2wk from the onset of pancreatitis [B].
  - *Sterile necrosis*—should be managed conservatively if possible [B]. Surgical intervention should be reserved for individual cases [B].
  - *Septic necrosis*—requires radiological and/or surgical drainage depending on available experience and the individual case [B].
  - *Current surgical options*—should aim at an 'organ-preserving approach'. Options include radiological drainage, percutaneous necrosectomy with closed continuous lavage of the pancreatic bed, laparoscopic necrosectomy with or without cyst gastrostomy, endoscopic drainage or open necrosectomy.
  - *Pancreatic fluid collection and pseudocyst*—can be treated conservatively if remains symptom-free.

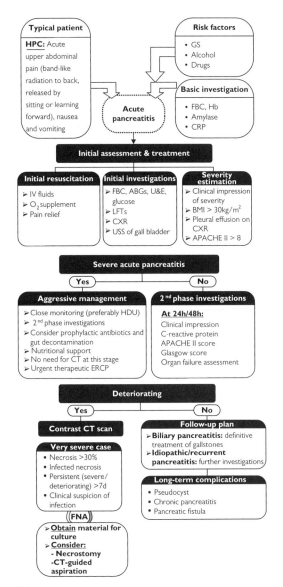

Fig. 39.1 Recommended approach to patients with acute pancreatitis.

Box 39.4 Supportive management—special considerations

- *Oxygen management*—usually required as hypoxia is common. Pleural effusion can be treated conservatively unless affecting pulmonary function.
- *Fluid management*—crystalloids are preferred over colloids. Aggressive fluid resuscitation (even for mild cases) is preferable if no contraindications exist (better outcome). A CVP line may be required if fluid management is compromised by poor cardiac function.
- *Hypocalcaemia*—is common (due to hypoalbuminaemia) and does not require treatment (unless severe or symptomatic).
- *Hypomagnesaemia*—is common.
- *Hypo- or hyperglycaemia*—are common as well.

Further reading

Working Party of the British Society of Gastroenterology, Association of Surgeons of Great Britain and Ireland, Pancreatic Society of Great Britain and Ireland, Association of Upper GI Surgeons of Great Britain and Ireland (2005). UK guidelines for the management of acute pancreatitis. Gut 54 (Suppl 3:iii), 1–9.

National Institute for Health and Clinical Excellence (2003). Percutaneous pancreatic necrostomy. Available from: https://www.nice.org.uk/guidance/ipg384

Forsmark CE, Baillie J; AGA Institute Clinical Practice and Economics Committee, AGA Institute Governing Board (2007). AGA Institute technical review on acute pancreatitis. Gastroenterology 132, 2022–44.

Uhl W, Warshaw A, Imrie C et al. (2002). IAP guidelines for the surgical management of acute pancreatitis. Pancreatology 2, 565–73.

Sanders G, Kingsnorth AN (2007). Gallstones. BMJ 335, 295–9.

Venneman NG, Buskens E, Besselink MG et al. (2005). Small gallstones are associated with increased risk of acute pancreatitis: potential benefits of prophylactic cholecystectomy? Am J Gastroenterol 100, 2540–50.

Tenner S, Dubner H, Steinberg W (1994). Predicting gallstone pancreatitis with laboratory parameters: a meta-analysis. Am J Gastroenterol 89, 1863–6.

Ammann RW, Heitz PU, Klöppel G (1996). Course of alcoholic chronic pancreatitis: a prospective clinicomorphological long term study. Gastroenterology 111, 224–31.

Fortson MR, Freedman SN, Webster PD 3rd (1995). Clinical assessment of hyperlipidaemic pancreatitis. Am J Gastroenterol 90, 2134–9.

Balthazar EJ, Freeny PC, van Sonnenberg E (1994). Imaging and intervention in acute pancreatitis. Radiology 193, 297–306.

Peter A Banks, Thomas L Bollen, Christos Dervenis, et al (2013)Acute Pancreatitis Classification Working Group Classification of acute pancreatitis—2012: revision of the Atlanta classification and definitions by international consensus (Gut) 62, 102-111.

Villatoro E, Bassi C, Larvin M (2010). Antibiotic therapy for prophylaxis against infection of pancreatic necrosis in acute pancreatitis. Cochrane database Syst Rev 5, CD002941.pub3.

Marik PE, Zaloga GP (2004). Meta-analysis of parenteral nutrition versus enteral nutrition in patients with acute pancreatitis. BMJ 328, 1407.

McClave SA, Chang WK, Dhaliwal R, Heyland DK (2006). Nutrition support in acute pancreatitis: a systematic review of the literature. JPEN J Parenter Enteral Nutr 30, 143–56.

Banks PA, Freeman ML, the Practice Parameters Committee of the American College of Gastroenterology (2006). Practice guidelines in acute pancreatitis. Am J Gastroenterol 101, 2379–400.

Luiten EJ, Hop WC, Lange JF, Bruining HA (1995). Controlled clinical trial of selective decontamination for the treatment of severe acute pancreatitis. Ann Surg 222, 57–65.

T S. E. Roberts, A. Akbari, K. Thorne. M. et al (2013) he incidence of acute pancreatitis: impact of social deprivation, alcohol consumption, seasonal and demographic factors AP&T 38, 539-546 18.

Scott Tenner ,John Baillie , John DeWitt et al (2013). American College of Gastroenterology Guideline: Management of Acute Pancreatitis. American J Gastroenterology DOI 10.1038

Hjalmar C. van Santvoort,, Marc G. Besselink, Olaf J. Bakker,(2010). A Step-up Approach or Open Necrosectomy for Necrotizing Pancreatitis NEJM 362, 1491-1502

Chronic pancreatitis*

Basic facts 380
Recommended investigations 382
Recommended treatment 384
Further reading 386

Key guidelines

- Whitcomb DC, Yadav D, Adam S et al. (2008). Multicentre approach to recurrent acute and chronic pancreatitis in the United States: the North American Pancreatitis Study 2 (NAPS2).
- BMJ ABC of diseases (2001). ABC of diseases of liver, pancreas, and biliary system: chronic pancreatitis.
- Society for Surgery of the Alimentary Tract (2013). Operative treatment of chronic pancreatitis. Available from http://ssat.com/guidelines/Chronic-Pancreatitis.cgi.
- National Institute for Health and Care Excellence (2010). Pancreatitis-chronic available from http://cks.nice.org.uk/pancreatitis-chronic.

* The guidelines on this chapter have been sourced and summarized from different UK, Europe, and international government sources, professional organizations, and medical specialty societies. Leading guidelines have been listed in the further reading section at the end of this chapter.

Basic facts

- *Definition*—syndrome characterized by progressive long-standing and irreversible inflammatory changes and/or fibrosis in the pancreas with consequent permanent structural damage and resultant pain and impairment of exocrine and endocrine functions.
- *Incidence*—affects 5–10 persons per 100,000 population per year with a prevalence of 14–33 per 100,000.
- *Risk factors*—see Box 40.1.
- *Clinical manifestations*—commonly presents with abdominal pain (Box 40.2) and pancreatic insufficiency (fat malabsorption, vitamin deficiency, and pancreatic diabetes) at a later stage.
- *Complications*—include pseudocyst formation (10% of cases), bile duct or duodenal obstruction (5–10% of cases), pancreatic ascites or pleural effusion (due to pancreatic fistula or rupture of pseudocyst), splenic vein thrombosis, and pancreatic cancer.

Box 40.1 Risk factors for chronic pancreatitis

- Alcohol abuse—accounts for most cases (70–80%). Other factors play important role in alcohol-induced chronic pancreatitis, e.g. only ~5–10% of alcoholics will suffer from chronic pancreatitis. Cigarette smoking and genetic factors might predispose alcoholics to serious hyper-reaction to alcohol.
- Other risk factors—include hereditary pancreatitis (autosomal dominant trait affecting younger ages and increasing the risk of pancreatic adenocarcinoma), persistent pancreatic ductal obstruction (trauma, pseudocysts, stones, or tumours), tropical pancreatitis. In a few tropical areas, most notably Kerala in southern India, malnutrition and ingestion of large quantities of cassava root are implicated in the aetiology. The disease affects men and women equally, with an incidence of up to 50/1,000 population), systemic diseases (hypertriglyceridemia, hyperparathyroidism, cystic fibrosis, and systemic lupus erythematosus), and idiopathic pancreatitis (majority of cases not related to alcohol abuse). Work on genetic and molecular factors is progressing.

Box 40.2 Pain types in chronic pancreatitis

- Type A pain—short episodes of <10d separated by long pain-free intervals. Predominant pattern in idiopathic senile or late onset chronic pancreatitis (ISCP) and hereditary pancreatitis. Can successfully be managed without invasive procedures.
- Type B pain—≥1–2mo intermittent intervals. Occurs in ~60% of idiopathic juvenile or early onset chronic pancreatitis (IJCP). Usually requires surgery and is commonly associated with local complications (e.g. pseudocysts and obstructive cholestasis). This has a major implication on the widespread recommendation of endoscopic therapy in chronic pancreatitis.

Recommended investigations

- See Fig. 40.1.
- *Confirmation of diagnosis*—can be challenging. Clinical manifestations may be atypical, laboratory tests may be normal, and imaging investigations might be inconclusive. A proper combination of clinical, functional, histologic, or morphologic criteria can be helpful (Box 40.3). The diagnosis has often to be made on the exclusion of other diseases.

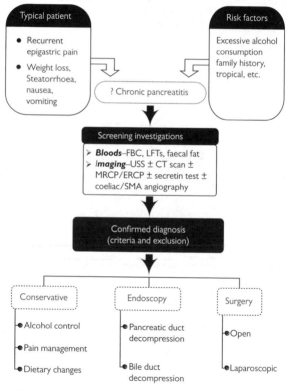

Fig. 40.1 An algorithm showing the steps in approaching patients with chronic pancreatitis.

Box 40.3 Diagnosis of chronic pancreatitis

- *Confirmed chronic pancreatitis (within appropriate clinical setting)*—
  presence of pancreatic stones on screening KUB, USS, or CT scan;
  scattered irregular dilatation of pancreatic duct branches (chain of
  lakes) or main duct with proximal obstruction on ERCP/MRCP;
  decreased pancreatic enzyme and bicarbonate output on secretin
  test; irregular fibrosis and loss of exocrine parenchyma on histologic
  examination; and/or the presence of protein plugs or cyst formation.
- *Probably chronic pancreatitis*—coarse hyper-reflectivity on USS;
  pancreatic deformity on CT scan; irregular isolated dilatation on
  ERCP; decreased pancreatic enzyme or bicarbonate output on
  secretin test; and atypical chronic changes on histologic specimens.

Recommended treatment

- See Fig. 40.1.
- As a general rule, a multidisciplinary approach is required to treat chronic pancreatitis, preferably in specialist centres.
- *Objectives*—management of excessive alcohol consumption, pain relief, correction of pancreatic insufficiency, and management of complications.
- *Alcohol consumption*—should be avoided as a first step (consensus opinion). Stopping alcohol consumption has clear benefits and can prevent further injury to the pancreas and other organs.
- *Smoking cessation*—smoking is an established but under-recognized risk factor for chronic pancreatitis. It is an equally potent cause of chronic pancreatitis as alcohol and the combination of alcohol and smoking particularly toxic.
- *Pain management*—follow a stepwise approach with judicious use of analgesics. (See Chapter 21). Placebo effect has significant role in those patients (effective in up to 30% of cases).
- *Tramadol*—more effective than morphine at reducing pain within 4d, but is associated with more adverse gastrointestinal effects.
- *Coeliac plexus block/ablation*—reserved for patients with refractory pain to opioid analgesics. Supportive evidence of consistent efficiency is weak. Best performed on patients with small duct pancreatitis (large duct patients may benefit more from surgical drainage as a last option). Using endoscopic ultrasound-guided plexus block/ablation may be more effective in managing the pain at 4wk compared with CT-guided nerve blocks.
- *Dietary changes*.
  - *Low-fat diet*—there is no supporting evidence of any significant beneficial effect on pain management or progression of chronic pancreatitis. A low-fat diet may help in alleviating steatorrhoea by decreasing the overall amount of ingested fat.
  - *Pancreatic enzyme supplement*—not been shown to be more effective when compared with placebo in reducing the pain at 2–32wk of follow-up. Pancreatic enzyme supplements have a significant effect in reducing steatorrhoea.
  - *Oral citrate*—is less effective than placebo in reducing pain at 18mo. However, it is more effective at reducing the calcification within the same time period.
- *Endoscopic procedures*.
  - *Endoscopic pancreatic duct decompression*—is recommended as the first-line therapy for painful, uncomplicated, chronic pancreatitis and has been shown to be effective in reducing pain in 60–70% of patients when done selectively. Obstructive calcification in the head of pancreas, short disease duration, low frequency of pain attacks as well as discontinuation of alcohol and tobacco are predictive factors for long-term pain relief following endoscopic decompression. It has a relatively quick recovery, but has slightly lower results compared to surgery in controlling the pain and helping in gaining weight. However, views have been expressed that the quality of studies

has been limited and the benefits limited, with further evidence from a recent randomized trial showing better results with surgical procedures.

- *Endoscopic biliary duct decompression*—may be required in 5–10% of patients to treat jaundice and prevent cholangitis. It is recommended in the case of biliary stones, progressive biliary stricture, or cases of secondary biliary cirrhosis

- *Surgical interventions.*
  - *Indications*—usually reserved for patients with complications, patients who failed to control symptoms with adequate analgesia and/or endoscopic measures, and patients who would prefer to avoid the risk of addiction to opioid analgesia.
  - *Benefits*—with careful selection, can control the pain in 75% of patients who failed endoscopic procedures and increase the body weight at 5y follow-up.
  - *Harm*—no significant difference in complication rates compared to endoscopic procedures.
  - *Technique*—most common are the duodenal preserving resection of the pancreatic head (Beger's procedure) and Frey's ductal decompression (pancreatico-jejunostomy). There is no significant difference in outcome between the two procedures. Occasionally total and subtotal pancreatectomies are necessary. NICE have supported laparoscopic distal pancreatectomy under careful clinical governance conditions.

Further reading

Whitcomb DC, Yadav D, Adam S et al. (2008). Multicentre approach to recurrent acute and chronic pancreatitis in the United States: the North American Pancreatitis Study 2 (NAPS2). Pancreatology 8, 520–31.

Bornman PC, Beckingham IJ (2001). ABC of diseases of liver, pancreas, and biliary system: chronic pancreatitis. BMJ 322, 660–3.

Etemad B, Whitcomb DC (2001). Chronic pancreatitis: diagnosis, classification, and new genetic developments. Gastroenterology 120, 682–707.

Society for Surgery of the Alimentary Tract (2013). Operative treatment for chronic pancreatitis available from http://ssat.com/guidelines/Chronic-Pancreatitis.cgi

National Institute for Health and Care Excellence (2010) Pancreatitis-chronic available from http://cks.nice.org.uk/pancreatitis-chronic

Kocher HM, Froeling FE (2011). Chronic pancreatitis. BMJ Clin Evid (online) Dec 21;2011 pii0417

Maisonneuve P, Lowenfels AB, Mullhaupt B et al. (2005). Cigarette smoking accelerates progression of alcoholic chronic pancreatitis. Gut 54, 510–4.

DiMagno MJ, DiMagno EP (2006). Chronic pancreatitis. Curr Opin Gastroenterol 22, 487–97.

Homma T, Harada H, Koizumi M (1997). Diagnostic criteria for chronic pancreatitis by the Japan Pancreas Society. Pancreas 15, 14–5.

Warshaw AL, Banks PA, Fernández-Del Castillo C (1998). AGA technical review: treatment of pain in chronic pancreatitis. Gastroenterology 115, 765–76.

Gress F, Schmitt C, Sherman S, Ikenberry S, Lehman G (1999). A prospective randomized comparison of endoscopic ultrasound and computed tomography-guided coeliac plexus block for managing chronic pancreatitis pain. Am J Gastroenterol 94, 900–5

Endoscopic treatment of chronic pancreatitis:European Society of Gastrointestinal Endoscopy (ESGE), Clinical Guideline

Rösch T, Daniel S, Scholz M et al. (2002). Endoscopic treatment of chronic pancreatitis: a multicentre study of 1,000 patients with long-term follow-up. Endoscopy 34, 765–71.

Cahen DL, Gouma DJ, Nio Y et al. (2007). Endoscopic versus surgical drainage of the pancreatic duct in chronic pancreatitis. N Engl J Med 356, 676–84.

Strate T, Taherpour Z, Bloechle C, et al (2005) Long-term follow-up of a randomized trial comparing the beger and frey procedures for patients suffering from chronic pancreatitis. Ann Surg. Apr; 241(4):591-8.

National Institute for Health and Clinical Excellence (2007). Laparoscopic distal pancreatectomy. Available from: http://www.nice.org.uk/nicemedia/pdf/IPG204guidance.pdf.

Pancreatic cancer*

Basic facts *388*
Recommended investigations *390*
Recommended initial assessment *392*
Recommended further investigations *394*
Recommended treatment *396*
Further reading *398*

Key guidelines

- European Society for Medical Oncology (2015). Cancer of the Pancreas: ESMO Clinical Practice Guidelines.
- National Comprehensive Cancer Network (2011). Practice guidelines in oncology for pancreatic adenocarcinoma.
- Cancer Research UK (2014). Pancreatic cancer.

---

* The guidelines on this chapter have been sourced and summarized from different UK, Europe, and international government sources, professional organizations, and medical specialty societies. Leading guidelines have been listed in the further reading section at the end of this chapter.

Basic facts

- *Incidence*— the tenth most common cancer in the UK but fifth most common cause of cancer death. The majority of cases are diagnosed after the age of 65. Incidence in the UK is fairly stable at 10.8 and 8.7 new cases per 100,000 of the population in men and women, respectively. Periampullary carcinomas and distal cholangiocarcinomas are less common, but may present with the same symptoms. Neuroendocrine tumours of the pancreas are not considered in this chapter. (See ⮕ Chapter 31, PP. 296–302).
- *Risk factors*—smoking accounts for 1 in every 5 cases of pancreatic cancer. Other risk factors include chronic pancreatitis (RR ×13.3) type 1 or 2 diabetes, obesity, and familial cancers (Box 41.1). Underlying pancreatic cancer should be excluded in adult onset of non-familial diabetes and in unexplained attack of pancreatitis (5% of pancreatic cancer presentations).
- *Pathology*— pancreatic ductal adenocarcinoma accounts for >80% of pancreatic neoplasms of which 75% occur in the head or neck of the pancreas. The majority (80%) exhibit KRAS mutations and develop from premalignant pancreatic intraepithelial neoplasms (PanINs). Other common mutations are seen in the *CDKN2* gene, tumour suppressor p53, and SMAD4. Each pancreatic cancer has on average over 60 genetic mutations.
- *Clinical presentation*— presentation varies dependent on tumour size and location. Tumours of the head and neck may present with jaundice due to biliary obstruction. Many patients with pancreatic cancer report non-specific symptoms such as back pain and dysphagia up to a year before diagnosis. Both endocrine (new-onset diabetes) and exocrine (pancreatic exocrine insufficiency) disturbances may be present. Weight loss is a frequent presenting symptom. Only 15–20% of new diagnoses can be treated with curative intent (Box 41.2).

Box 41.1 Risk factors for pancreatic cancer

- *Smoking*—very important risk factor (RR ×1.4–2.4). Smoking accounts for 25–30% of cases, and risk reduces by 48% within 2y of stopping smoking
- *Genetic susceptibility*—has a role in 10% of patients. Risk increases in families with hereditary pancreatitis (RR ×50–70), familial pancreatic cancer (OR ×1.5–5.25), and other familial-related cancers (familial atypical multiple mole melanoma, Peutz–Jeghers syndrome, hereditary non-polyposis colorectal carcinoma (HNPCC), familial breast-ovarian cancer syndromes, and familial adenomatous polyposis (FAP).
- *Medical diseases*—include chronic pancreatitis (RR ×5–15), adult onset diabetes of <2y duration (RR ×2.1) and obesity.
- *Other factors*—of unproven correlation, includes diet (high fat and protein, low fruit and vegetable intake), coffee and alcohol consumption, and occupation
- *Primary prevention*—includes educational programmes in smoking cessation, the role of secondary screening for high-risk patients is not yet established.

Box 41.2 Symptoms and signs of pancreatic cancer

- *Main symptoms*—weight loss (90–100% of cases at presentation), abdominal pain (70–85% of cases), and jaundice (82% of cancers in the head and 7% of cancers in the body and tail).
  - *Other symptoms*—include nausea (45%), anorexia (33–66%), malaise (40%), and vomiting (35%).
  - *Advanced disease*—may present with back pain, marked and rapid weight loss, abdominal mass, migratory thrombophlebitis, ascites, and supraclavicular lymphadenopathy.
- *Physical examination*—may be non-specific.
  - *Courvoisier's sign*—distended, palpable, but non-tender gall bladder in a jaundiced patient.
  - *Lymphadenopathies*—are late signs in pancreatic cancer. Left supraclavicular (Virchow's node) or umbilical (Sister Mary Joseph's nodule), and recurring superficial thrombophlebitis (Trousseau's sign).
  - *Other findings*—tender enlarged liver, ascites, palmar erythema, and spider angioma.

Recommended investigations

- *Abdominal USS*—a useful initial investigation for jaundiced patients but has been superseded by more advanced techniques for pancreatic imaging. Is user dependent and images of the pancreas (particularly the body and tail) may be obscured by overlying structures.
- *MD-CT/MRI*—contrast enhanced multi-detector computerized tomography (MD-CT) or MR imaging are the modalities of choice to investigate pancreatic masses. Both provide additional information on tumour size, infiltration, resectability, and the presence of metastatic disease. MRCP is useful for further investigation of the biliary tree.
- *Tissue diagnosis*—is not considered necessary in the presence of highly suspicious imaging findings for pancreatic cancer amenable to surgical resection. Equivocal findings are best investigated with EUS; transperitoneal techniques should be avoided in potentially resectable cancers due to the risk of seeding. In locally advanced or metastatic patients tissue diagnosis may guide chemotherapeutic selection.
- *Serum markers*—although a number may be raised with pancreatic cancer, none are diagnostic. The most useful of them is the carbohydrate antigen 19-9 (CA 19-9). However, CA 19-9 levels may be raised secondary to obstructive jaundice, chronic pancreatitis, and biliary or gastrointestinal cancers. Therefore, CA 19-9 is not recommended as a screening test for pancreatic cancer. It may have a role to play in assessing treatment response/ relapse.

Recommended initial assessment

- See Fig. 41.1.
- *Resectability*—metastatic disease or locally advanced disease (major arterial involvement) are contraindications to curative surgery. Resectability should be assessed according to NCCN criteria (see https://academic.oup.com/view-large/35533906/Cancer%20of%20 the%20pancreas:%20ESMO%20Clinical%20Practice%20Guidelines%20 for%20diagnosis,%20treatment%20and%20follow-up†).
- *Surgical fitness*—despite improvements in post-operative care and surgical technique, mortality following a major pancreatic resections is up to 5%, careful patient selection is therefore of paramount importance. In the elderly or patient with significant co-morbidities cardiopulmonary exercise (CPEX) testing may help to objectively assess fitness for surgery.
- *MDT discussion*—an essential requirement prior to commencing any definitive staging or treatment. Decisions are taken in the context of predicted prognosis and expected effect of any investigation or treatment intervention on quality of life. The MDT team should typically include physicians, surgeons, oncologists, radiologists, histopathologists, specialist nurses, research personnel (for clinical trials), and representatives from palliative care, and nutritional services.
- *Breaking bad news*—an essential step to ensure adequate compliance. Should be done in a professional and effective way and ideally with a specialist cancer care nurse present. Confirmation of diagnosis, treatment options, expected perioperative period experience, contact details, and sources for further information (including patient support groups) should all be discussed. This discussion should be documented and communicated to other members of the team (e.g. GP, oncologists, and cancer care nurses).

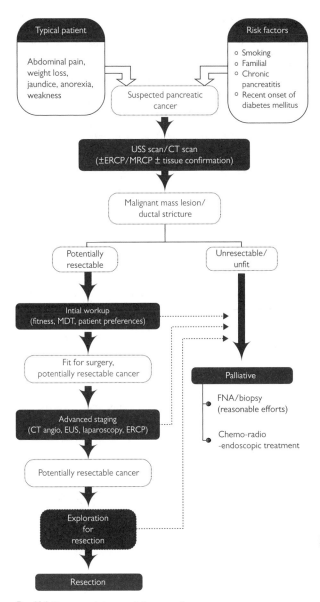

Fig. 41.1 Recommended approach for pancreatic cancer.

Recommended further investigations

- *MD-CT*—of the thorax is recommended to assess for lung metastases that would rule out curative surgery.
- *PET-CT* may improve sensitivity and specificity of staging and influence management of patients. It may soon be recommended for routine use.
- *EUS*.
  - *Indications*—to assess pancreatic masses of unknown pathology and in some cases assess resectability. It is the modality of choice for obtaining biopsy or fine needle aspiration cytology samples. Results vary between centres, reflecting in part differences in the standards against which EUS is compared and also expertise.
  - *Benefits*—ideal for the assessment of small tumours (<2cm in diameter), lymph node metastases, and involvement of the portal venous system, with an accuracy reaching 94–100% in some series. Fluid aspirate can be sent for CEA and amylase to aid the diagnosis of pancreatic cystic lesions.
- *Laparoscopy*—diagnostic laparoscopy including laparoscopic ultrasound, can detect occult metastatic lesions in the liver and peritoneal cavity which have not been identified by other imaging modalities. In some patients this will prevent futile laparotomy but should be used selectively where available.
- *ERCP*.
  - *Indications*—therapeutic intervention in biliary obstruction. In the pre-operative setting it is only indicated for the relief of jaundice if surgery cannot be performed expeditiously. ERCP does have a role to play in obtaining histological samples for periampullary masses and biliary strictures where pathology is uncertain.
  - *Delayed operation*—should not routinely be used for relief of jaundice prior to resection. However, if definitive surgery must be delayed for more than 10d, biliary drainage should be performed and the operation should be delayed for 3–6wk to allow the jaundice to resolve.
  - *Surgical incurable cases*—short metal stents can relieve the symptoms of obstructive jaundice effectively in advanced cancer cases and are recommended in patients with >3mo life expectancy as they need to be changed less frequently than plastic stents.
- *Cancer staging*—based on the International Union Against Cancer (UICC) tumour node metastasis (TNM) classification (2010).

Recommended treatment

- *Surgery.*
  - *Resection with intent to cure*—should be recommended for patients with localized tumours, who are fit enough to tolerate major surgery. Pancreatic resections should only take place in a specialist centre with appropriate workload to maximize benefits and minimize harm. The aim of surgery is to achieve an R0 resection as this has been shown to confer significant survival advantages.
- *Standards for surgical resection.*
  - *Options*—include proximal pancreaticoduodenectomy with antrectomy (Kausch–Whipple procedure), pylorus preserving pancreaticoduodenectomy, total pancreaticoduodenectomy, and left (distal) pancreatectomy.
  - *Kausch–Whipple procedure*—involves resection of the pancreatic head, duodenum, first part of the jejunum, common bile duct, and gall bladder (with partial gastrectomy). Anastomoses are performed between the pancreas, biliary tree (bile duct bypass is preferable to gall bladder bypass), and the gastrointestinal tract. Portal vein involvement is no longer a contraindication to resection provided clear margins can still be obtained. Involvement of the splenic vein or artery is not considered a contraindication for resection.
  - *Laparoscopic pancreatic surgery*—although not routine, current evidence is adequate to support the use of this procedure within appropriate clinical governance framework.
- *Chemotherapy.*
  - *Adjuvant*—all patients should be offered postoperative chemotherapy. The combination of gemcitabine (GEM) and capecitabine is recommended on the basis of the ESPAC-4 randomized trial (A). Adjuvant chemoradiation is popular in the USA but within Europe, on the basis of the ESPAC-1 trial, chemoradiation in the adjuvant or additive setting should only be performed within randomized controlled clinical trials (B).
  - *Neoadjuvant*—some studies suggest a benefit of neoadjuvant therapy in patients with borderline resectable pancreatic cancer but currently this treatment should only be used in the context of a clinical trial.

Recommendation for palliative treatment

- *Palliative chemotherapy*— FOLFIRINOX should be offered to patients with Eastern Cooperative Oncology Group (ECOG) performance status 0-1. Gemcitabine should be considered for people not well enough to tolerate FOLFIRINOX.
- *Pancreatic endocrine insufficiency (PEI)*—all patients with blockage of the main pancreatic duct (due to tumour or stent) will have PEI and benefit from enzyme replacement.

- *Interventional options.*
  - *Palliative duodenal bypass surgery*—should be considered to relieve symptoms of duodenal obstruction.
  - *Endoscopic stent placement*—is indicated to relieve obstructive jaundice and is preferable over percutaneous stenting, and also can be used to stent duodenal obstruction.
  - Percutaneous transhepatic biliary draining—is indicated to relieve obstructive jaundice when endoscopic methods have failed. It is usually reserved for more proximal biliary obstruction.
- *Pain management*—pain is a frequent and disabling symptom of pancreatic cancer and responds best to opioid analgesia.
- *Other measures*—include nutrition and involvement of palliative care physicians.

Further reading

Lynch SM, Vrieling A, Lubin JH, et al. Cigarette smoking and pancreatic cancer: a pooled analysis from the pancreatic cancer cohort consortium. American journal of epidemiology 2009; 170(4): 403–13.

CRUK. Pancreatic Cancer Key Facts June 2014 2014. http://publications.cancerresearchuk.org/cancerstats/statspancreas/keyfactspancreas.html. (accessed 21st August 2014).

Micames C, Jowell PS, White R, et al. Lower frequency of peritoneal carcinomatosis in patients with pancreatic cancer diagnosed by EUS-guided FNA vs. percutaneous FNA. Gastrointestinal endoscopy 2003; 58(5): 690–5.

CRUK. Cancer Incidence in the UK in 2011. 2014. http://publications.cancerresearchuk.org/downloads/Product/CS_REPORT_INCIDENCE.pdf (accessed 21st August 2014).

Klein AP, Hruban RH, Brune KA, Petersen GM, Goggins M. Familial pancreatic cancer. Cancer journal 2001; 7(4): 266–73.

Cancer of the Pancreas: ESMO Clinical Practice Guidelines (2015). Available from http://www.esmo.org/Guidelines/Gastrointestinal-Cancers/Cancer-of-the-Pancreas

Raimondi S, Lowenfels AB, Morselli-Labate AM, Maisonneuve P, Pezzilli R. Pancreatic cancer in chronic pancreatitis; aetiology, incidence, and early detection. Best Pract Res Clin Gastroenterol 2010; 24(3): 349–58.

Renehan AG, Tyson M, Egger M, Heller RF, Zwahlen M. Body-mass index and incidence of cancer: a systematic review and meta-analysis of prospective observational studies. Lancet 2008; 371(9612): 569–78.

Huxley R, Ansary-Moghaddam A, Berrington de Gonzalez A, Barzi F, Woodward M. Type-II diabetes and pancreatic cancer: a meta-analysis of 36 studies. British journal of cancer 2005; 92(11): 2076–83.

Larsson SC, Wolk A. Red and processed meat consumption and risk of pancreatic cancer: meta-analysis of prospective studies. British journal of cancer 2012; 106(3): 603–7.

Everhart J, Wright D. Diabetes mellitus as a risk factor for pancreatic cancer. A meta-analysis. Jama 1995; 273(20): 1605–9.

NHS treated cancer patients receiving major surgical resections. Major Surgical Resections 2004–2006. Online: National Cancer Intelligence Network; 2011.

National Comprehensive Cancer Network. Practice Guidelines in Oncology for Pancreatic Adenocarcinoma. 2011.

Neoptolemos JP, Russell RC, Bramhall S, Theis B. Low mortality following resection for pancreatic and periampullary tumours in 1026 patients: UK survey of specialist pancreatic units. UK Pancreatic Cancer Group. The British journal of surgery 1997; 84(10): 1370–6.

Snowden CP, Prentis JM, Anderson HL, et al. Submaximal cardiopulmonary exercise testing predicts complications and hospital length of stay in patients undergoing major elective surgery. Ann Surg 2010; 251(3): 535–41.

Pisters PW, Lee JE, Vauthey JN, Charnsangavej C, Evans DB. Laparoscopy in the staging of pancreatic cancer. The British journal of surgery 2001; 88(3): 325–37.

van der Gaag NA, Rauws EA, van Eijck CH, et al. Preoperative biliary drainage for cancer of the head of the pancreas. N Engl J Med 2010; 362(2): 129–37.

Birkmeyer JD, Siewers AE, Finlayson EV, et al. Hospital volume and surgical mortality in the United States. N Engl J Med 2002; 346(15): 1128–37.

Verbeke CS, Leitch D, Menon KV, McMahon MJ, Guillou PJ, Anthoney A. Redefining the R1 resection in pancreatic cancer. The British journal of surgery 2006; 93(10): 1232–7.

Neoptolemos JP, Stocken DD, Bassi C, et al. Adjuvant chemotherapy with fluorouracil plus folinic acid vs gemcitabine following pancreatic cancer resection: a randomized controlled trial. JAMA 2010; 304(10): 1073–81.

Neoptolemos JP, Stocken DD, Friess H, et al. A randomized trial of chemoradiotherapy and chemotherapy after resection of pancreatic cancer. N Engl J Med 2004; 350(12): 1200–10.

Oettle H, Post S, Neuhaus P, et al. Adjuvant chemotherapy with gemcitabine vs observation in patients undergoing curative-intent resection of pancreatic cancer: a randomized controlled trial. JAMA 2007; 297(3): 267–77.

Sultana A, Smith CT, Cunningham D, Starling N, Neoptolemos JP, Ghaneh P. Meta-analyses of chemotherapy for locally advanced and metastatic pancreatic cancer. Journal of clinical oncology : official journal of the American Society of Clinical Oncology 2007; 25(18): 2607–15.

Conroy T, Desseigne F, Ychou M, et al. FOLFIRINOX versus gemcitabine for metastatic pancreatic cancer. N Engl J Med 2011; 364(19): 1817–25.

Neoptolemos JP, Palmer DH, Ghaneh P, et al. Comparison of adjuvant gemcitabine and capecitabine with gemcitabine monotherapy in patients with resected pancreatic cancer (ESPAC-4): a multicentre, open-label, randomised, phase 3 trial. Lancet. 2017 Mar 11;389(10073):1011–1024

Part 8

Hepatobiliary

Gallstone disease*

Basic facts *402*
Recommended investigations *404*
Recommended treatment *406*
Other issues to consider *410*
Management of common bile duct stones *412*
Further reading *414*

Key guidelines

- National Institute for Health and Clinical Excellence (2014). Gallstone disease.
- BMJ Clinical Review (2007). Gallstones.
- BMJ Clinical Evidence (2008). Acute cholecystitis.
- The Society for Surgery of the Alimentary Tract (2006). Treatment of gallstone and gall bladder disease.

---

* The guidelines on this chapter have been sourced and summarized from different UK, Europe, and international government sources, professional organizations, and medical specialty societies. Leading guidelines have been listed in the further reading section at the end of this chapter.

Basic facts

- *Incidence*—very common and costly medical condition in developed countries. The estimated prevalence is ~15% of adults with a female to male ratio of ~2:1. Over 5 million people have gallstones in the UK, resulting in over 50,000 cholecystectomy operations performed each year.
- *Pathogenesis*—failure to maintain biliary solutes, primarily cholesterol, and calcium salts in a solubilized state (Box 42.1).
- *Clinical presentation*.
  - *Incidental (asymptomatic) gallstones*—can be found unexpectedly on USS during evaluation for abdominal pain, pelvic diseases, or abnormal LFTs.
  - *Biliary colic*—usually results from a stone or sludge being forced against the gall bladder outlet (or cystic duct) during contraction of the gall bladder
  - *Cholecystitis*—inflammation of the gallbladder (Box 42.2).
  - *Atypical symptoms*—uncommon presentation. May present with non-specific abdominal pain, fat intolerance, nausea, and early satiety. These symptoms may be due to chronic dysfunction of the gall bladder (chronic cholecystitis). However, in the majority, such symptoms are unlikely to be due to gall bladder disease, even in the presence of gall bladder stones. The less consistent the symptoms are with biliary colic, the higher the likelihood that they will not respond to cholecystectomy.
  - *Complications*—the initial presentation may be with a complication. Examples include acute pancreatitis due to small stones, cholangitis, or obstructive jaundice in the elderly due to a large bile duct stone.

Box 42.1 Risk factors

Patient demographics.
- *Age*—major risk factor. The incidence increases significantly after the age of 40.
- *Females*—much more affected than males. The female to male ratio is 2.9:1 in patients younger than 40, and 1.2:1 in patients over the age of 50.
- *Ethnicity*—Western Caucasian, Hispanic, and Native Americans.

Reproductive factors.
- *Pregnancy*—established risk factor for cholesterol gallstones. More common in multiparous patients (12%) compared to nulliparous (1.3%). Following delivery, over 30% of small gallstones (<10mm) found during pregnancy disappear completely.
- *Oestrogen replacement therapy*—increases the risk of developing symptomatic gallstone disease by about 3.7 times compared to non-users. Cholecystectomy rate in HRT is significantly higher (RR ×2.1).
- *Oral contraceptives*—increase slightly the risk of gallstone formation at the beginning of its use.

Medical conditions.
- *Obesity (BMI >30)*—established risk factor for cholesterol gallstones (up to 3-fold increase in risk).
- *Rapid weight loss*—gallstones occur in ~35% of patients after proximal gastric bypass, and other types of bariatric surgery.

Box 42.2 Clinical features of biliary colic
- Dull pressure-like discomfort.
- Sudden onset in epigastrium or right upper quadrant. May radiate round to the back and right shoulder blade.
- Persists from 15min up to 24h, and subsides spontaneously or with opioid analgesics.
- Accompanied by nausea or vomiting.
- Classically occurs 1–2h following the ingestion of fatty meals, and occurs in a characteristic pattern and timing known to the individual patient.
- Pain does not usually change with movement, squatting, passing of flatus or faeces.

Recommended investigations

- *USS*—the initial investigation of choice in clinically suspected gallstone disease [C]. USS is a non-invasive, relatively inexpensive, and safe modality (Box 42.3).
- *Other imaging modalities (suchas MRCP scan, EUS)*—may be required in some occasions, where no objective evidence of gallstones is found despite the presence of classic biliary pain.

Box 42.3 USS for gallstones

- *Accuracy*—can identify gallstones with a sensitivity ranging from 76 to 99% (average 84%) and specificity of 99% (95% CI 97–100%).
- *Findings*—gallstones present with acoustic 'shadowing' of opacities lying within the gall bladder lumen and typically change with the patient's position (gravitational dependency).
- Gall bladder sludge is an echogenic shadow that has no acoustic shadow, more viscous than surrounding bile, and does not move with the change in a patient's position.
- *Preparation*—patients should keep fasting (ideally >8h) to allow the gall bladder to be at its maximum distension. The examiner should use both sagittal and axial planes to visualize the gall bladder, and should look specifically at Hartmann's pouch as well as at the cystic duct down to the porta hepatis. CBD and peri-gall bladder spaces should all be examined thoroughly.

Recommended treatment

- *General approach.*
  - The pure finding of gallstones on USS does not confirm the diagnosis of gallstone-related pain unless it has been associated with a proper clinical scenario (see Fig. 42.1).
- *Asymptomatic gallstones.*
  - *Reassurance*—asymptomatic gallstones can be safely managed conservatively. Surgical removal is not recommended [C].
  - *Natural history*—the majority of patients remain asymptomatic over the years. The risk of developing symptoms is 1–4% per year, and when symptoms occur, they usually present with a self-limiting biliary colic rather than a life-threatening major complication.
  - *Prophylactic cholecystectomy*—diabetic patients have a higher risk of developing severe complications, but no data support the benefits of prophylactic cholecystectomy in this group. However, prompt surgery is recommended if symptoms develop. Prophylactic cholecystectomy is practised in patients living in endemic regions to reduce the gall bladder cancer risk (e.g. Peru). There is no guidance for prophylactic cholecystectomy in the UK
  - *Gall bladder cancer*—the risk in the presence of gallstones is <0.01%. The risk is higher in certain cases such as the presence of porcelain gall bladder (25% risk), gall bladder adenoma (larger polyps greater than 1cm are more likely to contain foci of invasive cancer), and in certain ethnic groups and endemic regions. Prophylactic cholecystectomy is recommended in such individual cases for this reason.
- *Symptomatic gallstones.*
  - *Biliary colic*—the management is mainly directed at relieving pain. (Box 42.4).
  - *Medical curative treatment of gallstones*—can be used in carefully selected patients with a functioning gall bladder and radiolucent stones <10mm in diameter. Complete dissolution occurs in ~50% of such patients within 6mo to 2y with ursodeoxycholic acid (UDCA). However stone recurrence is high This practice is most commonly used in the USA in post-bariatric surgery patients (as a prophylactic measure) as these patients are at increased risk of developing gallstones but is not routine practice in the UK as there is no evidence of benefit. [B].
- *Laparoscopic cholecystectomy*—is the gold standard treatment for the majority of patients with symptomatic disease [B].
  - *Natural history*—about 70% of patients with symptomatic gallstones are expected to develop further symptoms or complications within 2y of initial presentation. Life-threatening complications are very uncommon in mildly symptomatic patients, and ~30% of patients may not experience any more episodes of biliary colic or complications in the long term.
  - *Benefits*—laparoscopic cholecystectomy is a cost-effective treatment option for patients with symptomatic gallstones who are willing to prevent another episode of pain in the future. The procedure has a low rate of complication (2–4%), bile duct injury (0.3–0.8%),

bile leak (~1%), retained stone(s) (2–3%), and mortality (<0.1%), and it is effective in completely relieving the biliary colic in over 90% of patients. Laparoscopic cholecystectomy is now increasingly performed as a day case procedure.

- *Side-effects*—commonly accepted to have no long-lasting physiologic effects, but can cause increased frequency of less formed stool in 750% of patients in some studies; 10–15% develop post-cholecystectomy syndrome.
- *Decision-making*—the decision between immediate intervention and expectant management in patients not keen on taking the risk of surgery to prevent another pain attack may become a matter of personal choice or convenience.
- *Open cholecystectomy*—Open surgery has been shown to have no significant difference in terms of long-term complications and mortality rate compared to the laparoscopic approach. Open cholecystectomy is only indicated as a conversion procedure for difficult laparoscopic procedure or may be entertained in certain individual cases (e.g. repair of a fistula from the gall bladder into the bile duct or intestine, and perforation and abscess formation) if the procedure cannot be done laparoscopically.

Box 42.4 Management of biliary colic

- Clear/free fluids
- *Analgesia*—best achieved by:
  - Opiods if required are safe and there is no evidence that morphine should not be used due to effects on sphincter of Oddi motility.
  - *NSAIDs*—also effective with expected complete pain relief in >75% of cases. NSAIDs can also reduce the progression of biliary colic to cholecystitis, possibly due to its effect on prostaglandins and the role of the latter in the pathogenesis of acute cholecystitis.
- *IV fluids*—should be considered in the presence of nausea/vomiting where there is reduced oral intake.

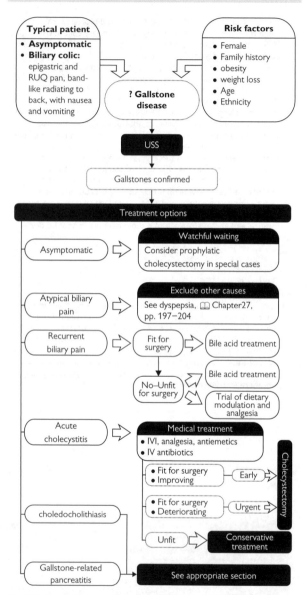

Fig. 42.1 Recommended approach to patients with gallstone disease.

Other issues to consider

- *Biliary dyskinesia*—attributed to the sphincter of Oddi dysfunction or gallbladder dysmotility is defined as a gall bladder ejection fraction of <50% on cholecystokinin hepatobiliary imino-diacetic acid scintigraphy (HIDA) scan, associated with typical biliary colic. Most patients with dyskinesia associated with microlithiasis or sludge can be successfully treated with cholecystectomy.
- *Management of bile duct stones*—will be considered later in this chapter (p.412).

Acute cholecystitis

- *Definition*—acute inflammation of the gall bladder wall, usually following obstruction of the cystic duct by a stone.
- *Mechanisms*—three factors invoke the inflammatory response:
  - Mechanical inflammation produced by increased intraluminal pressure.
  - Chemical inflammation caused by the release of lysolecithin.
  - Bacterial inflammation in 50–85% of patients.
- *Organisms*—most frequently isolated organisms are *Escherichia coli*, *Klebsiella* spp., *Streptococcus* spp., and *Clostridium* spp.
- *Clinically*—prolonged, more generalized biliary colic with low-grade fever, chills and rigors, late jaundice, nausea, and vomiting.
- *Diagnosis*—usually made on the basis of characteristic history and physical examination. USS is required to confirm the diagnosis.
- *Management.*
  - *First-line treatment.* Admission to hospital, patients require IV fluids, analgesia, and antibiotics, and abdominal US. NGT may be required when vomiting is excessive. *Surgery*—if fit enough, patients should be offered cholecystectomy, within 1 week of diagnosis.

Management of bile duct stones (CBDS)

Basic facts

- CBDS originate mainly in the gall bladder and migrate. De novo CBDS (those arising primarily in the CBD) have a different composition and may result from infection or stasis.
- The prevalence of CBDS in symptomatic gallstone patients ranges from 10 to 20%. CBDS is less common (<5%) with normal LFTs and non-dilated duct on USS.
- CBDS can pass spontaneously to the duodenum and cause no symptoms. CBDS that are able to cause symptoms have a high risk of causing further complications, and therefore should be extracted [B].

Recommended investigations

- *Recommended investigations.*
- *Transabdominal USS*—is the primary investigation of choice [B].
  - No one test can be relied upon to exclude the presence of CBDS. The combination of relevant clinical, biochemical and/or imaging tests should be used to identify high risk patients for CBDS [B], e.g. the presence of age >55, bilirubin >30, and dilated CBD on USS in patients with known gallstones correlate with a 70% chance of finding CBDS on ERCP. The absence of all of these factors decreases the risk of CBDS to <5%.
- *MRCP*—has a high accuracy in detecting (and excluding) the presence of CBDS. Different studies have shown an MRCP accuracy of >90% when compared to ERCP, with decreasing accuracy in small (<5mm) CBD stones.
- *Other tests*—include CT cholangiography (sensitivity of 65–95% and specificity of 85–100%), and EUS (comparable accuracy to ERCP and superior accuracy to MRCP).
- *Intra-operative cholangiography (IOC)*—is recommended for patients with medium to high risk of CBDS where other diagnostic tests have failed to confirm this or as an adjunct to laparoscopic cholecystectomy [B].
- *ERCP*—should NOT be used as a purely diagnostic tool, but only in patients who are likely to require intervention [B].

Recommended management

- *ERCP*—is the gold standard non-operative treatment for CBDS.
  - *Selection of patients*—should be based on the clinical, biochemical, and non-invasive imaging tests. ERCP should not be used as a purely diagnostic tool [B], e.g. dilated CBD on USS with normal LFTs should be investigated with MR first. Patients should be properly consented, and FBC and clotting screen should be checked no more than 72h prior to the procedure [B]. Aspirin and LMWH are not contraindications to ERCP and/or sphincterectomy [B].
  - *High-risk patients for complications*—include younger ages (<60), female gender, the presence of comorbidities (coagulopathy, cirrhosis, etc.), and where the indication for ERCP is less clear (e.g. normal CBD diameter).
  - *Sphincterectomy (using pure cut)*—in patients with high risk for ERCP-induced pancreatitis (who have low risk of bleeding) may be preferable [A].

- *Achieving adequate biliary drainage*—is essential [B]. Using biliary stents (temporarily or permanently in high-risk end-of-life patients) is advisable where appropriate, but not as a routine management for CBDS [A]. Short-term pancreatic stenting for patients at high risk for post-ERCP pancreatitis is advisable [A].
- *Surgical extraction of CBDS*—usually takes place during laparoscopic cholecystectomy.
  - Laparoscopic common bile duct exploration (LCBDE).
  - *Patient selection*—for common bile duct exploration should be based on a clear risk–benefit balance. LCBDE has reached a comparable morbidity (2–17%) and mortality (1–5%) rate to that for ERCP in many centres, and both approaches are deemed acceptable. ERCP is preferable where the surgical risk (due to technical difficulties or lack of resources) is considered higher [B].

Beyond the guidelines and the future

Laparoscopic cholecystectomy has revolutionized the management of symptomatic gallstone disease. The indications for laparoscopic cholecystectomy have broadened. At present disseminated intravascular coagulation is regarded as the only absolute contraindication for laparoscopic cholecystectomy. Laparoscopic bile duct exploration is increasingly practised and in centres with expertise a 'one stop approach' has become the first line treatment for patients with gallbladder stones and concomitant bile duct stones. Intraoperative ultrasound is practiced as a complementary procedure to laparoscopic cholangiography to facilitate the detection of bile duct stones.

The technological advancements have resulted in the development of newer laparoscopes with superb resolution and illumination that produce excellent three-dimensional images. Miniaturization of laparoscopes and production of miniature instruments which are sturdy has refined the dexterity and precision of the technique of laparoscopic cholecystectomy. The traditional four port technique is giving way to three and two port techniques. The 12mm ports have been replaced with 2mm ports. The bile duct injury rate following laparoscopic approach is still approximately twice that of the open procedure and this issue continues to be a concern.

Robotic laparoscopic cholecystectomy and computer assisted surgery (CAS) is practiced in some centres but there is no evidence that such developments offer real advantages over conventional laparoscopic cholecystectomy. However the availability of digitized data and the ability to transmit over a distance may open a new era of surgical practice in the future. Minimal access endoscopic surgery has now become the first line of treatment for bile duct stones.

Increasingly, laparoscopic surgery is being used to treat CBD stones in patients who have undergone obesity surgery such as gastric bypass. In these instances, specialist centres are performing laparoscopically-assisted ERCP where an enterotomy/gastrotomy is made to facilitate passage of the endoscope. *Mr S. S. Jaunoo*

Further reading

Sanders G, Kingsnorth AN (2007). Gallstones. BMJ 335, 295–9.

Beckingham IJ (2001). ABC of diseases of liver, pancreas, and biliary system. Gallstone disease. BMJ 322, 91–4.

Fialkowski E, Halpin V, Whinney R (2008). Acute cholecystitis. BMJ ClinEvid 12, 411.

Bellows CF, Berger DH, Crass RA (2005). Management of gallstones. Am Fam Physician 15, 637–42.

British Columbia Guidelines and Protocols (2007). Gallstones—treatment in adults. Available from: http://www.spitalmures.ro/_files/protocoale_terapeutice/gastro/gallstone.pdf.

American College of Physicians (1993). Guidelines for the treatment of gallstones. Ann Intern Med 119, 620–2.

Venneman NG, Buskens E, Besselink MG et al. (2005). Small gallstones are associated with increased risk of acute pancreatitis: potential benefits of prophylactic cholecystectomy? Am J Gastroenterol 100, 2540–50.

Kraag N, Thijs C, Knipschild P (1995). Dyspepsia—how noisy are gallstones? A meta-analysis of epidemiologic studies of biliary pain, dyspeptic symptoms, and food intolerance. Scand J Gastroenterol 30, 411–21.

DavideFesti, Ada Dormi, Simona Capodicasa, TommasoStaniscia, Adolfo F Attili, Paola Loria, Paolo Pazzi, Giuseppe Mazzella, Claudia Sama, Enrico Roda, Antonio Colecchia. Incidence of gallstone disease in Italy: Results from a multicenter, population-based Italian study (the MICOL project). World J Gastroenterol 2008 September 14; 14(34): 5282–5289.
URL: https://www.ncbi.nlm.nih.gov/pmc/articles/PMC2744058/

Thompson DR (2001). Narcotic analgesic effects on the sphincter of Oddi: a review of the data and therapeutic implications in treating pancreatitis. Am J Gastroenterol 96, 1266–72.

Thune A, Baker RA, Saccone GT, Owen H, Toouli J (1990). Differing effects of pethidine and morphine on human sphincter of Oddi motility. Br J Surg 77, 992–5.

Akriviadis EA, Hatzigavriel M, Kapnias D, Kirimlidis J, Markantas A, Garyfallos A (1997). Treatment of biliary colic with diclofenac: A randomized double-blind, placebo-controlled study. Gastroenterology 113, 225–31.

Thistle JL, Cleary PA, Lachin JM, Tyor MP, Hersh T (1984). The natural history of cholelithiasis: the National Cooperative Gallstone Study. Ann Intern Med 101, 171–5.

Keus F, de Jong JA, Gooszen HG, van Laarhoven CJ (2006). Laparoscopic versus open cholecystectomy for patients with symptomatic cholecystolithiasis. Cochrane Database Syst Rev 4, CD006231.

Vetrhus M, Soreide O, Solhaug JH, Nesvik I, Sondenaa K (2002). Symptomatic, non-complicated gall bladder stone disease. Operation or observation? A randomized clinical study. Scand J Gastroenterol 37, 834–9.

Zakko SF, Guttermuth MC, Jamali SH et al. (1999). A population study of gallstone composi- tion, symptoms, and outcomes after cholecystectomy. Gastroenterology 116, A43.

Bateson MC (2000). Gallstones and cholecystectomy in modern Britain. Postgrad Med J 76, 700–3.

The Rome Group for Epidemiology and Prevention of Cholelithiasis (GREPCO) (1988). The epidemiology of gallstone disease in Rome, Italy. Part I. Prevalence data in men. Hepatology 8, 904–6.

Maringhini A, Ciambra M, Baccelliere P et al. (1993). Biliary sludge and gallstones in pregnancy: Incidence, risk factors, and natural history. Ann Intern Med 119, 116–20.

Grodstein F, Colditz GA, Stampfer MJ (1994). Postmenopausal hormone use and cholecystec- tomy in a large prospective study. ObstetGynecol 83, 5–11.

Kalimi R, Gecelter GR, Caplin D et al. (2001). Diagnosis of acute cholecystitis: sensitivity of sonography, cholescintigraphy, and combined sonography-cholescintigraphy. J Am CollSurg 193, 609–13.

Brink JA, Simeone JF, Mueller PR, Richter JM, Prien EL, Ferrucci JT (1988). Physical character- istics of gallstones removed at cholecystectomy: implications for extracorporeal shock-wave lithotripsy. AJR Am J Roentgenol 151, 927–31.

Dill JE, Hill S, Callis J et al. (1995). Combined endoscopic ultrasound and stimulated biliary drainage in cholecystitis and microlithiasis—diagnoses and outcomes. Endoscopy 27, 424–7.

Reiss R. Nudelman I. Gutman C. Deutsch AA (1990). Changing trends in surgery for acute chole- cystitis. World J Surg 14, 567–70.

Vollmer C, Strasberg S (2002). Biliary surgery. In: Washington manual of Surgery, 3rd ed. Lippicott Williams & Wilkins, Philadelphia.

Bateson MC (2000). Gallstones and cholecystectomy in modern Britain. Postgrad Med J 76, 700–3.

Okamoto M, Okamoto H, Kitahara F, Kobayashi K (1999). Ultrasonographic evidence of association of polyps and stones with gall bladder cancer. Am J Gastroenterol 94, 446–50.

Williams EJ, Green J, Beckingham I, Parks, R, Martin D, Lombard M; British Society of Gastroenterology (2008). Guidelines on the management of common bile duct stones (CBDS). Gut 57, 1004–21.

Jaunoo SS, Mohandas S, Almond LM (2010) Postcholecystectomy syndrome (PCS). Int J Surg 8 (1): 15–17

Chapter 43

Surgical management of liver metastasis

Basic facts *416*
Recommended investigations *417*
Recommended treatment *418*
Further reading *420*

Key guidelines
- National Comprehensive Cancer Network Oncologic Guidelines (2015). Colon cancer.
- Adam, R. et al. (2012). The oncosurgery approach to managing liver metastases from colorectal cancer: a multidisciplinary international consensus.
- National Institute for Health and Care Excellence. Colorectal Cancer: NICE clinical guideline 131. Managing advanced and metastatic colorectal cancer (2017).
- ESMO consensus guidelines for the management of patients with metastatic colorectal cancer (2016).

Basic facts

- *Incidence*—the liver is the most common site for cancer metastasis, and over 50% of patients who die from cancer have liver metastasis.
- *Pathophysiology*—common sites of primary cancer are colorectal, bronchial, pancreas, breast, stomach, and cancers of unknown origin. Surgical resection is the mainstay of treatment for colorectal and neuroendocrine liver metastasis offering a 5y survival ranging from 40% to 60%.
  - Colorectal cancer is the third most common cancer in the UK after breast and lung and the second most common cause of cancer death. Liver is a common site of metastatic disease. Approximately 25% of patients develop detectable liver metastases at the time of the initial diagnosis with a further 50% of patients developing liver metastases after resection of the primary tumour. Colorectal cancer metastasis is the single most common indication for liver resection with a steady rise in resection rates over the last decade in the UK.
  - Neuroendocrine tumours (NETs) arise from the neuroectoderm, and most commonly from gastrointestinal and bronchopulmonary tracts. With a rising incidence (5/100,000), NETs arising from pancreas and colon have the highest risk of synchronous liver disease (60% and 30%). Metachronous liver metastases are seen in 40% of patients.
  - Metastatic malignant disease with an unknown primary origin (MUO) is the fourth most common cause of cancer deaths in England and Wales. Liver metastasis of unknown primary comprises 3–5% of all cancer diagnosis and typically present with non-specific features of malignancy such as malaise and weight loss. The benefit of liver resection for non-colorectal, non-neuroendocrine metastatic disease is unproven. However, in selected breast cancer patients with minimal extra-hepatic disease, resection has shown a median 5y survival of 40% and may play a role in a toolbox of multimodal management.
- *Clinical presentation*—most patients with early liver metastasis remain asymptomatic. Metastases are usually found incidentally during disease staging, in patients undergoing surveillance with raised carcinoembryonic antigen (CEA), neuroendocrine hormone levels, or presenting with the consequences of deranged liver function in advanced disease. Advanced liver metastasis is usually accompanied by fatigue, fever, weight loss, jaundice, pain, and a palpable hepatomegaly.

Recommended investigations

- *Detection of liver metastasis*—best achieved by combining a thorough history and physical examination.
  - *LFTs*—found abnormal in 65% of patients with liver metastasis and in 80% with advanced liver disease.
  - *Colorectal cancer metastasis*—raised *CEA* (>5ng/mL) has an overall sensitivity of 78% in detecting disease relapse in patients with completely resected colorectal cancer. Patients undergoing intensive screening with serial CEA monitoring and imaging (CT) provides an increased chance curative treatment in the follow-up period. However, the benefits of routine serial CEA measurements remain unproven [C]. A stepwise imaging approach is the recommended [B] and should comprise first of an abdominal/pelvic and thoracic CT scan (primary modality for staging and surveillance). A contrast-enhanced US (CEUS) or MRI can be used to further characterize liver lesions and a PET/CT scan for extra-hepatic disease [B]. There is no evidence for routine use of PET in all patients.
  - *Neuroendocrine tumours secreting serotonins* (5HT) with liver metastasis give rise to carcinoid syndrome (flushing and diarrhoea) with less common features heart failure and bronchoconstriction. Other gastrointestinal neuroendocrine tumours include insulinoma, gastrinomas, glucagonoma, somatostatinomas, and tumours secreting vasoactive intestinal peptide. Metastases are hypervascular and a contrast CT provides a sensitivity of 70–85% (similar to MRI). Somatostatin receptor scintigraphy (SRS) is often used with CT in the detection of metastatic disease.
  - *Metastatic disease of unknown origin*—investigations are guided by a comprehensive history and physical examination including breast, skin, nodal areas, testes, rectal and pelvic examination. Further investigations include symptom-directed endoscopy, prostate-specific antigen (PSA), cancer antigen 125 (CA125), alpha-fetoprotein (AFP), human chorionic gonadotrophin (hCG), and testicular ultrasound.
- *Preoperative assessment*—an assessment of cardiopulmonary fitness is undertaken in context of the oxygen demands expected following major surgery. Objective assessment of cardiopulmonary function and perioperative risk prediction derived from Cardiopulmonary Exercise Testing (CPET) has now superseded more subjective forms of assessment (POSSUM, Revised Cardiac Risk Index), but are being used in conjunction at various stages of preoperative workup to inform and guide therapies.

Recommended treatment

- *General approach to resection surgery*—surgical resection offers the greatest chance of cure for patients with liver metastasis from colorectal cancer. Oncological (prognostic) and technical (surgical) criteria are considered in patient selection.
  - *Technical considerations*—absolute contraindication when R0 resection is not possible without ≥30% future liver remnant (FLR) or presence of unresectable extra-hepatic disease. Relative contraindication when R0 resection possible only with complex procedure (portal vein embolisation, two-stage hepatectomy, hepatectomy combined with ablation) or R1 resection.
  - *Oncological considerations*—adverse factors contraindicating resection include concomitant unresectable extra-hepatic disease, number of lesions ≥5, and tumour progression.
  - Decision-making should include patients' characteristics and preferences [B].

Recommended management of metachronous colorectal liver metastasis

- Multidisciplinary treatment is essential for improving clinical and survival outcomes [B].
- Both technical criteria for resection and prognostic considerations define the need for systemic peri-operative therapy [B].
- In patients with clearly resectable disease and favourable prognostic criteria, perioperative treatment may not be necessary and upfront resection is justified [C].
- In patients with technically resectable disease where the prognosis is unclear or unfavourable, perioperative combination chemotherapy (FOLFOX or CAPOX) should be administered [B].
- In situations where the criteria for prognosis and resectability are not clearly defined, peri-operative therapy should be considered [B]. Patients who have not received previous chemotherapy, adjuvant treatment with FOLFOX or CAPOX is recommended [B].
- In potentially resectable patients (conversion therapy), a regimen of a cytotoxic doublet plus an anti-EGFR antibody provides a high resection rate in patients with RAS wild-type disease [A]. A cytotoxic doublet plus bevacizumab or FOLFOXIRI plus bevacizumab may also be considered in patients with RAS wild-type and RAS mutant disease [A].
- In patients with unresectable liver metastases only, local ablation techniques can be considered based on local experience, tumour characteristics, and patient preference [B].

Recommended management of synchronous colorectal liver metastasis

- No consensus exists on sequence of resection or timing of perioperative therapies for patients presenting with synchronous colorectal liver metastasis.
- Oncological (prognostic) and technical (surgical) criteria are considered with the staged approach of 'liver first' or 'bowel first' approach. A synchronous colorectal and hepatic resection can be undertaken combining a major bowel/hepatic with a minor bowel or hepatic resection (Fig. 43.1).

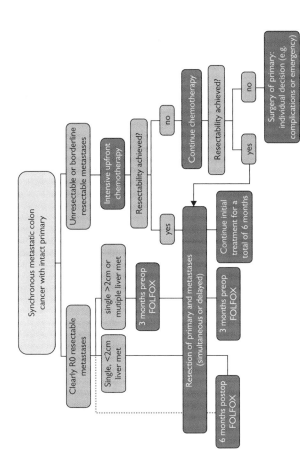

Fig. 43.1 Treatment algorithm for synchronous metastatic colon cancer

Further reading

Garden OJ, Rees M, Poston GJ, et al. (2006). Guidelines for resection of colorectal cancer liver metastases. Gut 55 (Suppl 3), iii1–8.

Nordlinger B, Sorbye H, Glimelius B, et al. (2008). Perioperative chemotherapy with FOLFOX4 and surgery versus surgery alone for resectable liver metastases from colorectal cancer (EORTC Intergroup trial 40983): a randomised controlled trial. Lancet; 371: 1007–1016.

National Institute for Health and Care Excellence (2010). Diagnosis and management of metastatic malignant disease of unknown primary origin: NICE clinical guideline 104. https://www.nice.org.uk/guidance/cg104.

Adam R, De Gramont A, Figueras J et al. (2012). The oncosurgery approach to managing liver metastases from colorectal cancer: a multidisciplinary international consensus. Oncologist 2012; 17: 1225–1239.

Tan MC, Jarnagin WR, (2014). Surgical management of non-colorectal hepatic metastasis. J Surg Oncol. Jan; 109(1):8-13.

Primrose JN, Perera R, Gray A et al. (2014). Effect of 3 to 5 years of scheduled CEA and CT follow-up to detect recurrence of colorectal cancer: the FACS randomized clinical trial. JAMA. 15;311(3):263-70.

National Comprehensive Cancer Network Oncologic Guidelines (2015). Colon cancer. http://www.nccn.org/professionals/physician_gls/pdf/colon.pdf.

Van Cutsem E, Cervantes A, Adam R et al. (2016). ESMO consensus guidelines for the management of patients with metastatic colorectal cancer. Annals of Oncology 27: 1386–1422, 2016

National Institute for Health and Care Excellence (2017). Colorectal Cancer: NICE clinical guideline 131. Managing advanced and metastatic colorectal cancer. http://pathways.nice.org.uk/pathways/colorectal-cancer

Hepatocellular carcinoma (HCC) and hepatic hydatid disease (HHD)*

Basic facts *422*
Recommended investigations *424*
Recommended treatment *426*
Hepatic hydatid disease (HHD) *428*
Basic facts *428*
Recommended investigations *428*
Recommended treatment *429*
Further reading *430*

Key guidelines
- NICE (2017). Liver Disease.
- British Society of Gastroenterology (2003). Guidelines for the diagnosis and treatment of hepatocellular carcinoma (HCC) in adults.
- American Association for the Study of Liver Diseases (2010). Management of hepatocellular carcinoma an update.
- European Association for the study of the Liver (2012). Management of hepatocellular carcinoma.

---

* The guidelines on this chapter have been sourced and summarized from different UK, Europe, and international government sources, professional organizations, and medical specialty societies. Leading guidelines have been listed in the further reading section at the end of this chapter.

Basic facts

- *Incidence*—wide geographical variation. Affects approximately 4.5 per 100,000 population in Europe (and >60 per 100,000 population in some areas of Africa and Asia) and accounts for 1,500 death per year in the UK. The overall incidence has been rising over the years.
- *Pathogenesis*—strongly associated with cirrhosis (90–95% of cases of HCC). High-risk groups include patients with cirrhosis due to hepatitis B (HBV) or C (HCV) virus (annual risk of 3–5%), cirrhosis due to genetic haemochromatosis (annual risk of 7–9%), primary biliary cirrhosis, alcoholic cirrhosis or other autoimmune cirrhosis
- *Surveillance programmes*—should be considered in high-risk patients using 6-monthly abdominal USS [B]. High risk groups are defined as: Patients with cirrhosis, non-cirrhotic HBV carriers with active hepatitis or family history of HCC, non-cirrhotic HCV carriers with chronic hepatitis and advanced fibrosis (METAVIR score F2 or greater).
- *Clinical manifestations*—vague and usually related to the underlying liver disease. HCC should be suspected in patients with previously compensated liver cirrhosis who develop symptoms and signs of decompensation such as jaundice, ascites, encephalopathy, or variceal bleeding.

Recommended investigations

- See Fig. 44.1.
- *Imaging tests*—US is the accepted radiological modality for both screening of high-risk groups and initial investigation where there is clinical suspicion of HCC.
- *Diagnosis*—can be confirmed using spiral chest and abdominal CT scan together with contrast MRI, if the lesion appearance proved typical for HCC (i.e. hypervascular with washout in the portal/venous phase) [B].
  - AFP levels are no longer recommended for diagnosis or surveillance due to poor sensitivity/specificity except in patients with cirrhosis due to hepatitis B and significant fibrosis [B].
  - Other imaging modalities (contrast US or angiography)—can support the diagnosis in suspicious cases.
- *Indefinite cases*—lesions <2cm in diameter has a probability of 75% to be HCC. If the diagnosis cannot be made using appropriate scanning techniques, a repeated examination should be performed at monthly intervals to detect any suspicious changes [C].
- *Confirmation biopsy*—Should be avoided especially if disease is potentially operable as seeding can occur in 1–3% [B].

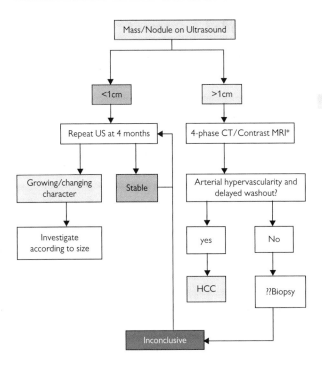

*Forlesions of 1-2cm there should be 2 postive ra diological modalities
for lesion >2cm 1 positive modality is accepted

Fig 44.1 Algorithm for diagnosing HCC.
*For lesions of 1–2cm, there should be two positive radiological modalities. For lesions >2cm, one
positive modality is accepted.

Recommended treatment

- See Fig. 44.2.
- *General concept*—management is determined by the BCLC staging system and /or HAP score. Surgery is the only proven curative therapy. Unfortunately, most patients are not eligible for surgery due to tumour stage.
- *Surgical options.*
  - *Surgical resection*—should be offered to suitable patients who have a single lesion of <2cm diameter and no (or mild) cirrhosis and well-preserved liver function, normal bilirubin, and acceptable hepatic vein pressure gradient (<10mmHg). 5y survival of approximately 66%. Tumour recurrence occurs in 70% of cases in 5y [B].
  - *Liver transplantation*—should be offered to patients with solitary tumour of <5cm in diameter, or patients with up to three cancer nodules of <3cm in diameter and cirrhosis(Milan Criteria). 5y survival of approximately 70%. Neo-adjuvant chemotherapy should be considered if waiting time for transplant is likely to exceed 6mo [B].
  - *Radiofrequency ablation*—for patients who cannot tolerate surgical resection, or as a bridge to later transplantation. Works by causing coagulative necrosis of lesions. Most suitable lesions are peripheral smaller nodules (<3cm in diameter). 5y survival of approximately 50% [B].
- *Transarterial chemoembolization*—recommended as a first-line palliative treatment for Intermediate (stage B) disease, with a median survival benefit of 4mo.
- *Sorafenib*—recommended as systemic chemotherapy for palliative treatment of Advanced (stage C) disease with a median survival benefit of 2.9mo.
- *Other treatment options*—include radiotherapy, SIRT, and immunotherapy.

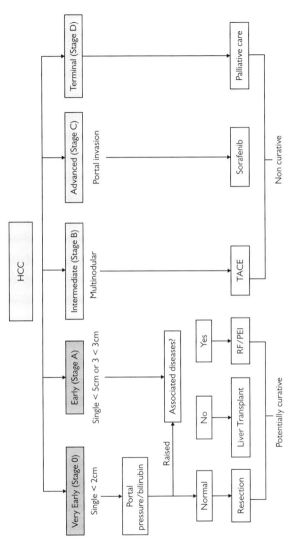

Fig. 44.2 Algorithm for treatment of HCC.

Hepatic hydatid disease (HHD)

Cystic echinococcosis (CE) and alveolar echinococcosis (AE) of the liver are caused by the metacestode stages of *Echinococcus granulosus* and *Echinococcus multilocularis*, respectively.

Basic facts

- *Epidemiology*—extremely rare in northern Europe and the USA (<1 case per 1 million). CE is endemic in Mediterranean countries, Australia, and parts of China, Africa, and South America (1–220 cases per 100,000). AE cases are less common even in endemic areas (0.03–1.2 cases per 100,000).

Recommended investigations

Laboratory tests

- *The enzyme-linked immunosorbent assay (ELISA)*—is the initial test of choice (~90% sensitivity, approaching ~100% with novel antigens). ELISA is also useful in follow-up to detect recurrence.
- *The indirect hemagglutination antibody test*—has a sensitivity of 85–90%.
- *Casoni skin test*—is largely abandoned because of low sensitivity (~70%).
- *USS*—is the initial and most productive diagnostic modality in both suspected and asymptomatic cases.
- *CT*—is the imaging modality of choice with ~94–98% sensitivity in demonstrating the daughter cysts (hydatid sand), revealing bilobar involvement (seen in ~15% of cases), and excluding other causes of hepatic cysts.
- *CXR*—is mandatory to rule out concomitant pulmonary disease (present in ~10% of cases).

Recommended treatment

- *Medical treatment*—is reserved for small cysts or inoperable cases. Benzimidazole compounds (albendazole or mebendazole) are expected to be curative in ~30% of CE cases, with only partial improvement in 30–50% of patients. Praziquantil has recently been suggested, but with limited data on efficacy.
- *PAIR procedure (puncture-aspiration-injection-reaspiration)*—is considered in imaging-accessible unilocular cysts that are 5–10cm in diameter, with >80% response rate.
- *Conservative surgery*—open or laparoscopic cystectomy is practised in endemic areas. Surgery is generally contraindicated in dead, calcified, or very small cysts which should be kept under surveillance.
- *Radical surgery*—pericystectomy or liver resection is recommended is associated with a lower incidence of local recurrence but higher incidence of complications. Total hepatectomy with liver transplantation may even be considered in advanced cases.

Further reading

Ryder SD; British Society of Gastroenterology (2003). Guidelines for the diagnosis and treatment of hepatocellular carcinoma (HCC) in adults. Gut 52 (Suppl 3), iii1–8.

American Association for the Study of Liver Diseases (2010). Management of hepatocellular carcinoma an update. Available from: www.aasld.org/sites/default/files/guideline_documents/HCCUpdate2010.pdf.

European Association for the study of the Liver. Management of hepatocellular carcinoma. http://www.easl.eu/medias/cpg/issue7/English-Report.pdf

Grosso G, Gruttadauria S, Biondi A, et al. Worldwide epidemiology of liver hydatidosis including the Mediterranean area. World J Gastroenterol. 2012 April 7; 18(13): 1425–1437.

Pektaş B, Altintaş N, Akpolat N, et al. Evaluation of the diagnostic value of the ELISA tests developed by using EgHF, Em2 and EmII/3-10 antigens in the serological diagnosis of alveolar echinococcosis. Mikrobiyol Bul. 2014 Jul;48(3):461-8.

Jiao W, Fu C, Liu WL, et al. Diagnostic potential of five natural antigens from Echinococcusgranulosus in the patients of cystic echinococcosis with different clinical status. Chinese journal of parasitology & parasitic diseases. 2014 Apr;32(2):116-22.

Marrone G, Crino F, Caruso S, et al. Multidisciplinary imaging of liver hydatidosis. World J Gastroenterol. 2012 Apr 7; 18(13): 1438–1447.

Gómez R, Moreno E, Loinaz C, et al. Diaphragmatic or transdiaphragmatic thoracic involvement in hepatic hydatid disease: surgical trends and classification. World J Surg 1995; 19:714-719.

Stojkovic M, Zwahlen M, Teggi A, et al. Treatment response of cystic echinococcosis to benzimidazoles: a systematic review. PLoSNegl Trop Dis. Sep 29 2009;3(9):e524.

Bygott JM, Chiodini PL. Praziquantel: neglected drug? Ineffective treatment? Or therapeutic choice in cystic hydatid disease?.Acta Trop. Aug 2009;111(2):95-101.

Golemanov B, Grigorov N, Mitova R, et al. Efficacy and safety of PAIR for cystic echinococcosis: experience on a large series of patients from Bulgaria. Am J Trop Med Hyg. Jan 2011;84(1):48-51.

Expert consensus for the diagnosis and treatment of cystic and alveolar echinococcosis in humans. Brunetti E, Kern P, Vuitton DA, Writing Panel for the WHO-IWGE. Acta Trop. 2010 Apr; 114(1):1-16.

Martel G, Ismail S, Bégin A, et al. Surgical management of symptomatic hydatid liver disease: experience from a Western centre. Canadian Journal of Surgery. 2014 Oct; 57(5)320-326.

Mamarajabov S, Kodera Y, Karimov S, et al. Surgical alternatives for hepatic hydatid disease. Hepatogastroenterology. Oct 12 2011;58(112).

Part 9

Spleen

Prevention of post-splenectomy sepsis (PSS)*

Basic facts *434*
Recommended investigations *434*
Recommended treatment *436*
Further reading *440*

Key guidelines

- Review of guidelines for the prevention and treatment of infection in patients with an absent or dysfunctional spleen: Prepared on behalf of the British Committee for standards in Haematology (BCSH) by a Woking Party of Haemato-Oncology Task Force (2011).
- British National Formulary (2017). Vaccines and asplenia.
- Adults and children summary for patients with absent or dysfunctinoal spleen. Nottingham University Hospitals Antimicrobial Committee (Jan 2014).

---

* The guidelines on this chapter have been sourced and summarized from different UK, Europe, and international government sources, professional organizations, and medical specialty societies. Leading guidelines have been listed in the further reading section at the end of this chapter

Basic facts

- *Definition of PSS*—fulminant, potentially lethal, infection affecting post-splenectomy patients.
- *Incidence*—about 4.4% of splenectomized children under the age of 16y (mortality rate 72.2%) and 70.9% of splenectomized adults (mortality rate 70.8%). The risk of late septicaemia in patients undergoing splenectomy increases by 12.6-fold (and 8.6-fold in traumatic cases) compared to the general population.
- *Lifetime risk*—most PSS attacks occur within 2y of splenectomy. About one third of all pneumococcal infections occur after 5y. The risk of subsequent severe infection among survivors of a first episode is more than 6-fold above average, and the risk of a third episode among second-time survivors is more than 2-fold.
- *Pathogens in PSS*—most commonly are encapsulated organisms, including *Streptococcus pneumoniae* (~60%), *Haemophilus influenzae*, and *Neisseria meningitidis*. The mortality rate ranges from 60% in *Streptococcus pneumoniae* to 30% in the other two.

Recommended investigations

- *High index of suspicion*—any fever developing in patients with known splenectomy should be considered as possible PSS attack. Deterioration can occur over few hours if treatment has not been commenced immediately.
- *Clinical presentation*—varies from headache, gastrointestinal symptoms, rigors, and high fever to rapid development of severe sepsis with petechiae, purpura, and meningitis (more common in children).

Recommended treatment

General approach

- Early recognition and following the principles of managing severe sepsis (see Chapter 18) is the mainstay of effective treatment. Prophylactic oral antibiotics should be changed into systemic [C]. Consultation with the ICU team and microbiologist is essential.

Prevention

- Avoid splenectomy when possible.

Immunisation:

- *Choice of vaccine*.
  - *Pneumococcal polysaccharide vaccine*—to all splenectomized patients and to those with functional hyposplenism[B]. This includes patients with homozygous sickle cell disease and coeliac disease which could lead to splenic dysfunction. The vaccine protects against infection with *Streptococcus pneumoniae* (pneumococcus); the vaccines contain polysaccharide from capsular pneumococci.
  - *Haemophilus influenza type b vaccine*—to all patients not previously immunized [C].
  - *Meningococcal groups A with C and W135 and Y vaccine and meningo-coccal group B vaccine (rDNA, component, adsorbed);* —to all patients not previously immunized [C].
  - *Influenza vaccine*—which should be undertaken yearly.
- *Timing (see Fig. 45.1)*—at least 14d prior to the scheduled splenectomy, where possible. Otherwise, delay immunizations until after the 14th post-operative day (to get the best functional antibody response).
  - *Patients on immunosuppressive chemotherapy or radiotherapy*—delayed immunization is recommended for at least 3mo after completion of their treatment.
  - *Re-immunization*—currently recommended every 5y. Responses to pneumococcal vaccination and the timing of pneumococcal revac-cination may, where validated assays are available, be determined by levels of protective antibody.
- *Vaccination regime*—comes in different forms and combinations. It is advisable to check local guidelines as to which the patient should be immunized with. They depend on the age of the patient at presentation and previous vaccination status. The BHSA guideline review (2011) and Nottingham Antimicrobial Guideline (2014) discuss this at great depth.

Antibiotic prophylaxis

- Lifelong prophylactic antibiotics with oral phenoxymethylpenicillin (penicillin V) [B] or erythromycin [C] are still recommended. Evidence-based local protocols should be followed where appropriate (e.g. minimum 2y prophylactic antibiotics for adults in general and lifelong for patients with lymphoproliferative disease or sickle cell disease).
- *Dosing*—phenoxymethylpenicillin adult and child over 5y, 250mg twice daily; child under 1y 62.5 mg twice daily, 1–5y 125mg twice daily—if cover also needed for *H. influenzae* in child give amoxicillin instead

(1mo–5y 125mg twice daily, 5–12y 250mg twice daily, 12–18y 500mg twice daily). If penicillin-allergic, erythromycin adult and child over 8y, 500mg twice daily; child 1mo–2y 125mg twice daily, 2–8y 250mg twice daily (clarithromycin 250mg BD alternate regime). This advice must be reviewed with up to date BNF guidance and local microbiology teams in light of pneumococcal resistance patterns.

- All patients should carry a supply of appropriate antibiotics for emergency use.
- Factors associated with high risk of invasive pneumococcal disease in hyposplenism include: age of less than 16y or greater than 50y, inadequate serological response to pneumococcal vaccination, a history of previous invasive pneumococcal disease, and splenectomy for underlying haematological malignancy particularly in the context of on-going immunosuppression [B][C].

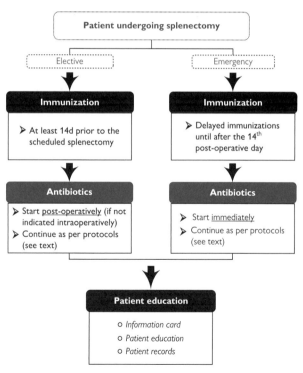

Fig. 45.1 Algorithm for the prevention of post-splenectomy sepsis.

- Lifelong antibiotic prophylaxis is appropriate for high-risk groups. Low-risk patients should be counselled as to the risks and benefits of prophylaxis particularly where adherence is an issue.

Patient information

- *Information card or bracelet*—should be given to all patients to alert caring health care professionals of the high susceptibility for overwhelming infection [C]. (A patient card and information leaflet for patients with asplenia are available from the Department of Health UK, published Jan 2015.)
- *Patient education*—should be effective, including advice on the potential risk of overseas travel to epidemic areas [B] and the risk of animal bites [C]. Consideration must be taken to areas where malaria is prevalent as patients with an absent or dysfunctional spleen are at increased risk of severe falciparum malaria. Guidance should be given on appropriate malaria prophylaxis and the need for close adherence to this.
- *Patient records*—should be clearly labelled as high risk for infection [C]. Vaccination and re-vaccination status should be clearly documented.

Further reading

Davies JM, Barnes R, Milligan D; British Committee for Standards in Haematology. Working Party of the Haematology/Oncology Task Force (2002). Update of guidelines for the prevention and treatment of infection in patients with an absent or dysfunctional spleen. Clin Med 2, 440–3.

British National Formulary (2017). Available from: https://bnf.nice.org.uk/treatment-summary/vaccines.html. Last Accessed: Sep 2017.

Holdsworth RJ, Irving AD, Cuschieri A (1991). Post-splenectomy sepsis and its mortality rate: actual versus perceived risks. Br J Surg 78, 1031–8.

Cullingford GL, Watkins DN, Watts AD, Mallon DF (1991). Severe late postsplenectomy infection. Br J Surg 78, 716–21.

Kyaw MH, Holmes EM, Toolis F et al. (2006). Evaluation of severe infection and survival after splenectomy. Am J Med 119, 276.

Foxon P & Hills T. Adults and children summary for patients with absent or dysfunctinoal spleen. Nottingham University Hospitals Antimicrobial Committee (Jan 2014). Available from: https://www.nuh.nhs.uk/handlers/downloads.ashx?id=60984.

John M. Davies, Michael P. N. Lewis, Jennie Wimperis, Imran Rafi, Shamez Ladhani and Paula H. B. Bolton-Maggs. Review of guidelines for the prevention and treatment of infection inpatient with an absent or dysfunctional spleen: Prepared on behalf of the British Committee for standards in Haematology by a Woking Party of Haemato-Oncology Task Force. 2011. British Journal of Haematology, 155, 308–317

Part 10

Vascular

Chronic limb ischaemia*

Basic facts 444
Recommended investigations 446
Recommended management 448
Further reading 452

Key guidelines

- Inter-Society consensus for the management of peripheral arterial disease (TASC II). 2007.
- An Update on Methods for Revascularization and Expansion of the TASCII guidelines (2015).
- NICE (2014). Peripheral arterial disease.
- ESC (2017). Peripheral arterial diseases (diagnosis and treatment of).
- American Family Physician (2013). Diagnosis and management of peripheral arterial disease.
- ACCF/AHA (2016). Guidelines for the management of patients with peripheral artery disease.

---

* The guidelines on this chapter have been sourced and summarized from different UK, Europe, and international government sources, professional organizations, and medical specialty societies. Leading guidelines have been listed in the further reading section at the end of this chapter.

Basic facts

- *Incidence*—common overlooked syndrome in Western countries. Affects 73–10% of the population on objective non-invasive tests, and ~15–20% of those over 70y of age.
- *Risk factors*—see Box 46.1.
- *Anatomical classification*—of chronic limb ischaemia (also called peripheral arterial disease (PAD)) is useful for descriptive as well as planning purposes. Aorto-iliac occlusive segmental disease occurs when the infrarenal aorta, common, and/or external iliacs are affected (also called inflow disease). Femoro-popliteal segmental disease occurs when the common femoral, superficial, profunda, and/or popliteal arteries are affected. Tibial-peroneal segmental disease (run-off or outflow disease) occurs when distal arteries (tibials and/or peroneal arteries) are affected.
- *Clinical presentation*—most patients have limited walking ability and exercise performance (Box 46.2). Critical limb ischaemia (CLI) is the presence of ischaemic rest pain, ulceration, or gangrene in objectively proven PAD patients.
- *Physical examination*—should include measuring BP in both arms, examining carotid pulses, abdomen, and legs. Pulse examination should include brachial, radial, ulnar, femoral, popliteal, dorsalis pedis, and posterior tibial pulses. Pulse characteristics and arterial bruits (over subclavian arteries, carotid arteries, abdominal aorta, and femoral arteries) are traditionally examined as well.
- *Differential diagnosis*—should be considered and other diseases should be identified in each individual case (Box 46.3).

Box 46.1 Risk factors for PAD

- *General*—male (OR ×1.1–2.1) and elderly (OR ×2–3 per 10y ageing) patients
- *Smoking*—the most important risk factor (OR ×3–4). The number of cigarettes smoked correlates strongly with the severity of PAD. Risk declines gradually upon smoking cessation (RR drops from 73.5 to 71.5 within 5y).
- *Diabetes*—significant risk factor (OR ×3). Risk of having PAD increases by 26% for every 1% chronic increase in HbA1c.
- *Hypertension*—OR ×2.
- *Dyslipidaemia*—OR ×2. Incidence of symptomatic PAD doubles if fasting cholesterol level were >7mmol/L (270mg/dL).
- *Hyperhomocysteinaemia*—occurs commonly in PAD patients compared to the general population, and is associated with increased risk of PAD (OR ×1–3).
- *Others*—chronic kidney disease (OR ×2) and raised CRP (OR ×2).

Box 46.2 Clinical features of chronic limb ischaemia

- *Intermittent claudication*—fatigue, aching or cramping pain, commonly in the calf, thigh, or buttocks, brought on by walking (typically within the same distance), and relieved by rest within 10min. Pain increases significantly by walking uphill or against a wind, and changes with the change in the speed of walking. Pain is reproduced by exercise and does not present on taking the first step. Pain varies slightly from day to day in the same person, and may become prominent if significant changes in general health (severe anaemia, heart failure) occur.
- *Ischaemic rest pain*—severe intolerable pain, affects the most distal part of the limbs, commonly awakes the patient up from sleep, and typically relieved by hanging the foot out of bed or even sleeping in a chair.
- *Arterial-type leg ulcers*—are sharp, small, superficial erosions over the bony prominences of the leg (head of metatarsals, malleolus, and heel).
- *Digital gangrene*—blackened, mummified areas of skin that cannot be mistaken by the observer.

Box 46.3 Differential diagnosis of intermittent claudication

- *Nerve root compression*—sharp, lancinating pain, radiates down the leg posteriorly, starts immediately on commencing exercises (or even without doing any movement), and is not relieved easily with rest. Changing back position may help.
- *Arthritis and inflammatory processes*—aching pain, affects foot and joints predominantly, starts after variable degree of exercises, not relieved quickly on rest. May be relieved by taking certain positions.
- *Others*—spinal stenosis (weakness more than pain, body positions have significant effect), hip arthritis (pain usually localized to hip and gluteal region), and peripheral arthritis.

Recommended investigations

Basic investigations

- *Handheld Doppler examination*—should support the clinical impression
  [C], especially in suspected critically ischaemic legs [B].
  - Handheld Doppler can reliably detects the presence, type, and
    strength of blood flow signals in peripheral arteries.
- *Ankle brachial pressure index (ABPI)*—quick and cost-effective method
  to confirm or exclude the presence of significant lower limb PAD, and
  is indicated for any patient with suspected chronic limb ischaemia as an
  objective baseline measurement [B] (Box 46.4).

Advanced investigations

- *General approach*—patients with established PAD (based on clinical
  history and basic investigations), which has no significant effect on their
  quality of life, require no further advanced investigations and should be
  managed conservatively (i.e. risk factor optimization etc.) [A]. Advanced
  investigations are indicated for critically ischaemic legs, intermittent
  claudicants with significant effect on quality of life who have failed the
  more conservative measures, and where a clear favourable risk–benefit
  ratio for intervention exists [A].
- *Toe brachial index (TBI)*—measures the digital perfusion and requires
  small cuffs and well-trained investigators. TBI is useful in patients with
  non-compressible arteries (long-standing diabetes, renal failure, or
  advanced age) [B].
- *Colour flow duplex USS*—is a reliable, non-invasive, and reproducible
  investigation for PAD patients. In experienced hands, a duplex scan
  can accurately map the diseased artery and identify the haemodynamic
  properties of each lesion [A], identify candidates for endovascular
  interventions [B], and reliably select candidates for surgical bypass [B].
  Duplex scan is recommended for the routine surveillance of the patency
  of femoro-popliteal/distal bypass grafts [A]. The accuracy of duplex

---

Box 46.4 Ankle brachial pressure index

- *Technique*—systolic pressure in posterior tibial and/or dorsalis pedis
  arteries is measured for each leg using a sphygmomanometer cuff
  and a handheld Doppler. These are compared against the higher
  brachial pressure of either arm (using handheld Doppler) to formulate
  the ABPI.
- *Findings*.
  - *Resting ABPI <0.90*—correlates well with a haemodynamically
    significant arterial stenosis, and is often used as a cut-off point
    for the definition of PAD, with a sensitivity of ~95% in detecting
    arteriogram-positive PAD, and specificity of ~100% in identifying
    healthy persons (when combined to the signal type).
  - *6min walk test*—can provide an objective assessment of functional
    capacity in selected cases when normal resting ABPI measurements
    do not correlate with the clinical findings [B].

scan is highest in outflow (sensitivity of ~85% and specificity of ~95%) and slightly lower in inflow disease (sensitivity of ~89% and specificity of ~90%).

- *MRA*—is a reliable and accurate modality for localizing stenotic lesions and estimating the degree of stenosis [A]. MRA can identify lesions suitable for endovascular interventions [B] and can reliably select candidates for surgical bypass [B].
- *CT angiogram*—can be considered to obtain an accurate map of the arterial tree, especially in more proximal inflow lesions [B]. CT angiogram can provide high-quality images that are comparable to those from angiogram or MRI scan.
- *Digital subtraction arteriography (DSA)*—remains the gold standard technique for investigating PAD patients and plan for surgical treatment (Box 46.5).
- *Other investigations*—may be useful in selected cases, including leg segmental pressure measurement [B], pulse volume recordings [B], and continuous wave form (CWF) Doppler ultrasound [B].

Box 46.5 DSA—facts and figures

- *Technique*—arterial access is gained using a modified Seldinger technique (floppy guidewire passing through a hollow puncture needle). This is followed by the injection of contrast material to obtain detailed images in different angles.
- *Benefits*—provides detailed map of the arterial system, estimation of arterial inflow and outflow, and allows for therapeutic interventions (angioplasty, stent insertion, coil insertion) via the same access [B].
- *Quality standards*—a full history and complete vascular examination should be performed prior to referral for angiography [C]. Iliacs, femorals, and tibials should be visualized [B]. A history of contrast allergy should be documented clearly [B]. Hydration should be provided prior to angiography in patients with renal impairment [B]. Follow-up clinical examination and renal tests are recommended after 2wk [C]. Metformin (Glucophage®), an oral agent used in the management of diabetes mellitus, has been associated with the development of severe lactic acidosis following administration of IV contrast media. It is recommended by many experts to stop the metformin therapy pre-procedure, and for at least 48h following the administration of contrast material.

Recommended management

- *Natural history*—in 5 years' time, 70–80% of patients with non-critical ischaemic lower legs will remain stable. Claudication will get worse in 10–20%, and will develop into critical ischaemia (rest pain, ulcer, or gangrene) in 5–10% of cases with a high probability of amputation within 6mo. The main causes of morbidity and mortality in symptomatic PAD patients remain in cardiovascular events rather than vascular events. About 20% of symptomatic non-critical PAD patients will sustain a non-fatal MI or stroke, and a further 10–15% will die of cardiovascular (75%) or non-cardiovascular (25%) event. In 1 year's time, 25% of CLI patients will be dead and 30% will end up with an amputation. Of the remaining pool of patients, less than 50% will have their critical ischaemia resolved satisfactorily.

Intermittent claudication

- *Overall strategy*—patients with intermittent claudication who have no significant life-limiting symptoms should be offered conservative management (control of risk factors, exercises, and consideration for drug therapy) as a first-line treatment [A].
  - Deteriorating or resistant symptoms require further advanced investigations and consideration for endovascular or surgical revascularization where benefits clearly outweigh risks [A].
- *Management of risk factors*—is an essential first step (Box 46.6).
- *Supervised structured exercises*—effective and safe modality and is a recommended option for all patients with intermittent claudication [A]. An effective programme should be performed in sessions (30–45min each), three times (2h) a wk or more for 3mo. Each session should contain a proper exercise (treadmill, track walking) that is able to bring the claudication pain on (to its maximum) before taking a rest [A]. Structured exercise can result in increased maximum walking time (mean difference 6.5min), which may sometimes exceed that seen with angioplasty at 6mo (mean difference 3.3min).
- *Pharmacotherapy*—is not widely adopted as part of the initial management for intermittent claudication. Level 1 evidence supports the use of cliostazole [A] and naftidrofuryl [A], especially where risk factors have been modified and patient is unfavourable for intervention.
- *Endovascular treatment*—should be considered for those who fail the conservative management where claudication is significantly affecting their quality of life [A]. Arterial lesions should be of the types that will most likely benefit from endovascular intervention [A].
  - *TASC II classification of PAD lesions*—may be used for descriptive and research purposes. Lesions are classified according to their site (in-flow, outflow), length (short, long), number (single, multiple), and exact location (critical, preferred site) into types A to D. Angioplasty results are best in type A and not as favourable in type D.
  - *Stent placement*—should be considered for iliac, femoral, popliteal, or tibial lesions with suboptimal (or failed) angioplasty results [B]. The effectiveness of distal stents has not been fully established yet.
  - *Other modalities of treatment* (including atherectomy, cutting balloons, thermal devices, and lasers)—are yet to be established.

- *Surgery*—is rarely required (or justifiable) in pure intermittent claudication. Surgery remains an option in selected patients where intermittent claudication has a significant effect on the mobility, effective conservative management has failed to improve symptoms, and the lesion is likely to benefit from surgical intervention [B].

Critically ischaemic leg

- *Basic treatment*—includes effective pain control (see ➔ Chapter 21), appropriate management of ulcers and wounds (see ➔ Chapter 10), and control of infection (see ➔ Chapter 20).
- *Pharmacological therapy*—includes the use of parenteral prostaglandin E1 or ileoprost for 7–28d (limited efficiency to some patients) [A], and possible use of angiogenic growth factors within a trial context [C].

Box 46.6 Risk factor modification

- *Smoking cessation*—essential for improving symptoms and reducing cardiovascular risks as well as improving the success rate of any revascularization intervention [B]. Smoking cessation is best achieved by advising patients on behavioural modification techniques, frequent follow-ups (1y smoking cessation success rate is 75% vs 0.1% when no formal follow-up by health care professionals has been arranged), and providing patients with nicotine replacement therapy (1y success rate increases up to ~16%) and/or bupropion (1y success rate ~30%).
- *Antiplatelets*—aspirin (75mg od) is recommended to reduce the risk of cardiovascular death [A]. Aspirin can significantly reduce the risk of subsequent vascular events (non-fatal MI, non-fatal stroke, and vascular death) by ~22%. Clopidogrel (75mg od) is a safe and effective alternative to aspirin (~5%) of aspirin-intolerant patients) in reducing cardiovascular death [B]. Oral anticoagulants are NOT indicated for cardiovascular prophylactic purposes [C].
- *Statins (simvastatin 40mg od)*—have been shown to significantly reduce the risk of stroke, MI, or the need for revascularization by ~25%. The 2007 TASC II guidelines provide no graded recommendations pending further analysis of trials.
- *Hypertension*—should be well controlled (140/90 or 130/80 for diabetic and renal insufficiency patients) [A]. ACE inhibitors are a reasonable first option [B] and their effect appears to extend to non-hypertensive PAD patients [C].
- *Hyperlipidaemia*—all patients with PAD should have their LDL cholesterol lowered to <100mg/dL (2.6mmol/L) [B]. In patients with PAD and atherosclerosis in other vital organs, it is advisable to lower the LDL cholesterol to <70mg/dL (1.8mmol/L) [B].
- *Control of diabetes*—aggressive management of blood glucose levels with a HbA1c goal of <7.0% (or as close to 6.0% as possible) is currently recommended to reduce microvascular complications and potentially improve cardiovascular outcomes [C]. Proper care of the diabetic foot is essential [B].

- *In general terms, TASC II recommends endovascular treatment of inflow lesions*—as the preferred initial treatment of choice [B]. Outflow lesions should be addressed if the inflow lesion correction is not expected to lead to acceptable improvement in symptoms and signs [B].
- *Surgery*—is indicated where endovascular procedure is not expected (or has failed) to achieve adequate inflow and/or outflow results [B].
  - *Examples of inflow procedures*—include aorto-bifemoral bypass procedure iliac endarterectomy, aorto-iliac or aorto-femoral by-pass, femoro-femoral cross-over bypass, axillofemoral bypass, and axillofemoral-femoral bypass graft.
  - *Examples of outflow procedures*—include fem-above knee (AK) pop-liteal vein graft, fem-AK popliteal prosthetic graft, fem-below knee (BK) popliteal vein graft, fem-BK popliteal prosthetic graft, fem-tibial vein graft, fem-tibial prosthetic graft.
  - *Amputation*—should be considered primarily for unsalvageable limbs or where surgical intervention carries a significant risk. Amputation may be the only effective option to manage the pain. The decision to proceed with amputation should take into consideration the ability of the amputation wound to heal, the rehabilitation requirements, and the overall quality of life [C].

Further reading

Norgren L, Hiatt WR, Dormandy JA et al. (2007). Inter-Society consensus for the management of peripheral arterial disease (TASC II). Eur J Vasc Endovasc Surg 33 (Suppl 1), S1–75.

An Update on Methods for Revascularization and Expansion of the TASCII guidelines (2015). NICE (2014) Peripheral arterial disease

American Family Physcian (2013) Diagnosis and Management of Peripheral arterial disease

ESC (2017). Peripheral Arterial Diseases (Diagnosis and Treatment of). Available from: https://www.escardio.org/Guidelines/Clinical-Practice-Guidelines/Peripheral-Artery-Diseases-Diagnosis-and-Treatment-of. Last accessed Sep 2017

ACCF/AHA (2016) Focused Update of the Guidelines for the Management of Patients With Peripheral Artery Disease

American College of Cardiology/American Heart Association. Guidelines. Peripheral Arterial Disease, 2006. Available from: http://circ.ahajournals.org/cgi/reprint/113/11/e463. Accessed May 2009.

Scottish Intercollegiate Guidelines Network (2006). Diagnosis and management of peripheral arterial disease. Available from: http://www.nhstaysideadtc.scot.nhs.uk/wound%20Formulary/Pdf%20docs/Sign%2089%20PAD.pdf.

Moneta GL, Yeager RA, Antonovic R et al. (1992). Accuracy of lower extremity arterial duplex mapping. J Vasc Surg 15, 275–84.

Jorenby DE, Leischow SJ, Nides MA et al. (1999). A controlled trial of sustained-release bupropion, a nicotine patch, or both for smoking cessation. N Engl J Med 340, 685–91.

Antithrombotic Trialists' Collaboration (2002). Collaborative meta-analysis of randomized trials of antiplatelet therapy for prevention of death, myocardial infarction, and stroke in high risk patients. BMJ 324, 71–86.

Collins R, Armitage J, Parish S, Sleight P, Peto R; Heart Protection Study Collaborative Group (2004). Effects of cholesterol-lowering with simvastatin on stroke and other major vascular events in 20,536 people with cerebrovascular disease or other high-risk conditions. Lancet 363, 757–67.

Leng GC, Fowler B, Ernst E (2000). Exercise for intermittent claudication. Cochrane Database Syst Rev 2, CD000990.

Thompson PD, Zimet R, Forbes WP, Zhang P (2002). Meta-analysis of results from eight randomized, placebo-controlled trials on the effect of cilostazol on patients with intermittent claudication. Am J Cardiol 90, 1314–9.

McCartney MM, Gilbert FJ, Murchison LE, Pearson D, McHardy K, Murray AD (1999). Metformin and contrast media—a dangerous combination? Clin Radiol 54, 29–33.

Carotid artery stenosis[*]

Basic facts 454
Recommended investigations 456
Recommended management 458
Further reading 460

Key guidelines

- ESC (2017). Peripheral arterial diseases (diagnosis and treatment of) including carotid artery stenosis.
- NICE (2015). Diagnosis and initial management of acute stroke and transient ischaemic attack (TIA).
- NHS Standard Contract (2014). Specialised vascular services.
- Cochrane Database Systematic Reviews. (2011). Carotid endarter- ectomy.
- American 14 Societies' Guidelines on Extracranial Carotid and Vertebral Artery Disease (2011).
- National Institute for Health and Clinical Excellence (2011). Carotid artery stent placement for carotid stenosis.

[*] The guidelines on this chapter have been sourced and summarized from different UK, Europe, and international government sources, professional organizations, and medical specialty societies. Leading guidelines have been listed in the further reading section at the end of this chapter.

Basic facts

- *Definitions*—transient ischaemic attack (TIA) is a medical emergency, indicating an unstable brain ischaemia with a high risk of imminent, potentially preventable, stroke. See Box 47.1 for definitions.
- *Incidence*—TIA affects ~66 per 100,000 population every year and precedes ischaemic stroke in 15–25% of patients. Stroke is the third most common cause of death in developed countries, affecting ~0.2% of population every year.
- *Pathogenesis*—of all strokes, 10–15% follow thromboembolism from a 50–99% internal carotid artery stenosis. Other causes of TIA are cardiogenic embolism (20% of TIA cases), small artery disease (25%), and haematologic or non-atheromatous diseases (10%).
- *Clinical presentation*—varies widely depending on the area of the brain involved (Box 47.2).

Box 47.1 Definitions

- *Stroke*—a clinical syndrome consisting of 'rapidly developing clinical signs of focal (at times global) disturbance of cerebral function, lasting more than 24h or leading to death with no apparent cause other than that of vascular origin'.
- *Transient ischaemic attack (TIA)*—stroke symptoms and signs that resolve within 24h (arbitrary cut-off time).

Box 47.2 TIA/stroke clinical presentation

- *TIA common presentation*—temporary monocular blindness (amaurosis fugax), difficulty speaking (dysphasia), weakness on one side of the body (hemiparesis), and numbness or tingling (paraesthesia), usually on one side of the body.
- *Stroke*—presents with total anterior circulation infarction (TACI: extensive sensory, motor, and higher cortical dysfunction), partial anterior circulation infarction (PACI: more localized and less extensive neural dysfunction), posterior circulation infarction (POCI: blindness, diplopia, vertigo, ataxia, etc.), and lacunar infarction (LACI: pure motor or sensory dysfunctions).

Recommended investigations

- *Obtain ABCD score* (see Fig. 47.1) and estimate the risk of a major subsequent stroke.
- *Basic investigations for TIA/minor stroke*—include basic blood tests (FBC, CRP, U&E, blood sugar, lipid profile, and clotting screen if on warfarin), ECG, and CXR. Echocardiography is indicated if a cardiogenic embolism is suspected (and 24h ambulatory ECG for paroxysmal cardiac arrhythmias if necessary) [C].
- *Coagulopathy screening*—is required for cases with no identifiable risk factors. Screening tests include coagulation screen, thrombophilia screen, anti-cardiolipin antibody, and screening for vasculitis auto-antibody and plasma homocysteine.
- *Carotid imaging*—first-line specialist vascular investigation for patients with suspected hemispheric (carotid territory) TIA who are fit for surgery (Fig. 47.1, Box 47.3) [B]. Carotid stenosis are expressed differently between the European and American trials centres and this should be taken into consideration.
- *When CEA is considered, it is recommended to corroborate the duplex estimation by either MAR, CTA, or a repeated duplex* by an expert scientist [B].

Box 47.3 Carotid duplex scan

- *Technique*—a two-dimensional image (B-mode) of the carotid is obtained using real time USS. A waveform analysis of the blood flow within the artery lumen is then performed and displayed diagrammatically.
- *Diagnostic criteria*—an accurate estimation of the carotid stenosis depends on the judicious and validated use of B-mode images and spectral analysis. The use of peak systolic velocity (PSV) and end diastolic velocity (EDV) are of special use in estimating the degree of narrowing. For example, a PSV value of >125cm/s and EDV value of 140m/s predict a carotid stenosis of >50% with ~89% accuracy (sensitivity of ~96% and specificity of ~85%). A PSV value of >270m/s and EDV value of >110m/s predict a carotid stenosis of >70% with ~93% accuracy (sensitivity of ~96% and specificity of ~91%).

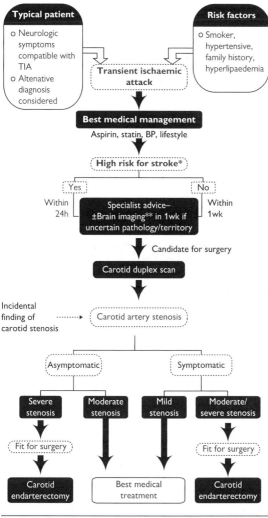

* for example, using the ABCD scoring system: **age** >60 = 1 point; **BP** >140/90 = 1 point; **clinical features** (speech disturbance = 1 point, unilateral weakness = 2 points); **duration** (<60min = 1 point, >60 min = 2 points). Score ≥4 is high risk for stroke[5]

** preferably diffusion-weighted MRI[5]

Fig. 47.1 Recommended approach to carotid artery stenosis.

Recommended management

Best medical treatment
- See Box 47.4.
- *Smoking*—should be completely discontinued (within a lifestyle changing approach) [A].
- *High blood pressure and high lipids*—should be well controlled. [A].
- *Other comorbidities (e.g. cardiac, diabetes)*—should be optimized.

Surgical treatment
Carotid stenosis in symptomatic patients
- *Key trials*—recommendations are mainly based on two international randomized trials.
  - North American Symptomatic Carotid Endarterectomy Trial (NASCET).
  - European Carotid Surgery Trial (ECST).

Current recommendations
- *Severe stenosis*—carotid endarterectomy (CEA) has established safety and effectiveness for recently symptomatic patients (within 2wk) with 70–99% internal carotid artery (ICA) stenosis when performed by an experienced surgeon [A]. CEA significantly reduces the risk of disabling stroke (from 28 to 9% (NASCET) or 19 to 11% (ECST); RRR ×45–70%).
- The majority of recently symptomatic patients will gain maximum benefit when carotid interventions are performed within 14 days of symptom onset [A].
- *Moderate stenosis*—CEA may be beneficial for patients with 50–69% symptomatic stenosis, and should be considered for patients with expected life expectancy of minimum 5y by a centre/surgeon with reported perioperative stroke/death rate of <6% for symptomatic patients [A]. CEA moderately reduces the risk of disabling stroke or death (RRR ×27%).

Box 47.4 Best medical management for carotid stenosis
- *BP control is essential*—two RCTs (PROGRESS and HOPE) showed significant relative risk reduction (RRR ×20–30%) in stroke rate in patients using ACE inhibitors. Nevertheless, no specific recommendation on their routine use has been published.
- *Aspirin* (300mg for first 2wk, then long-term antithrombotic treatment)—first-line agent. Significantly reduces the risk of stroke (by about 25–30%). People with a history of dyspepsia should have PPI protection.
- *Clopidogrel*—is a good alternative or additional treatment to aspirin.
- *Control of other risk factors*—include smoking, hyperlipidaemia, diabetes, and optimization of cardiovascular and respiratory condition.

- *Mild stenosis*—CEA has established harm for symptomatic patients with <50% stenosis and should not be considered [A]. The risk of a disabling stroke or death increases by 20%. Best medical management is recommended [A].

Carotid stenosis in asymptomatic patients
- Key trials
  - Endarterectomy for asymptomatic carotid artery stenosis (ACAS).
  - Asymptomatic Carotid Stenosis Trial (ACST).

Current recommendations
- *Severe stenosis*—it is reasonable to consider CEA for youngish patients (age 40–75y) with asymptomatic stenosis of 60–99% (ACST) who has an expected life expectancy of minimum 5y, where the centre/surgeon has a reported perioperative stroke/death rate of <3% for asymptomatic patients [A]. CEA moderately reduces the risk of disabling stroke or death (from 11 to 5% (ACAS) or 12 to 6% (ACST) at 5y; RR ×0.71).
- *Factors increasing risk of stroke in asymptomatic patients include the presence of contralateral TIA/stroke, silent infarction on MRI, stenosis progression (>20%), spontaneous embolization on transcranial Doppler, impaired cerebral vascular reserve, large plaques, echolucent plaques, increased juxta-luminal black (hypoechogenic) area, intraplaque haemorrhage on MRI, and lipid-rich necrotic core on MRI.*

Prognosis
- The risk of stroke, myocardial infarction, or vascular death after a TIA event is ~9% per year. Most patients die from heart disease (~40%) or other disorders (30%) rather than another stroke (25%).

Further reading

ESC (2017). Peripheral Arterial Diseases (Diagnosis and Treatment of). Available from: https://www.escardio.org/Guidelines/Clinical-Practice-Guidelines/Peripheral-Artery-Diseases-Diagnosis-and-Treatment-of. Last accessed Sep 2017

NICE (2015) Diagnosis and initial management of acute stroke and transient ischaemic attack (TIA)

NHS Standard Contract (2014) Specialised Vascular Services

Cochrane Database Systematic Reviews. (2011). Carotid endarter- ectomy

American 14 Societies' Guidelines on Extracranial Carotid and Vertebral Artery Disease (2011)

CREST (2006). Guidelines for investigation and management of transient ischaemic attack.

National Institute for Health and Clinical Excellence (2011). Carotid artery stent placement for carotid stenosis.

Cina C, Clase C, Haynes RB (1999). Carotid endarterectomy for symptomatic carotid stenosis. Cochrane Database Syst Rev 3, CD001081

Chambers BR, Donnan G (2005) Carotid endarterectomy for asymptomatic carotid stenosis. Cochrane Database Syst Rev 4, CD001923.

Chaturvedi S, Bruno A, Feasby T et al. (2005). Carotid endarterectomy—an evidence-based review: report of the Therapeutics and Technology Assessment Subcommittee of the American Academy of Neurology. Neurology 65, 794–801.

National Institute for Health and Clinical Excellence (2011). Carotid artery stent placement for carotid stenosis. Available from: https://www.nice.org.uk/Guidance/ipg389.

National Institute for Health and Clinical Excellence (2017). Stroke. Available from: https://www.nice.org.uk/guidance/cg68

Scottish Intercollegiate Guidelines Network (2002). Management of patients with stroke: rehabilitation, prevention and management of complications, and discharge planning. Available from: http://www.sign.ac.uk/pdf/sign64.pdf;

Scottish Intercollegiate Guidelines Network (2008) Management of patients with stroke or TIA: assessment, investigation, immediate management and secondary prevention. Available from: http://www.sign.ac.uk/assets/sign108.pdf.

Lip GYH, Kalra L (2008). Stroke prevention. BMJ Clin Evid 9, 207.

Wikipedia. Stroke. Available from: http://en.wikipedia.org/wiki/Stroke;

Wikipedia. Transient ischaemic attack. Available from: http://en.wikipedia.org/wiki/Transient_ischemic_attack.

Naylor AR, Gaines PA (2006). Extracranial cerebrovascular disease. In: Vascular and endovascular surgery, 3rd ed, Elsevier Saunders, London.

Rothwell PM, Giles MF, Flossmann E et al. (2005). A simple score (ABCD) to identify individuals at high early risk of stroke after transient ischaemic attack. Lancet 366, 29–36.

Rothwell PM, Coull AJ, Silver LE et al. (2005). Population-based study of event rate, incidence, case fatality, and mortality for all acute vascular events in all arterial territories (Oxford Vascular Study). Lancet 366, 1773–83.

Van Wijk I, Kappelle LJ, van Gijn J et al. (2005). Long-term survival and vascular event risk after transient ischaemic attack or minor ischaemic stroke: a cohort study. Lancet 363, 2098–104.

North American Symptomatic Carotid Endarterectomy Trial Collaborators (1991). Beneficial effect of carotid endarterectomy in symptomatic patients with high-grade carotid stenosis. N Engl J Med 325, 445–53.

European Carotid Surgery Trialists' Collaborative Group (1991). MRC European Carotid Surgery Trial: interim results for symptomatic patients with severe (70–99%) or with mild (0–29%) carotid stenosis. Lancet 337, 1235–43.

Executive Committee for the Asymptomatic Carotid Atherosclerosis Study (1995). Endarterectomy for asymptomatic carotid artery stenosis. JAMA 273, 1421–8.

Halliday A, Mansfield A, Marro J et al. (2004). Prevention of disabling and fatal strokes by successful carotid endarterectomy in patients without recent neurological symptoms: randomised trial. Lancet 363, 1491–502.

Hatano S (1976). Experience from a multicentre stroke register: a preliminary report. Bull World Health Organ 54: 541–53.

PROGRESS Collaborative Group (2001). Randomized trial of a perindopril-based blood-pressure-lowering regime among 6,105 individuals with previous stroke or transient ischaemic attack. Lancet 358, 1033–41.

The Heart Outcomes Prevention Evaluation Study Investigators (2000). Effect of an angiotensin-converting enzyme inhibitor, ramipril, on cardiovascular events in high- risk patients. N Engl J Med 342, 145–53.

Antiplatelet Trialists' Collaboration (1988). Secondary prevention of vascular disease by prolonged antiplatelet treatment. Br Med J 296, 320–31.

CAPRIE Steering Committee (1996). A randomized blinded trial of clopidogrel versus aspirin in patients at risk of ischaemic event (CAPRIE). Lancet 348, 1329–39.

Abdominal aortic aneurysm (AAA)*

Basic facts *462*
Recommended investigations *464*
Recommended management *466*
Further reading *468*

Key guidelines
- NHS Standard contract for specialist vascular Services (2014).
- National Institute for Health and Clinical Excellence (2016). Endovascular aneurysm sealing for abdominal aortic aneurysm.
- American Society for Vascular Surgery practice guidelines (2009). The care of patients with an abdominal aortic aneurysm.
- ACC/AHA (2005). Practice guidelines for the management of patients with peripheral arterial disease.

* The guidelines on this chapter have been sourced and summarized from different UK, Europe, and international government sources, professional organizations, and medical specialty societies. Leading guidelines have been listed in the further reading section at the end of this chapter

Basic facts

- *Definition*—abnormal, persistent, localized dilatation of the aorta. An anteroposterior aortic diameter of ≥3cm (1.5 times the diameter measured at the level of the renal arteries) is considered aneurysmal, based on epidemiologic information of normal sizes of aorta in healthy adults adjusted to age and gender. AAA can be classified as small (<4.0cm), medium (4.0–5.5cm), large (>5.0cm), and very large (>6.0cm). Rapid expansion (potential marker for increased risk of rupture) is defined as an increase in maximal aortic diameter ≥5 mm over a 6mo or >10mm over 1yr, using the same radiographic method of measurement.
- *Prevalence*—occult AAA can be found on ultrasound screening studies in 4–8% of elderly population. Large aneurysms, however, are in only found in 0.4–0.6% of screened population.
- *Pathogenesis*—appears to be multifactorial (Box 48.1). The combination of aortic wall degenerative changes (associated with abnormal elastolytic and proteolytic activities), chronic inflammatory process (correlated with raised CRP and interleukin (IL)-6), and the haemodynamic forces progressively applied on the aortic wall play a major role in the formation and development of AAA. Most cases are associated with, but not necessarily caused by, atherosclerotic changes. Most (95%) are infrarenal aneurysms.
- *Clinical presentation*—the majority are asymptomatic until they rupture. Usually detected incidentally during investigations for other reasons (Box 48.2). About 15–25% of patients have multiple aneurysms (e.g. popliteal and iliac). Only 30% of AAA <4cm can be detected clinically, rising to 75% when AAA reaches 5cm or more.
- *Natural history*—only 10% of untreated AAA patients (depending on the aneurysm size) would be alive in 8 years' time (compared to 65% of non-AAA age-matching population). Ruptured AAA accounts for ~30–50% of death in this group (Table 48.1). The risk of rupture increases in higher aneurysm diameter, expanding aneurysm (>0.5cm/6mo), females (OR ×4.5), HTN, severe COPD, and possible recent surgery.

Box 48.1 Risk factors for AAA

- *Ageing process*—significant increase in prevalence with advancing age (~1.5% for men aged 45–55y, rising to 12.5% for men aged 75–85y). Screening (abdominal physical examination and one-time USS) should be offered to male patients at age 65, (and to those aged 65–75y who have never smoked as per US recommendations [B]).
- *Genetic*—higher risk (×4–10) in patients with affected first-degree relative. Risk rises to 20 times if a sister is affected. Screening (abdominal physical examination and USS) should be offered to first-degree male relatives of AAA patients [B]. Proper advice on stopping smoking (including smoking cessation interventions) should be offered to patients with a family history of aneurysms [B].
- *Smoking*—major risk factor (OR ×5.6) for the formation, growth, and rupture of AAA. Proper smoking cessation interventions (e.g. behavioural modification and nicotine replacement) should be offered to AAA patients [C].
- *Atherosclerosis*—more common in AAA patients (MI, carotid stenosis, peripheral arterial disease), and vice versa.
- *Others*—hypertension (relatively small effect OR ×1.2), Caucasian ethnicity, increased waist circumference (OR ×1.2), and other large vessel aneurysms.

Box 48.2 Symptoms of AAA

- *Asymptomatic*—detected incidentally or on rupture.
- *Symptomatic*—worsening abdominal or back pain (steady hypogastric gnawing pain for hours or days) and tender aneurysm are usually associated with recent expansion or inflammatory process and high risk for rupture. Distal embolization can also occur.
- *Ruptured aneurysm*—presents (if patient survives long enough to get medical attention) with abdominal or back pain, hypotension, and/or a pulsatile abdominal mass.

Table 48.1 Estimated risk of AAA rupture*

Size (cm)	Risk of rupture per year (%)
<3.9	0
4.0–4.9	0.5–5
5.0–5.9	3–15
6.0–6.9	10–20
7.0–7.9	20–40
≥8.0	30–50

* Based on a meta-analysis of 13 studies and Joint Council of the American Association for Vascular Surgery and Society for Vascular Surgery (2009)

Recommended investigations

- *USS*—highly reliable for detecting AAA (accuracy ~97–100%) [B].
  - USS is less reliable in screening iliac aneurysms and obese patients.
- *Abdominal contrast spiral CT scan/MRI/CT angiography*—should be used selectively (e.g. excluding other causes of abdominal pain, thorough assessment of aorta and iliacs, planning for open or endovascular aortic procedures).
- *Screening recommendations for AAA*—see Box 48.3.

Box 48.3 Screening recommendations for AAA

- Key trial—the Multicentre Aneurysm Screening Study (MASS) trial: four centres (7,000 men); screening (and treatment) vs control group. The screening arm had AAA-related mortality reduction by 42%; emergency ruptured AAA mortality reduction by 70%; reduced disruption to elective work; and better management of risk factors and ICU/HDU beds.
- Cost-effectiveness—estimated at ~£28,500 per QALY (quality adjusted life year) after 4y, and at ~£10,000 per QALY after 10y (cost-effective NHS screening programme should be less than £30,000 per QALY).
- Estimated increase in workload—one extra AAA repair per month for a general hospital serving ~400,000 population.
- Current recommendations—screening (abdominal physical examination and one-time USS) should be offered to male patients at the age of 65 (Table 48.1) [B]. This should be repeated in appropriate intervals to detect progression.

Recommended management

Best medical treatment

- *Smoking*—should be completely discontinued [C].
- *High BP and high lipids*—should be well controlled [C].
  - β-*blockers*—may be considered for AAA patients who are being followed non-operatively [B]. Patients undergoing AAA repair have been recommended to consider β-blockers in the perioperative period (if no contraindications exist) [A].
  - *POISE trial*—is the largest trial to date. A total of 8,351 patients with or at risk of atherosclerotic disease undergoing non-cardiac surgery (42% vascular surgery) were randomly assigned to either fixed dose metoprolol or placebo given 2–4h before surgery and repeated 0–6h after surgery. POISE results as well as two other meta-analyses confirmed that β-blockers decreases the risk of MI (RR=0.73), but increases the risk of death (RR=1.29) due to other causes (mainly stroke).

Follow-up surveillance for small aneurysms

- *Asymptomatic AAA (3.0–5.5cm)*—should be managed conservatively (watchful waiting) to balance the risks of rupture (Table 48.1) with the risk of operation (Box 48.4) [A]. Monitoring with regular USS (or CT scan) is recommended 3–12 monthly (depending on the initial size and expansion rate of the aneurysm) [A].

Surgical treatment

- *General approach*—factors to be considered include the size and rate of growth of the aneurysm, perioperative expected risk (see Chapter 6, p. 59), quality of life issues, and patient's wishes and expectations.
- *Aneurysm key trials*—include the UK Small Aneurysm trial and VA Aneurysm Detection and Management (ADAM) Trial (US). EVAR 1 and 2 trials (see Box 48.4) and their updates are key cornerstones for the current recommendations of AAA repair.
- *Large-sized infrarenal asymptomatic AAA (>5.5cm)*—benefits from elective repair (endovascular or open) in fit (good or average) and willing patients [B]. Elective repair for screen-detected AAA can offer an extra 9y of life to over 3,000 men per year in the UK (Box 48.4).
- *Symptomatic AAA*—requires surgical repair (endovascular or open) regardless of the size in fit and suitable candidates [C]. Aneurysms increasing by ≥0.5cm in diameter per year should also be considered for repair.
- *Surgical options*—include open and endovascular surgical repair (Box 48.4). EVAR patients should undergo immediate and long-term surveillance to detect endoleaks, displacement, and any need for further intervention [B].

Box 48.4 Surgical treatment of AAA

- *Elective open repair.*
  - Surgical technique—involves full laparotomy, assessment of the aneurysm, full control of proximal, distal and collateral ends, and placement of appropriate aortic bypass graft.
  - Risks—recorded in-hospital mortality rate is 2–8% depending on the surgeon and the centre. Operative non-fatal morbidity (CVA, MI, renal failure, ischaemic bowel, ischaemic legs) differs between centres as well (5% on average). Graft infection and impotence can also occur.
- *Elective endovascular aneurysm repair (EVAR).*
  - *Surgical technique*—collaboration of vascular surgeons and interventional radiologists. Bilateral groin access allows wires, catheters, and graft delivery systems to be delivered into the aorta and the bypass graft to be deployed under X-ray guidance.
  - *Risks*—recorded in-hospital mortality rate is <3%. Operative non-fatal morbidity (CVA, MI, renal failure, ischaemic bowel, ischaemic legs) is ~3% on average. Graft infection and endoleak (persistent flow into aneurysm sac after deployment of graft) can also occur.
- *Laparoscopic repair of AAA*—can be performed using a hand-assisted or total laparoscopic surgery. Current evidence on safety and efficacy supports the use of this procedure by well-trained surgeons in appropriate clinical governance setting and multidisciplinary patient selection.

Further reading

NHS Standard contract for specialist vascular Services (2014)

National Institute for Health and Clinical Excellence (2009). Stent-graft placement in abdominal aortic aneurysm.

American Society for Vascular Surgery practice guidelines (2009) The care of patients with an abdominal aortic aneurysm

Hirsch AT, Haskal ZJ, Hertzer NR et al. (2006). ACC/AHA 2005 Practice guidelines for the management of patients with peripheral arterial disease (lower extremity, renal, mesenteric, and abdominal aortic): a collaborative report from the American Association for Vascular Surgery/Society for Vascular Surgery, Society for Cardiovascular Angiography and Interventions, Society for Vascular Medicine and Biology, Society of Interventional Radiology, and the ACC/AHA Task Force on Practice Guidelines (Writing Committee to develop guidelines for the management of patients with peripheral arterial disease): endorsed by the American Association of Cardiovascular and Pulmonary Rehabilitation; National Heart, Lung, and Blood Institute; Society for Vascular Nursing; TransAtlantic Inter-Society Consensus; and Vascular Disease Foundation. Circulation 113, e463–654.

Vascular Society of Great Britain and Ireland (2004). Screening for abdominal aortic aneurysm. Available from: https://legacyscreening.phe.org.uk/aaa.

National Institute for Health and Clinical Excellence (2006). Stent-graft placement in abdominal aortic aneurysm. Available from: http://www.nice.org.uk/nicemedia/pdf/ip/IPG163guidance.pdf.

Lederle FA, Johnson GR, Wilson SE et al. (2000). The aneurysm detection and manage- ment study screening program: validation cohort and final results. Aneurysm Detection and Management Veterans Affairs Cooperative Study Investigators. Arch Intern Med 160, 1425–30.

Powell JT, Greenhalgh RM (2003). Clinical practice. Small abdominal aortic aneurysms. N Engl J Med 348, 1895–901.

Scott RA, Ashton HA, Kay DN (1991). Abdominal aortic aneurysm in 4,237 screened patients: prevalence, development and management over 6 years. Br J Surg 78, 1122–5.

Lederle FA, Johnson GR, Wilson SE et al. (1997). Prevalence and associations of abdominal aortic aneurysm detected through screening. Aneurysm Detection and Management (ADAM) Veterans Affairs Cooperative Study Group. Ann Intern Med 126, 441–9.

Chronic venous insufficiency (CVI)*

Basic facts *470*
Recommended investigations *472*
Recommended treatment *474*
Further reading *478*

Key guidelines
- NICE (2013). Varicose veins in the legs.
- National Clinical Guideline Centre (2013). Varicose veins in legs.
- Cochrane Evidence (2014). Varicose veins.

---

* The guidelines on this chapter have been sourced and summarized from different UK, Europe, and international government sources, professional organizations, and medical specialty societies. Leading guidelines have been listed in the further reading section at the end of this chapter.

Basic facts

- *Definitions*—CVI is the impairment of venous return in the lower limbs, presenting with a broad clinical spectrum, including varicose veins, skin changes, and venous ulceration (Box 49.1).
- *Incidence*—CVI affects ~2–9% of the population. Varicose veins affect ~40% of men and 16% of women aged 18–64y. Telangiectasis and reticular veins occur in ~80–85% of both genders. Ankle oedema is present in ~7% of men and 16% women. Venous leg ulcers (active or healed) occur in ~1% of the population.
- *Impact on health resources*—tremendous. Most venous leg ulcers require an average of 1y to heal satisfactorily, 20% require >2y, and 66% of patients complain of episodes of ulceration for >5y. The cost of care for chronic venous disease accounts for ~1–3% of the total health care budget in developed countries.
- *Pathophysiology*—not fully understood (Box 49.2).
  - Risk factors for venous insufficiency include multiple pregnancies (RR ×1.2 after two pregnancies), age, obesity in women (RR ×1.3), and a history of phlebitis or venous thrombosis.
- *Clinical presentation*—ranges from cosmetically upsetting, but otherwise asymptomatic, ectatic veins to severe skin changes, oedema, and ulcerations (Box 49.1).
- *Classification*—the Clinical, Etiologic, Anatomic, and Pathophysiologic (CEAP) classification was developed in 1994 by an international consensus conference and is widely accepted (Table 49.1). CEAP was developed

---

Box 49.1 Clinical presentation of varicose veins

- *Aching pain and heaviness*—fullness feeling, leg cramps during night, aching discomfort, or leg heaviness. Discomfort may be made worse upon standing, during menstrual cycle, and with the progression of pregnancy. Pain may interfere with normal daily activities and makes ambulation difficult.
- *Dilated veins*—vary in size and palpability.
  - Telangiectases are tiny (<1mm), bluish, ectatic, non-palpable venules located intradermally.
  - Reticular veins presents as small, tiny (<3mm), dilated, non-palpable veins located subdermally.
  - Varicose veins are larger (>3mm), dilated, palpable veins located subcutaneously.
- *Leg and ankle oedema*—usually associated with varicose veins at an early stage. Oedema is made worse with prolonged standing positions and improves significantly (at the initial stages of the disease) with leg elevation and walking. Oedema becomes persistent as the disease progresses.
- *Skin changes*—occur at a later stage; reddish brown colour skin changes on the medial aspects of leg and ankle. Lipodermatosclerosis (heavily pigmented skin with extensively fibrotic, and impeding lymphatic and venous flow) results from the fibrosing panniculitis of subcutaneous tissue.
- *Venous ulcer*—usually located on the medial shin over a perforating vein, or along the line of long or short saphenous veins. The ulcer is typically tender, varies in diameter, is shallow with sloping edges, and usually has irregular, but not undermined edges.

initially as a method to standardize reporting in venous disease. However, it was shown to have high interobserver/intraobserver variability and heterogeneity. VCSS (Venous Clinical Severity Score) was developed to allow more advanced and consistent reporting of venous disease severity (http://tinyurl.com/8ahqdcf). VCSS is composed of ten parameters (pain, varicose veins, oedema, pigmentation, inflammation, induration, number of ulcers, duration of ulcers, size of ulcers, compressive therapy) that escalate in severity with increased area of the limb involved and are graded 0 to 3 (absent, mild, moderate, severe).

Box 49.2 Pathophysiology of CVI

In most cases, CVI results from an obstruction to venous flow, dysfunction of venous valves, and/or failure of the venous pump. This results in an abnormal direction of the venous blood flow from the deep to the superficial system, with resultant local tissue anoxia, inflammation, white cell trapping, and occasionally, necrosis. The resulting 'subcutaneous fibrosing panniculitis' obstructs further the proximal lymphatic and venous flow.

Table 49.1 CEAP classification

Classification	Description/definition
C: Clinical	
(subdivided into A for asymptomatic, S for symptomatic)	
0	No venous disease
1	Telangectiases
2	Varicose veins
3	Oedema
4	Lipodermatosclerosis or hyperpigmentation
5	Healed ulcer
6	Active ulcer
E: aEtiologic	
Congenital	Present since birth
Primary	Undetermined aetiology
Secondary	Associated with post-thrombotic, traumatic
A: Anatomic distribution (alone or in combination)	
Superficial	Great and short saphenous veins
Deep	Cava, iliac, gonadal, femoral, profunda, popliteal, tibial, and muscular veins
Perforator	Thigh and leg perforating veins
P: Pathophysiological	
Reflux	Axial and perforating veins
Obstruction	Acute and chronic
Combination of both	Valvular dysfunction and thrombus

Recommended investigations

- *General approach*—the diagnosis of venous insufficiency and incompetent valve system is mainly based on thorough clinical history, detailed physical examination, and appropriate use of invasive and non-invasive investigations. The widespread use of the non-invasive Doppler and duplex scan has reduced the need for more time-consuming clinical tests such as Trendelenburg (selective occlusion) test.
- *Handheld Doppler*—can detect the presence of reflux in the saphenofemoral junction (SFJ), long saphenous vein, saphenopopliteal junction (SPJ), and occasionally, perforating veins. Reported accuracy is ~75%. Limitations include the inability to identify the specific veins and it is operator-dependent.
- *Duplex scanning*—(B-mode USS combined with wave Doppler scan) is the investigation of choice for CVI. Duplex scan can accurately delineate venous anatomy, including areas of venous reflux disease. Reported accuracy is ~95% when compared to traditional venography. There is strong evidence that Duplex scanning should be used for all varicose vein patients. RCTs (BJS 05, BJS 11) comparing routine vs selective preoperative duplex scan showed a significant difference in recurrence rate (14% vs 46%) and reoperation rate (14% vs 35%). Specific reasons for using Duplex scanning include: detecting DVTs; ruling out SPJ incompetency; marking SPJ; excluding the presence of duplicate/multiple veins; and for medico-legal reasons.
- *Other investigations*—may occasionally be required, including venography and functional calf volume measurements. A full description of available investigations for CVI with their benefits and limitations can be found in Nicolaides's review article.

Recommended treatment

- *General approach.*
  - *The main treatment goal in CVI*—is to improve the venous and lymphatic back flow. This in turn would improve the oxygen transport to the skin and subcutaneous tissues, and reduce the inflammatory process, which will allow for the reduction of oedema, elimination of fibrosing panniculitis of the subcutaneous tissue, and eventually healing of the venous ulcers, if present.
  - *Venous and lymphatic back flow can be improved* using general (leg elevation, muscle pump activation, etc.), pharmacologic (e.g. injection sclerotherapy), and operative measures (e.g. treatment of incompetent varicose veins, reconstruction of deep veins). The local treatment of chronic ulcers can be found in Chapter 9.
- *General measures*—include elevation of the legs above the heart level at rest, regular exercises (sensible option, but lack evidence), avoidance of long standing, and management of confounding factors such as obesity [G].
- *Graduated compression stockings*—is the primary effective management of CVI. Stockings that apply the highest pressure around the ankle (~30–40mmHg) and decreases proximally has been validated in a Cochrane systematic review to significantly increase the healing rate of leg ulcers, especially when multi-component systems (three or four layers of bandages) that contain an elastic bandage were used. Caution should be taken when applied in patients with concurrent arterial disease. The reported healing rate is ~93% in a mean duration of 5.3mo. Surgical correction of superficial venous reflux in addition to compression bandaging has been shown in ESCHAR trial **NOT** to be superior to compression bandaging alone in improving the ulcer healing, but was able to reduce the recurrence of ulcers at 4y and resulted in a greater proportion of ulcer-free time.
- *Injection sclerotherapy for varicose veins*—has been shown in a Cochrane review to have significant effect (improved symptoms and cosmetic appearance) when used for recurrent varicose veins following surgery and thread veins (such as telangectiasia or spider veins). Compared to surgery, injection sclerotherapy appears to have superior results in the short term, but inferior results after 5y, although the evidence is weak. Box 49.3 summarizes the technique, contraindications, and possible side-effects.

Box 49.3 Injection sclerotherapy—technique and side-effects

Technique—following marking the varicosities while patient is standing, a small (25–30G) needle is used to inject a small amount (0.25–0.50mL) of an appropriate sclerosing agent slowly into the lumen of the vein. Compression stockings are then applied for few weeks and the patient is asked to walk for half an hour daily.

Contraindications—include allergy to the agent in use, peripheral vascular disease, immobility, and acute thrombophlebitis.

Complications—are rare, including thrombosis, ulceration, and anaphylactic reactions.

- *Ultrasound-guided foam sclerotherapy* —current evidence on the safety and efficacy of this treatment for varicose veins appears adequate to support its use as a second-line treatment option (Box 49.4).
- Endovascular treatment of varicose veins.
  - *Endovenous laser therapy (EVLT)*—current evidence on the safety and efficacy of this treatment for incompetent long saphenous vein appears adequate to support its use (in addition to RFA) as a FIRST-line treatment option (Box 49.5).
- *Radiofrequency ablation of varicose veins*—this technique involves accessing the long saphenous vein (puncture or small incision) and heating the wall of the diseased vein using a bipolar generator and specially designed catheters. By manually withdrawing the catheter at 2.5–3cm/min, the vein wall temperature can be maintained at 85°C. Current evidence on the safety and efficacy of this treatment for incompetent long saphenous vein appears adequate to support its use as a first-line treatment option.

Box 49.4 Ultrasound-guided foam sclerotherapy

Technique—a variation of the traditional liquid sclerotherapy. Under ultrasound guidance, a sclerosant foam is injected into the vein and compression stockings are applied.

Safety—no major safety concerns according to current available evidence. Transient side-effects in a small proportion of patients have been noticed. Possible adverse effects include skin pigmentation (~30% of cases), skin necrosis (~1.5%), local neurological injury (<1%), transient visual disturbance (0–6%), and rare cases of stroke, MI, epilepsy, and DVT.

Efficiency—successful vein occlusion occurs in ~85% of cases. Compared to surgery, no significant difference was noticed. Recurrence rate ranged from 1–15%.

Terms of use—special arrangements should be undertaken for clinical governance, patient consent, audit, and review of all outcome results by a dedicated team.

Box 49.5 Endovenous laser therapy (EVLT) and Radiofrequency Ablation (RFA)

Technique—following injection of a local anaesthesia, a catheter is placed into the long saphenous vein under ultrasound guidance. The laser/RF catheter is passed through to just below (distal) the SFJ. Further local anaesthesia is injected, and then energy from a diode laser/RF machine is delivered while slowly withdrawing the catheter.

Safety—no major safety concerns were reported according to current available evidence. Possible complications include DVT, minor skin burns (~0.5%), and temporary paraesthesia (~2%).

Efficiency—appears to be more effective in the short term and at least as effective overall as the comparative procedure of junction ligation and vein stripping for the treatment of varicose veins.

Terms of use—special arrangements should be undertaken for clinical governance, patient consent, audit, and review of all outcome results by a dedicated team.

- *Open surgery for varicose veins*. This is currently recommended as a third-line treatment option for varicose veins.
  - *Technique*—ligation of the SFJ, stripping of the long saphenous vein, and avulsion of the remaining varicosities is the traditional varicose vein operation, and one of the commonest sources of litigation in the UK.
  - *Benefits*—a Cochrane systematic review has shown that open surgery has significantly reduced the risk of varicose vein recurrence and improved cosmetic appearance when compared with injection sclerotherapy alone.
  - *Standards of surgery*—include adequate preoperative investigation and marking, adequate and thorough patient consultation, using day surgery as a norm (see ➍ Chapter 4, pp.46–50), and appropriate stripping and avulsion techniques.
- Do not carry out interventional treatment for varicose veins during pregnancy other than in exceptional circumstances.

Further reading

NICE (2013) Varicose Veins in the Legs.National Clinical Guideline Centre (2013). Varicose Veins in Legs.

Cochrane Evidence (2014). Varicose veins. Tisi P (2007). Varicose veins. BMJ Clin Evid 10, 212.

Rigby KA, Palfreyman SJ, Beverley C, Michaels JA (2004). Surgery versus sclerotherapy for the treatment of varicose veins. Cochrane Database Syst Rev 4, CD004980.

National Institute for Health and Clinical Excellence (2007). Ultrasound-guided foam sclerotherapy for varicose veins. Available from: http://www.nice.org.uk/Guidance/IPG217.

National Institute for Health and Clinical Excellence (2004). Endovenous laser treatment of long saphenous vein. Available from: http://www.nice.org.uk/Guidance/IPG52.

National Institute for Health and Clinical Excellence (2003). Radiofrequency ablation of varicose veins. Available from: http://www.nice.org.uk/Guidance/IPG8.

National Institute for Health and Clinical Excellence (2004). Transilluminated powered phlebectomy for varicose veins. Available from: http://www.nice.org.uk/Guidance/IPG37.

Eberhardt RT, Raffetto JD (2005). Chronic venous insufficiency. Circulation 111, 2398–409.

Nicolaides AN (2000). Investigation of chronic venous insufficiency: a consensus statement. Circulation 102, e126–63.

Bergan JJ, Schmid–Schönbein GW, Smith PD, Nicolaides AN, Boisseau MR, Eklof B (2006). Chronic venous disease. N Engl J Med 355, 488–98.

Evans CJ, Fowkes FG, Ruckley CV, Lee AJ (1999). Prevalence of varicose veins and chronic venous insufficiency in men and women in the general population: Edinburgh Vein Study. J Epidemiol Community Health 53, 149–53.

Criqui MH, Denenberg JO, Bergan J, Langer RD, Fronek A (2007). Risk factors for chronic venous disease: the San Diego Population Study. J Vasc Surg 46, 331–7.

Scott TE, LaMorte WW, Gorin DR, Menzoian JO (1995). Risk factors for chronic venous insufficiency: a dual case-control study. J Vasc Surg 22, 622–8.

Chiesa R, Marone EM, Limoni C, Volonte M, Petrini O (2007). Chronic venous disorders: correlation between visible signs, symptoms, and presence of functional disease. J Vasc Surg 46, 322–30.

Porter JM, Moneta GL (1995). Reporting standards in venous disease: An update. J Vasc Surg 21, 635–45.

Campbell WB, Niblett PG, Ridler BM, Peters AS, Thompson JF (1997). Handheld Doppler as a screening test in primary varicose veins. Br J Surg 84, 1541–3.

Khaira, HS, Parnell, A (1995). Colour flow duplex in the assessment of varicose veins. Clin Radiol 50, 583–4.

Smith JJ, Brown L, Greenhalgh RM, Davies AH (2002). Randomized trial of preoperative colour duplex marking in primary varicose vein surgery: outcome is not improved. Eur J Vasc Endovasc Surg 23, 336–43.

The Alexander House Group (1992). Consensus paper on venous leg ulcer. J Dermatol Surg Oncol 18, 592–602.

Cullum N, Nelson EA, Fletcher AW, Sheldon TA (2002). Compression for venous leg ulcers. Cochrane Database Syst Rev 2, CD000265.

Mayberry JC, Moneta GL, Taylor LM Jr, Porter JM (1991). Fifteen year results of ambulatory compression therapy for chronic venous ulcers. Surgery 109, 575–81.

Tisi PV, Beverley C, Rees A (2006). Injection sclerotherapy for varicose veins. Cochrane Database Syst Rev 4, CD001732.

Rigby KA, Palfreyman SJ, Beverley C, Michaels JA (2004). Surgery versus sclerotherapy for the treatment of varicose veins. Cochrane Database Syst Rev 4, CD004980.

Medical Services Advisory Committee (2008). Endovenous laser treatment for varicose veins (ELT), MSAC application 1113. Available from: http://www.msac.gov.au/internet/msac/publishing.nsf/Content/7CAA933675966F4DCA25801000123B62/$File/1113-Assessment-Report.pdf.

Gohel MS, Barwell JR, Taylor M et al. (2007). Long-term results of compression therapy alone versus compression plus surgery in chronic venous ulceration (ESCHAR): randomized controlled trial. BMJ 335, 83.

Part 11

Breast

Chapter 50

Breast cancer[*]

Basic facts 482
Recommended investigations and diagnosis 484
Recommended initial staging 486
Recommended management 490
Further reading 496

Key guidelines

- National Institute for Health and Clinical Excellence.
  - Recognition and referral (2015).
  - Early and locally advanced breast cancer: Diagnosis and treatment CG80 (2017).
  - Advanced breast cancer: Diagnosis and treatment. CG81 (2017).
  - Improving outcomes in breast cancer – manual update (2002).
- Association of Breast Surgery at BASO.
  - Surgical guidelines for the management of breast cancer (2009).
  - Best practice diagnostic guidelines for patients presenting with breast symptoms (2010).
- Scottish Intercollegiate Guidelines Network. Guidance 134. Treatment of primary breast cancer.
- Cancer Research UK (2015). Breast cancer.

[*] The guidelines on this chapter have been sourced and summarized from different UK, Europe, and international government sources, professional organizations, and medical specialty societies. Leading guidelines have been listed in the further reading section at the end of this chapter

Basic facts

- *Incidence*—the commonest cancer affecting women and the commonest cause of cancer death in women worldwide. Over 50% increase in incidence since 1980 (more than 1% each year). In 2011 over 50,000 people were diagnosed with invasive breast cancer in the UK (49,936 women and 349 men), and nearly 6,000 women with in situ breast cancer in 2010.
- *Survival*—of women diagnosed with breast cancer 86% and 78% are expected to survive for more than 5 and 10 years, respectively. There were 1,716 deaths from breast cancer in 2012, which makes up 7% of the UK cancer deaths. Survival is linked to the stage at presentation. Improved survival is due to screening programmes, early presentation, and access to specialist care with improved treatment strategies.
- *Risk factors*—female gender, increasing age, previous breast cancer, or a significant family history of breast cancer are the main risk factors. Other risk factors relate to hormonal, reproductive, physical, and lifestyle factors. See Box 50.1.

Box 50.1 Risk factors for breast cancer

- *Patient age*—risk increases with increasing age. Rare under 30, estimated risk is 1 in 1,900, increasing to 1 in 50, under the age of 50). Most cases (8 out of 10) diagnosed in the screening 50–64 age group (estimated risk at age 70 is 1 in 10).
- *Personal and family history of breast cancer*—personal history increases the risk of a second primary breast cancer by 2–6 times. A positive family history of breast cancer in one first-degree relative (mother or sister) increases the risk of breast cancer by two. Two or more affected relatives increase the risk further. Note that over 85% of women with a close relative who had a breast cancer will never develop the disease.
- *Socioeconomic status*—more common in higher socioeconomic status females (up to 2-fold). More common in North America and Northern Europe. Possibly caused by the special modern reproductive lifestyle (parity, later age at first live birth).
- *Reproductive history*—more common in women with early age of menarche (each year menarche is delayed after age 12 reduces the risk by 3–7%), in women with late childbearing (risk increases by 3% for each year of delay), in nulliparous women (risk increases by 30% in nulliparous vs parous women), in women with no history of breastfeeding (each year of breastfeeding reduces the risk by 4.3%), and in women with delayed menopause (risk increases by 3% for each year delay in menopause).
- *Other risk factors*
  - *Oral contraceptives* confer a small increased risk with length of use (5y RR ×1.07, 10 y RR ×1.14,). HRT—some studies confer all HRT (oestrogen only and combined) with higher RR, increasing with length of exposure (Million Women Study, WHI), but unopposed oestrogens may infer no increased risk with use <5y (RR ×0.47) ESPRIT study.
  - *High BMI* increases the risk in post-menopausal women (30% increased risk for BMI >28 compared to BMI <21). Each 5kg increase in adult weight gain increases risk by 11% (RR ×1.11). Physically active women reduce their risk by 25%.
  - *Alcohol consumption* increases the risk by 7% for each daily alcoholic drink consumption. No proven link of tobacco to the risk of breast cancer. Exposure to ionizing radiation of the chest at a young age, as occurs with treatment of Hodgkin lymphoma.

Recommended investigations and diagnosis

- *Clinical presentation*—ranges from a highly suspicious breast lesion to a completely asymptomatic screen-detected cancer (Box 50.2). The estimated doubling time of breast cancer is 100–300d with frequent exceptions. A 1cm³ tumour usually requires ~30 doublings (≥7y) to become palpable clinically. Palpability depends also on the volume of breast, location of cancer, surrounding stromal reaction, and experience of the examiner. Breast screening detects many cancers at the pre-clinical stage (about 20–35% of all breast cancer cases in the UK).
- *Urgent referral to breast unit*—for all patients with a breast lump if age ≥30, skin ulceration or distortion, nipple eczema, retraction or unilateral discharge. All symptomatic patients are referred urgently within the '2 week rule', and ideally seen in a one stop clinic. Asymptomatic patients are referred routinely (e.g. those with a strong family history for risk assessment).
- *Triple assessment*—the mainstay of diagnosis [B]. This includes clinical history and examination, breast imaging (two-view digital mammography (most units ≥40y) and ultrasound), and pathological assessment of biopsy (core biopsy).
- *Accuracy*—depends on the quality of each constituent test. Reported sensitivity is 99% if all investigations concur. False negative rates are low, but higher in younger patients due to increased density of breast tissue. Concordance between tests is paramount, so if there remains doubt, further imaging (tomosynthesis, MRI) and pathological assessment (further cores or excision biopsy) is indicated.
- *Quality standards*—bilateral mammography prior to any definitive treatment is essential in any patient with early breast cancer [B]. Core biopsy also has the advantage of making the assessment of hormone receptor status possible.
- *Mammographic abnormalities*—detected in most cancers. The overall sensitivity and specificity is 80–85%, with increasing sensitivity in postmenpausal women (therefore, it cannot be the only diagnostic test for symptomatic breast patients).
  - *Most common findings*—suggestive of cancer are clustered microcalcifications and spiculated masses. Microcalcifications (calcium shadows measuring between 0.1 and 1mm in diameter, taking various shapes and sizes, and grouping as a cluster of more than 4–5/cm³) are found in about 60% of mammographically detected cancers. Spiculated masses are found in about a third of non-calcified breast cancer. Other suspicious findings include linear branching microcalcifications and granular calcifications.
  - *Summary of findings*—is best performed using the Royal College of Radiologists scoring system (Box 50.3), indicating the likelihood of a normal, benign, or malignant diagnosis.
- *USS*—complements the clinical examination and mammography, especially in undetermined cases (palpable masses with normal mammogram, breast masses in dense breasts, young ages, etc.).

Sensitivity, specificity, and negative predictive values when adding USS in such cases are around 97, 95, and 99%, respectively. Very beneficial in predicting (and downstaging) cancer size, and in guiding real-time FNA, core biopsy, or wire insertion in small or non-palpable lesions. Pretreatment assessment of axilla with USS and ultrasound-guided FNA is recommended.

- *Other imaging modalities (such as tomosynthesis and MRI scan)*—should be used in specific occasions after discussion at the MDT meeting. MRI scan is specifically useful for evaluating undetermined cases where a discrepancy between clinical and radiological assessments exists, in increased breast density, and as part of the assessment of the size of invasive lobular carcinoma, bilateral disease, and to consider if conservative surgery is possible.
- *Breast biopsy*—core biopsy is the standard of care.
  - *Core biopsy*—is able to distinguish invasive from in situ cancers in most cases. Findings should be reported using a standardized reporting system (Box 50.3).
  - *Other methods*—can occasionally be used for sampling purposes in certain cases, including open biopsy and stereotactic biopsy.

Box 50.2 Breast cancer—clinical features

- *Local features*—include breast lump (often hard, painless, can be immobile, fixed to surrounding tissues, to overlying skin, or to the underlying pectoral muscle), nipple discharge (usually unifocal, bloodstained, or clear), and skin changes (skin distortion, puckering, and peau d'orange sign).
- *Regional features*—include axillary and supraclavicular lymphadenopathy.
- *Distant features*—include hepatomegaly, ascites, and bone pain consistent with metastatic disease.

Box 50.3 Recommended reporting standards in breast cancer

- *Clinical findings*—P1: normal. P2: benign. P3: probably benign. P4: probably malignant. P5: malignant.
- *USS*—U1: normal. U2: benign. U3: probably benign. U4: probably malignant. U5: malignant.
- *Mammography*—R1: normal. R2: benign. R3: probably benign. R4: probably malignant. R5: malignant.
- *FNAc*—C1: inadequate. C2: benign. C3: atypia probably benign. C4: suspicious of malignancy. C5: malignant.
- *Core biopsy*—B1: unsatisfactory/normal tissue only. B2: benign. B3: lesions of uncertain malignant potential. B4: suspicion of malignancy. B5a: in situ malignancy. B5b: invasive malignancy. B5c: malignant, in situ/invasive status not assessable.

Recommended initial staging

- See Fig. 50.1.
- *MDT discussion*—essential prior to any definitive treatment [C*]. Main issues affecting treatment should be discussed, agreed, and documented (Box 50.4). Joint treatment recommendations should be documented and communicated to the patient as and when appropriate (see below).
- *Basic investigations*—should include baseline blood tests (FBC, LFTs, etc.) for all patients. Other staging tests (CXR, liver imaging or bone scan) are not required for early operable breast cancer [C], and only minimal investigations for asymptomatic patients with early breast cancer should be performed [A]. Agreed local protocols in well-established breast units should be followed.
- *Metastatic cancer*—should be suspected in locally advanced cancers, aggressive histologic and cellular cancer type (large tumours, inflammatory breast cancer, triple negative), and abnormal LFTs. Further staging with CT and bone radionuclide scan should be considered in such cases.
- *PET scan*—should only be used to make a new diagnosis of metastasis where imaging is suspicious, but not diagnostic.
- *Breaking bad news*—an essential step to ensure adequate compliance. Should be done in a professional and effective way (Box 50.5). The role of the cancer care nurse is essential.

Box 50.4 Points to discuss at MDT meeting

- *Surgeon's assessment*—includes clinical findings, patient's personal circumstances and preferences to treatment options, technical surgical considerations (including breast/cancer relative sizes), and any other relevant findings.
- *Radiologist's assessment*—includes the extent of breast disease, and axillary ultrasound findings, further ipsilateral or contralateral breast cancers, need for further radiological assessment or stereotactic histologic confirmation, axillary lymph gland USS assessment with FNAC if abnormal and preoperative requirement for localization of cancer.
- *Pathologist's assessment*—includes confirmation and histologic features of cancer, biological markers (including oestrogen receptors (ERs), progesterone receptors (PRs), and human epidermal growth factor receptor-2 (HER-2), lymphovascular invasion, genomics, and any other relevant issues.
- *Oncologist's assessment*—includes consideration of benefit from chemotherapy in the neoadjuvant or adjuvant setting, likelihood of need for radiotherapy and extent, and hormonal and biological treatment agents to be offered.
- *Breast care nurse*—a named breast care nurse is the essential advocate for the patient.

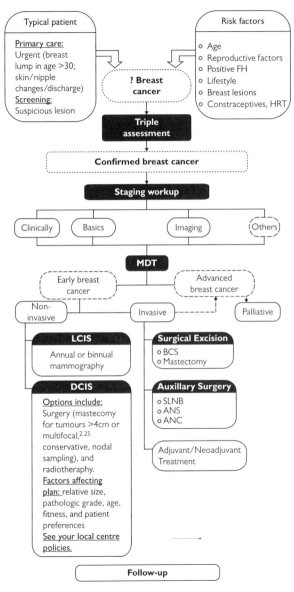

Fig. 50.1 Recommended approach to patients with breast cancer.

Box 50.5 Points to discuss with the patient in the result clinic

- Confirmation of diagnosis, available treatment options (including reconstruction options, with relative benefits and contraindications, undertaken locally and at allied level II oncoplastic units) expected perioperative period experience, contact details and sources for further information (including patient support groups) and further appointments or forums to explore and facilitate joint decision making .
- Discussion should be documented and communicated to other members of the team (GP, oncologists, plastic surgeon, breast care nurses, copy to patient.).

Recommended management

• See Fig. 50.1.

Operable (early stage) breast cancer

• *In general*—surgical excision is the treatment of choice irrespective of age with consideration of patient factors [A]. Neoadjuvant chemotherapy (NACT) should be considered if chemotherapy will be ultimately necessary and would allow downstaging of the breast cancer to achieve BCS rather than mastectomy. Even when mastectomy will be the ultimate surgery NACT may allow time to consider reconstructive options. HRT should be stopped.

• *Surgical options*—should be based on the individual patient needs following a thorough informed consent of benefits and risks of each option [A]. Breast-conserving surgery (BCS) is suitable for the majority if deemed acceptable by the patient (Box 50.6). Mastectomy is the option if BCS is contraindicated or not suitable [A].

Breast reconstruction

• *Should be discussed and offered* (preferably during the initial operation) to all patients undergoing mastectomy [C].

• *Oncoplastic breast surgery* (OPS) type II techniques (if 20–50% of the breast requires resection) can be used in BCS with local advancement flaps (e.g. LICAP, TDAP), or if large breast to tumour ratio therapeutic mammaplasty should be considered.

• *Mastectomy and immediate breast reconstruction* (IBR) or delayed reconstruction (DBR) should be offered, with consideration of patient preferences, surgical feasibility, and risks and benefits. Reconstruction techniques include, implant based (+/- ADM), local pedicled flap (latissimus dorsi), or free flap technique.

Margins

• *Axillary management*—aims to determine the extent of nodal disease and treat the axilla, whilst keeping morbidity to a minimum.

  • All patients with early operable breast cancer should have axillary staging using USS. All invasive operable breast cancer patients should undergo axillary surgery for staging and/or treatment purposes [A]. FNAC or core biopsy is indicated if abnormality such as eccentric cortical thickening or a uniform hypoechoic node with obliteration of the fatty hilum is detected.

  • If metastatic disease is detected, staging, neoadjuvant treatment and axillary node clearance should be considered.

  • If USS shows no nodal abnormalities or the FNAC is negative, sentinel lymph node biopsy is indicated, as 3 in 10 patients will have disease within the sentinel node.

    —Sentinel lymph node biopsy (SLNB)—is performed by selectively removing the first draining node/s following appropriate radio colloid mapping/methylene blue labelling. Nodal assessment can either be histological or techniques are available for upfront analysis (OSNA is NICE approved If the sentinel lymph node contains tumour, further treatment to the axilla, either axillary node clearance or axillary radiotherapy should be given.

—Axillary node clearance (ANC)—if there is proven axillary lymph node disease preoperatively then ANC should be undertaken.

—Macro- or micrometastases found following SLNB. There remains controversy as to the management of low-risk axillary nodal disease, as those with small low-grade tumours and minimal disease seen in the axilla may not benefit from further ANC, and ABS consensus guidance currently allows clinicians to stratify risk and treat appropriately following recent consensus statement guidance (Jan 2015).

- Further local treatment for the malignant sentinel lymph node in patients with early invasive breast cancer.
    —If the sentinel node(s) shows isolated tumour cells and/or micrometastases no further axillary treatment is required in addition to breast conserving surgery or mastectomy.
    —Further axillary treatment is no longer mandatory in patients with 1–2 sentinel nodes with macrometastases who are receiving breast conservation with whole breast radiotherapy, that are post-menopausal and have T1, grade 1 or 2, ER positive and HER2 negative tumours.
    —Further axillary treatment should usually be recommended for patients undergoing mastectomy, or with tumours with one or more of the following features: T3, grade 3, ER negative or HER2 positive.
    —Three or more sentinel nodes with macrometastases: patients should usually be recommended to have further axillary treatment.

Ductal carcinoma in situ (DCIS)

- See Box 50.7.
- *Presentation*—DCIS has shown an increase in incidence, due to the NHS breast cancer screening programme, and comprises 20% of all breast cancers. The majority are asymptomatic (90%) and impalpable, but associated with abnormal calcification on mammography, with a minority presenting symptomatically with a mass or associated with Paget's disease of the nipple.

Box 50.6 Management of early stage breast cancer—BCS benefits, risks, and contraindications

- Benefits and risks of BCS—10y outcome (cancer-related death, local and regional recurrence) is similar to that for mastectomy, good, long-term local control, and very acceptable cosmetic results (compared to mastectomy). BCS requires radiotherapy to reduce the possibility of recurrence in the breast. Radiation-related side-effects are a possibility. BCS may also require further surgery to clear margins.
- Contraindications—include mismatched tumour size to breast size (e.g. 4cm cancer can be treated with BCS in a large breast, and 3cm cancer requires mastectomy in a small breast), some multifocal lesion or extensive microcalcifications on mammography, and inability to tolerate radiotherapy [C].

Box 50.7 Management of DCIS

- Surgical resection is recommended. In general terms, image guided wide local excision with clear margins if amenable to BCS, otherwise (extensive disease or classically >4cm) warrants mastectomy (+/-IBR or DBR). Decisions should be based on the lesion/breast size ratio, pathological features of DCIS, age, fitness to surgery or radiotherapy, and patient preferences. Tamoxifen is not advised for those who have had breast-conserving surgery.
- Sentinel node biopsy is required if a mastectomy is undertaken as a small focus of invasive disease may be detected.
- Radiotherapy may be necessary depending on the Van Nuys Score, and individual risk–benefit analysis.

- *Biological features*—DCIS is a malignant precursor of invasive cancer, encompassing a wide range of pathology, and potential treatment strategies. High-grade DCIS has no precursor, is often ER negative and Her2 positive, and shows progression to grade 3 IDC at an undetermined, but more hasty rate. Low-grade and intermediate grade have precursors with a potentially indolent progression to grade 1 or 2 IDC, often ER positive breast cancer.
- *Management*—the aim is to prevent breast cancer. Surgical management of DCIS is similar to that of invasive breast cancer (see Boxes 50.6 and 50.7). The extent of DCIS needs careful preoperative work up with multiple stereotactic core biopsies and bracketing wires. Conservative management for low risk DCIS can be considered as part of the LORIS trial.
- *Radiotherapy* has been shown to reduce all ipsilateral breast events (HR=0.49) with nine women required to prevent one ipsilateral breast recurrence (NNT=9). All with high grade DCIS should have DXT, but benefit seen in those with low risk DCIS may not outweigh the risks.
- *Survival*—overall survival is excellent. Local recurrence is seen to be 50% DCIS and 50% invasive breast cancer, with further treatment requiring mastectomy.
- *Management*—see Box 50.7.

Lobular carcinoma in situ (LCIS)

- *Biological features*—risk of invasive cancer—not considered pre-malignant, but as a risk marker of potential to develop invasive cancer. 20–30% of patients develop invasive cancer of various types in both biopsied and opposite sides (RR is 2–18 times higher than average population).
- *Management*—see Box 50.8.

Breast reconstruction.

- Should be discussed and offered (preferably during the initial operation) to all patients undergoing mastectomy [C].

Surgical treatment of locoregional recurrence.

- *Recurrence in previously conservatively managed breast*—requires mastectomy (or conservative re-excision if safe and appropriate) and re-staging to exclude distant metastasis.

Box 50.8 Management of LCIS

- Optimal management is controversial. A policy of close surveillance (regular physical examination and annual or biennial mammography) is safe and acceptable [C].
- LCIS found coincidentally in biopsy for other lesions does not require further excision (even if margins contain LCIS).
- Prophylactic tamoxifen or raloxifene reduces the risk of invasive cancer by 38%, but is not currently licensed in the UK.
- Consideration of family history and risk assessment may lead to prophylactic bilateral mastectomy in individual cases, but is not generally recommended.

- *Recurrence in mastectomy patients*—should be managed with excision of recurrence (in solitary, confined, recurrent tumour) or as per the MDT decision.
- *Recurrence in regional lymph nodes*—should be managed with completion of axillary clearance or radiotherapy following local MDT recommendations.

Adjuvant systemic therapy

- *Adjuvant! Online (US data) and PREDICT (UK patient data) are online decision-making tools*—used widely by many MDT teams and centres to guide individual survival based on adjuvant treatment
- *Radiotherapy*—40Gy in 15 fractions (given over 3wk) can significantly reduce the risk of local or regional recurrence following breast conservative surgery (RR ×3.3) for all those with invasive breast cancer and the majority of those with DCIS, following MDT discussion [A]. Radiotherapy boost should be considered in those aged under 50 or those with high grade tumour. Post-mastectomy radiotherapy to chest wall should be considered if high risk of recurrence (4 or more involved lymph nodes, T3/4 disease) and considered in those at intermediate risk (high-risk node negative or those with 1–3 node positive disease).
- *Adjuvant chemotherapy*—should be based on a sound risk–benefit judgement [A]. It should start within 6wk of surgery. Docetaxel, and not paclitaxel, offered to node-positive patients with early breast cancer.
- *Neoadjuvant chemotherapy*—should be offered for large, but early, breast cancers if the patient's preference is for breast-conserving surgery [A].
- *Endocrine therapy*—is indicated for oestrogen-positive cancers. Tamoxifen is suitable for pre-menopausal women. Aromatase inhibitors (AI) are suitable for post-menopausal women, especially if tamoxifen has relative contraindications (e.g. high risk of thromboembolism). Patients starting on an AI should have baseline DEXA assessment of bone mineral density.
- Post-menopausal ER-positive patients not considered low risk should have initial adjuvant treatment with an AI (exemestane or anastrozole). Those on tamoxifen for 2–3y and those treated for 5y should be considered for transfer to letrozole.

- *Biological therapy*—trastuzumab (Herceptin®) should be given 3-weekly for 1y or until disease recurrence as adjuvant treatment for HER-2-positive patients following surgery, chemotherapy, or radio-therapy when appropriate. Requires cardiac function assessment pre-treatment and 3-monthly during treatment.

Follow-up

- Patients to have a written care plan with a copy to the GP. The need for clinical follow-up is debated, but the patient with early breast cancer should, after completion of radiotherapy and systemic adjuvant therapies, be given the options, and this includes primary, secondary, or shared care. Annual mammography—until a minimum age of 70 and this includes those treated for DCIS.
- *Lymphoedema*—patients must have access to specialized support.
- *Menopausal symptoms*—selective serotonin uptake inhibitors (paroxetine, fluoxetine) are useful for patients with hot flushes, but not if they are on tamoxifen. Clonidine, venlafaxine, and gabapentin should only be used if the patients understand the side-effects.
- *Survivorship management*—proven modifiable lifestyle risk factors associated with an impact on survival include, smoking, obesity, and lack of physical exercise.

Management of advanced disease

- Careful assessment of each individual patient's needs and circumstances, and close integration with the different clinicians involved in the management to avoid mixed messages.
- *Hormone therapy*—If ER-positive, the first-line therapy is hormone treatment unless life-threatening in which case chemotherapy followed with hormone therapy. Offer ovarian suppression to pre- and peri-menopausal patients who have previously been treated with tamoxifen. Treat male ER-positive patients with tamoxifen.
- *Chemotherapy*—use sequential single agent chemotherapy in the majority of patients, starting with anthracyclines, progressing to docetaxel as a single agent, second-line vinorelbine, or capecitabine, thirdly vinorelbine or capecitabine depending on what was used previously. Gemcitabine with paclitaxel have been used and paclitaxel in combination with trastuzumab can be offered to HER-2-positive patients scoring 3+.
- *Bone secondaries*—offer bisphosphonates to patients with bone secondaries and localized radiotherapy 8Gy to painful bone second-aries. Orthopaedic surgeons should be involved if there is a risk of long bone fracture.
- *Brain secondaries*—surgery in rare circumstances. Whole brain radiotherapy more often indicated.

Further reading

Cancer Research UK (2015). http://www.cancerresearchuk.org/cancer-info/cancerstats/types/breast/ accessed May 2015

Association of Breast Surgery (2005). Surgical guidelines for the management of breast cancer. Eur J Surg Oncol 35 (Suppl 1), 1–22.

Scottish Intercollegiate Guidelines Network (2013). Treatment of Primary Breast Cancer. Available from: http://www.sign.ac.uk/sign-134-treatment-of-primary-breast-cancer.html

National Institute for Health and Clinical Excellence (2002-2017). Improving outcomes in breast cancer

Breast Cancer Care. Available from: http://www.breastcancercare.org.uk/.

BMJ Clinical Evidence. Breast Cancer. 2009. Available from: http://clinicalevidence.bmj.com/x/systematic-review/0102/overview.html.

Kelsey JL, Fischer DB, Holford TR et al. (1981). Exogenous oestrogens and other factors in the epidemiology of breast cancer. J Natl Cancer Inst 67, 327–33.

Clavel-Chapelon F; E3N–EPICGroup (2002). Differential effects of reproductive factors on the risk of pre- and postmenopausal breast cancer. Results from a large cohort of French women. Br J Cancer 86, 723–7.

Ewertz M, Duffy SW, Adami HO et al. (1990). Age at first birth, parity and risk of breast cancer: a meta-analysis of 8 studies from the Nordic countries. Int J Cancer 46, 597–603.

Chen Y, Thompson W, Semenciw R, Mao Y (1999). Epidemiology of contralateral breast cancer. Cancer Epidemiol Biomarkers Prev 8, 855–61.

Collaborative Group on Hormonal Factors in Breast Cancer (2001). Familial breast cancer: collaborative reanalysis of individual data from 52 epidemiological studies including 58,209 women with breast cancer and 101,986 women without the disease. Lancet 358, 1389–99.

Collaborative Group on Hormonal Factors in Breast Cancer (1996). Breast cancer and hormonal contraceptives: collaborative reanalysis of individual data on 53,297 women with breast cancer and 100,239 women without breast cancer from 54 epidemiological studies. Lancet 347, 1713–27.

Key T, Appleby P, Barnes I, Reeves G; Endogenous Hormones and Breast Cancer Collaborative Group (2002). Endogenous sex hormones and breast cancer in postmenopausal women: re-analysis of nine prospective studies. J Natl Cancer Inst 94, 606–16.

Van den Brandt PA, Spiegelman D, Yaun SS (2000). Pooled analysis of prospective cohort studies on height, weight, and breast cancer risk. Am J Epidemiol 152, 514–27.

Hamajima N, Hirose K, Tajima K (2002). Alcohol, tobacco and breast cancer—collaborative reanalysis of individual data from 53 epidemiological studies, including 58,515 women with breast cancer and 95,067 women without the disease. Br J Cancer 87, 1234–45.

Greenall MJ, Wood WC (2001). Cancer of the breast. In: Oxford Textbook of Surgery, 2nd ed. Oxford University Press, Oxford.

Morrow M , Khan S (2006). Breast disease. In: Greenfield's surgery: scientific principles and practice, 2nd ed, Lippincott Williams & Wilkins, Philadelphia.

Querci della Rovere G, Warren R (2001). Detection of breast cancer. Mammography should be available. BMJ 322, 792–3.

Mittra I, Baum M, Thornton H, Houghton J (2000). Is clinical breast examination an acceptable alternative to mammographic screening? BMJ 321, 1071–2.

Smart CR, Hartmann WH, Beahrs OH, Garfinkel L (1993). Insights into breast cancer screening of younger women. Evidence from the 14-year follow-up of the Breast Cancer Detection Demonstration Project. Cancer 72, 1449–56.

The Royal College of Radiologists (1990). Quality assurance guidelines for radiologists. NHSBSP Publications, Oxford.

Flobbe K, Bosch AM, Kessels AG et al. (2003). The additional diagnostic value of ultrasonography in the diagnosis of breast cancer. Arch Intern Med 163, 1194–9.

Soo MS, Rosen EL, Baker JA, Vo TT, Boyd BA (2001). Negative predictive value of sonography with mammography in patients with palpable breast lesions. AJR Am J Roentgenol 177, 1167–70.

Tilanus-Linthorst MM, Obdeijn IM, Bartels KC (2005). MARIBS study. Lancet 365, 1769–78.

Saslow D, Boetes C, Burke W et al. (2007). American Cancer Society guidelines for breast screening with MRI as an adjunct to mammography. CA Cancer J Clin 57, 75–89.

Fisher ER, Land SR, Fisher B, Mamounas E, Gilarski L, Wolmark N (2004). Pathologic findings from the National Surgical Adjuvant Breast and Bowel Project: twelve-year observations concerning lobular carcinoma in situ. Cancer 100, 238–44.

Bradley SJ, Weaver DW, Bouwman DL (1990). Alternatives in the surgical management of in situ breast cancer. A meta-analysis of outcome. Am Surg 56, 428–32.

Abner AL, Connolly JL, Recht A et al. (2000). The relation between the presence and extent of lobular carcinoma in situ and the risk of local recurrence for patients with infiltrating carcinoma of the breast treated with conservative surgery and radiation therapy. Cancer 88, 1072–7.

Stolier AJ, Barre G, Bolton JS, Fuhrman GM, Looney S (2004). Breast conservation therapy for invasive lobular carcinoma: the impact of lobular carcinoma in situ in the surgical specimen on local recurrence and axillary node status. Am Surg 70, 818–21.

Cuzick J, Powles T, Veronesi U et al. (2003). Overview of the main outcomes in breast-cancer prevention trials. Lancet 361, 296–300.

Gump FE (1990). Lobular carcinoma in situ. Pathology and treatment. Surg Clin North Am 70, 873–83.

Morris A D, Morris RD, Wilson JF et al. (1997). Breast-conserving therapy vs mastectomy in early-stage breast cancer: a meta-analysis of 10-year survival. Cancer J Sci Am 3, 6–12.

Al-Ghazal SK, Blamey RW (1999). Cosmetic assessment of breast-conserving surgery for primary breast cancer. Breast 8, 162–8.

Wazer DE, DiPetrillo T, Schmidt–Ullrich R, Weld L et al. (1992). Factors influencing cosmetic outcome and complication risk after conservative surgery and radiotherapy for early-stage breast carcinoma. J Clin Oncol 10, 356–63.

Liljegren G, Holmberg L, Westman G (1993). The cosmetic outcome in early breast cancer treated with sector resection with or without radiotherapy. Uppsala–Orebro Breast Cancer Study Group. Eur J Cancer 29A, 2083–9.

Eltahir A, Jibril JA, Squair J et al. (1999). The accuracy of 'one-stop' diagnosis for 1,110 patients presenting to a symptomatic breast clinic. J R Coll Surg Edinb 44, 226–30.

Costantini M, Belli P, Lombardi R, Franceschini G, Mulè A, Bonomo L (2006). Characterization of solid breast masses: use of the sonographic breast imaging reporting and data system lexicon. J Ultrasound Med 25, 649–59.

The Royal College of Radiologists' Clinical Oncology Information Network (1999). Guidelines on the non-surgical management of breast cancer. Clin Oncol (R Coll Radiol) 11, S90–133.

Peters NH, Borel Rinkes IH, Zuithoff NP, Mali WP, Moons KG, Peeters PH (2008). Meta- analysis of MR imaging in the diagnosis of breast lesions. Radiology 246, 116–24.

Ljung BM, Drejet A, Chiampi N et al. (2001). Diagnostic accuracy of fine-needle aspiration biopsy is determined by physician training in sampling technique. Cancer 93, 263–8.

National Institute for Health and Clinical Excellence (2009). Breast cancer (early and locally advanced): diagnosis and treatment. Available from: http://www.nice.org.uk/guidance/CG80.

National Institute for Health and Clinical Excellence. Early and locally advanced breast cancer: Diagnosis and treatment CG80 (2009) https://www.nice.org.uk/guidance/cg80

Association of Breast Surgery at BASO. Surgical guidelines for the management of breast cancer (2009) http://www.associationofbreastsurgery.org.uk/media/4565/surgical_guidelines_for_the_management_of_breast_cancer.pdf

Patnaik JL et al, Br Cancer Treat Res 2011; 13: R64

Zhu et al 2012 Eur J Contraception and Reprod Health Care, 17: 402

(Million Women Study, WHI) ESPRIT

Xia X et al Sci Rep 2014; Keum N et al JNCI 2015

Lynch BM, Neilson HK, Friedenreich CM. Physical activity and breast cancer prevention. Recent Results Cancer Res. 2011;186:13-42

National GP guidelines and breast screening guidelines. Available at http://www.cancerscreening.nhs.uk/breastscreen/publications/nhsbsp69.pdf

https://associationofbreastsurgery.org.uk/media/63408/oncoplastic-breast-reconstruction-guidelines-for-best-practice-information-for-patients-2012.pdf

http://www.breastsurgeonsweb.com/wp-content/uploads/downloads/2012/10/515.pdf

Bedi DG, Krishnamurthy R, Krishnamurthy S, et al.. Cortical morphologic features of axillary lymph nodes as a predictor of metastasis in breast cancer: in vitro sonographic study. AJR Am J Roentgenol 2008;191(3):646–652.

http://www.bapras.org.uk/docs/default-source/commissioning-and-policy/final-oncoplastic-guidelines---healthcare-professionals.pdf?sfvrsn=0Post-operative radiotherapy for ductal carcinoma in situ of the breast--a systematic review of the randomised trials.Goodwin A, Parker S, Ghersi D, Wilcken N. Breast. 2009;18(3):143.

NICE guidance dg8. Intraoperative tests (RD-100i OSNA system and Metasin test) for detecting sentinel lymph node metastases in breast cancer.

https://associationofbreastsurgery.org.uk/media/63420/surgical-guidelines-for-the-management-of-breast-cancer-abs-baso-2009.pdf

Radiotherapy or surgery of the axilla after a positive sentinel node in breast cancer (EORTC 10981-22023 AMAROS): a randomised, multicentre, open-label, phase 3 non-inferiority trial Donker, Mila et al. The Lancet Oncology , Volume 15 , Issue 12 , 1303 - 1310

Benign breast diseases

Benign breast tumours *500*
Breast cyst *500*
Breast pain *501*
Gyanecomastia *502*
Breast infection *503*
Further reading *504*

Key guidelines

- Association of Breast Surgery (2010). Best practice diagnostic guidelines for patients resenting with breast symptoms.
- Association of Breast Surgery (2005). Guidelines for the management of symptomatic breast diseases.
- NICE (2016). Breast pain.
- Pearlman MD, Griffin JL; Benign breast disease. *Obstet Gynecol.* 2010. 116(3):747–58.
- BMJ Clinical Evidence (2014) Breast pain.

Benign breast tumours

Fibroadenoma

- *Epidemiology*—the most common benign lesion affecting women younger than 30. Peak incidence during the 2nd and 3rd decade of life. Juvenile fibroadenomas can occur in teenage girls.
- *Pathogenesis*—epithelial proliferation in a single terminal ductal unit and describes duct-like spaces surrounded by a fibroblastic stroma.
- *Clinical presentation*—well-defined, extremely mobile, solitary or multiple breast lumps. May increase in size during pregnancy or with oestrogen therapy, and regress after menopause. About 10% disappear each year.
- *Investigations*—triple assessment. In women <25y biopsy is not needed if clinically and radiologically benign.

Management options
- *Conservative management*—safe. Patients reassured and discharged.
- *Consideration for surgery if*—large size (>4mm), strong family history of breast cancer (patient requires follow-up in family history clinic) or patients insistence.
- *Newer methods of management.*
  - *Ultrasound-guided percutaneous excision* with a vacuum-assisted core biopsy device.
  - *Cryoablation.*

Phylloides

- Rare breast tumours that, like fibroadenomas, contain two types of breast tissue: stromal (connective) tissue and glandular (lobule and duct) tissue. Most common in women in their 30s and 40s, but they may be found in women of any age. Most are non-cancerous, but in rare cases they can be, therefore wide local excision is often performed.

Breast cysts

- *Epidemiology*—peak incidence between 35 and 50y of age. More often in premenopausal women.
- *Pathogenesis*—fluid-filled round or ovoid mass derived from the terminal duct lobular unit influenced by hormonal function and fluctuation. Therefore, occurs during lobular development, menstrual cyclic changes, and lobular involution in premenopausal and perimenopausal women.
- *Clinical presentation*—solitary mass or multiple masses with or without associated pain or discomfort.
- *Investigation*—triple assessment. Women >35y—mammogram and ultrasound to ensure no other lesions.
- *Management*—aspiration of cyst should abolish the lump. Patient can be reassured and discharged. Cyst fluid does not need to be sent for cytological examination unless it is blood stained. If the lump does not resolve completely following aspiration of cyst fluid then it should be treated like a suspicious breast lump.

Breast pain

- *Initial assessment*—full clinical history and examination.
- *Investigation*—if any incidental or focal clinical signs in the breast, imaging is required. If imaging normal, symptoms are treated based on the type of breast pain.

Cyclical breast pain

- *Epidemiology*—affects up to two thirds of women, with one in ten women having moderate-to-severe pain.
- *Clinical presentation*—pain that varies in intensity from one menstrual cycle to another, relating to the same time in the cycle, usually starting 1–3 days before the onset of menses and improving after menses.
- *Management*— eassurance of no underlying pathology. Better fitting/support bra. Oral analgesia.
  - If ongoing symptoms >6mo and severity confirmed on a minimum 2-mo pain chart, specialist referral for consideration of second-line treatment. These include danazol, tamoxifen, goserelin injections, gestrinon, or toremifene; however, can cause serious and unwanted side-effects.

Non-cyclical breast pain

- *Clinical presentation*—not associated with changes in pain intensity throughout the menstrual cycle and responds less well to drugs compared to cyclical mastalgia. Often confused with chest wall pain and is important to differentiate between the two. Non-cyclical mastalgia tends to be in the upper outer quadrant or behind the nipple without an obvious trigger spot.
- *Management*—same as cyclical mastalgia, but women should be warned that the response rates are not as good. Bra refitting.

Gynaecomastia

- *Epidemiology*—gynaecomastia peaks in teenagers (juvenile gynaecomastia) and males over the age of 65 (senile gynaecomastia). Both are benign conditions requiring reassurance and discharge. Idiopathic gynaecomastia accounts for approximately 20–25% of cases.
- *Clinical presentation*—men often present with breast formation or a breast lump.
- *Aetiology*.
  - *Excess oestrogens:* testicular tumours, adrenocortical tumours, hyperthyroidism.
  - *Disturbance in oestrogen metabolism:* alcoholism, chronic liver disease.
  - *Decreased androgens:* primary gonadal failure—Klinefelter, viral orchitis, secondary gonadal failure; pituitary or hypothalamic disease.
  - *Disturbance in androgen binding:* chronic renal failure, HIV.
  - *Side-effect from medication:* spironolactone digitalis, marijuana, alcohol, cimetidine, tricyclic antidepressants, phenothyazines.
  - All medications taken by the patient should be checked in the BNF to see if gynaecomastia is a known complication. Obviously any precipitating drugs should be reviewed by the patients GP and an alternative sought. In addition to marijuana, misuse of anabolic steroids in patients interested in body building can precipitate gynaecomastia.

Investigation

- *<20y*—exclude Klinefelter Syndrome, reassure patient and mother and discharge.
- *Age 20y–50y*—the following blood tests are recommended:
  - Testosterone & oestradiol levels.
  - *LH & FSH*— to check for hypogonadism.
  - *β-HCG*— to exclude choriocarcinoma, liver tumours.
  - *TSH*— check for thyroid disturbance.
  - *LFT & U&E*—to check for liver and renal disease.
  - Patient can be reassured and discharged if these tests are normal.
  - Routine use of breast ultrasound in these patients is not warranted.
- *Age 50y+*.
  - Blood tests as described above but β-HCG is not required.
  - Breast ultrasound and core biopsy if malignancy is suspected.

Treatment

- *Medical*.
  - Juvenile gynaecomastia is self-resolving and does not warrant treatment in the vast majority of cases.
  - Idiopathic gynaecomastia is usually self-limiting and warrants treatment only occasionally. Tamoxifen is not licenced for use in gynaecomastia but has some advocates. The use of danazol, clomiphene, and aromatase inhibitors is supported by very poor quality evidence.
  - Gynaecomastia secondary to hormonal imbalance should be dealt with in the medical endocrine clinic.
- *Surgical*.
  - Patients wanting gynaecomastia reduction surgery will need to obtain funding as it is not financed by the NHS

Breast infection

Lactational mastitis

- *Epidemiology*—a cohort study estimated that 2—10% of breast-feeding women get mastitis but only 0.4% develops an abscess.
- *Clinical presentation*—usually affects only one breast and symptoms can develop quickly. Presentation includes breast tenderness or warmth to the touch, general malaise or feeling ill, breast swelling, pain or a burning sensation continuously or while breast-feeding, fever, and skin redness often in a wedge-shaped pattern.
- *Management*—lactating women with mastitis should be prescribed appropriate oral antibiotics and encouraged to continue milk flow from the engorged segment (by continuation of breast feeding or use of a breast pump). Such measures reduce the rate of abscess formation and thereby relieve symptoms. Review the patient within 3–5d of commencing the antibiotic. If a woman chooses to stop breast feeding so that the breast infection can be controlled and the breast can heal, lactation can be suppressed using cabergoline.

Non-lactational (periductal mastitis)

- *Epidemiology*—the average age of this group of patients is 32y, and smoking is a major aetiology (90% of patients being smokers). Periductal mastitis and can also occur in men.
- *Clinical presentation*—periductal mastitis presents with either subareolar abscesses, mammary fistulae, nipple discharge, or transverse nipple retraction. Symptoms and signs are usually centred around the nipple areolar complex.
- *Management*—antibiotics and review the patient within 5–7d. Recurrence is common because the underlying duct pathology often persists and continuing to smoke increases recurrence rates up to 75%. Patients with recurrent symptoms may need definitive surgery to remove all underlying diseased ducts (total duct excision). These patients should be counselled regarding wound healing problems postoperatively. Clear documentation is important.

Breast abscesses

- *Investigation*—if an abscess is suspected an ultrasound scan should be done. This will reveal a uniloculated or multi-loculated collection.
- *Treatment*.
  - If the overlying skin is normal, there should be aspiration of the abscess under ultrasound guidance using adequate local anaesthesia.
  - If the overlying skin is compromised and is unhealthy or necrotic a mini-incision and drainage can be performed. Any necrotic skin can be debrided. Once the pus has drained, the cavity is thoroughly washed with local anaesthetic solution. The procedure is repeated every 2–3d until the wound closes and no further pus is draining. Pus is sent for culture and appropriate oral antibiotics and analgesia is continued until the abscess resolves.

Further reading

Association of Breast Surgery @ BASO, Royal College of Surgeons of England (2005). Guidelines for the management of symptomatic breast disease. Eur J Surg Oncol 31 (Suppl 1), 1–21.

Vaidyanathan L, Barnard K, Elnicki DM (2002). Benign breast disease: when to treat, when to reassure, when to refer. Cleve Clin J Med 69, 425–32.

American Society of Breast Surgeons. Available from: http://breastsurgeons.org/statements/ Management_of_Fibroadenomas_of_the_Breast_4-29-08.pdf. Accessed May 2009

NICE (2016). Breast Pain. Cyclical. Available from: https://cks.nice.org.uk/breast-pain-cyclical. Accessed Sep 2017.

Santen RJ, Mansel R (2005). Benign breast disorders. N Engl J Med 353, 275–85.

BMJ ClinicalEvidence. 2008. Available from: http://clinicalevidence.bmj.com/ceweb/conditions/ woh/0812.jsp. Accessed May 2009.

University of Michigan Health System (2013). Common breast problems. Guidelines. (US) Available rom:https://www.med.umich.edu/1info/FHP/practiceguides/breast/breast.pdf   Accessed Jan 2018.

Hartmann LC, Sellers TA, Frost MH et al. (2005). Benign breast disease and the risk of breast cancer. N Engl J Med 353, 229–37.

Dixon JM (1991). Cystic disease and fibroadenoma of the breast: natural history and relation to breast cancer risk. Br Med Bull 47, 258–71.

Hughes LE, Mansel RE, Webster DJ. Aberrations of normal development and involution (ANDI): a new perspective on pathogenesis and nomenclature of benign breast disorders. Lancet 1987; 2:1316.

Berg WA, Sechtin AG, Marques H, Zhang Z. Cystic breast masses and the ACRIN 6666 experience. Radiol Clin North Am 2010; 48:931.

Antibiotics for mastitis in breastfeeding women. Jahanfar S, Ng CJ, Teng CL. Cochrane Database Syst Rev 2009;1:CD005458

Gynaecomastia and breast cancer in men. Niewoehner CB, Schorer AE. BMJ, 2008; 336: 709–713

Gynecomastia: Pathophysiology, Evaluation, and Management. Johnson RE, Murad MH. Mayo Clin Proc, 2009, 84(11), 1010-1015

Evaluation and Management of Breast Pain. Smith RL, Pruthi S, Fitzpatrick LA. Mayo Clin. Proc., Mar 2004; 79: 353–372

NICE guideline breast pain management.

BASO guidelines.

Endocrine

Thyroid nodules and cancer*

Thyroid nodules *508*
Further reading *513*
Thyroid cancer *514*
Further reading *517*

---

* The guidelines in this chapter have been sourced and summarized from different UK, Europe, and international government sources, professional organizations, and medical specialty societies. Leading guidelines have been listed in the further reading section at the end of this chapter.

Thyroid nodules

Key guidelines

British Association of Endocrine Surgeons (2003). Guidelines for the surgical management of endocrine disease.

British Thyroid Association (2006/14). UK guidelines for use of thyroid function tests and management of thyroid cancer.

American Association of Clinical Endocrinologists and *Associazione Medici Endocrinologi* (2010). Medical guidelines for clinical practice for the diagnosis and management of thyroid nodules.

Basic facts

- *Incidence*—very common. Clinically apparent thyroid nodules present in 3–7% of women (<1% of men). True prevalence on ultrasound surveys or autopsy studies range from 37% to 57% of the population.
- *Risks of malignancy*—about 5% of all thyroid nodules, independent of their size.
- *Histologic classification*—four main types (Box 52.1).
- *Clinical presentation*—often discovered incidentally by patient, examining physician, or through imaging tests performed for other reasons. The absence of symptoms does not rule out the presence of malignancy [C]. Clinical history should include the onset and rate of growth, the presence of any compression symptoms (e.g. dysphagia, hoarseness), and any relevant medical or family history.
  - *Past medical history*—any previous disease or therapy involving the neck (history of head and neck irradiation during childhood), and any recent pregnancy.
  - *Family history*—the presence of benign or malignant thyroid diseases, familial adenomatous polyposis, Gardner's syndrome, and Cowden's disease.
  - *ALARM factors*—Box 52.2.

Recommended investigations

- *Blood tests*—all patients with thyroid nodule should have measurement of serum TSH concentration, using third generation high sensitive assay techniques, if available [B].
  - Free thyroxine (T4) and free triiodothyronine (T3) should be measured if the TSH level is low (<0.5μIU/mL) [C].
  - Free T4 and thyroid peroxidase antibody (TPOAb) should be measured if the TSH level is high (>5.0μIU/mL) [C].
  - There is no indication for routine measurement of thyroglobulin and no clear benefits of measuring serum calcitonin without any evidence of medullary thyroid cancer (MTC) on FNA or relevant family history [C].
- *FNAC (fine needle aspiration cytology)*—safe, reliable and simple outpatient procedure (Box 52.3). FNAC undertaken in the UK and Europe for all patients with solitary thyroid nodule or suspicious nodule in multinodular goitre. New BTA guidance recommends the use of

Box 52.1 Histologic classification of thyroid nodules

- *Simple, non-proliferative nodules*—colloid, cyst (simple or haemorrhagic).
- *Adenomas*—colloid adenomas, multinodular goitre, and follicular adenomas.
- *Thyroiditis-related nodules*—Hashimoto's thyroiditis.
- *Malignant nodules*—>80% differentiated (papillary and follicular), remainder medullary, anaplastic, lymphoma, and metastatic.

Box 52.2 ALARM factors in thyroid disease

- Any previous history of head and neck irradiation.
- Family history of thyroid cancer (MTC or MEN type 2).
- Patients younger than 20 (×2 risk) or older than 70, males (×2 risk).
- Suspicious nodule features—growing nodule with firm or hard consistency and fixed nodules.
- Any signs of invasion—cervical adenopathy, persistent hoarseness, dysphagia, and dyspnoea.

Box 52.3 Fine needle aspiration cytology

- *Technique*—with the patient supine, a 23–27G needle is inserted into the nodule without applying suction. Once in the nodule, suction is applied and the multiple needle passes made within the nodule. Rapidly the aspirate appears in the needle hub, suction is released, and the needle withdrawn. Smears are prepared by filling the syringe (after removing the needle) with air, reattaching the needle, and expulsing the material onto multiple slides, which are then stained appropriately. Similarly, cytospin 'blocks' are useful adjuncts.
- *Diagnostic usefulness*—sensitivity, specificity, and overall accuracy of FNA are excellent when performed by an experienced person (65–98, 70–100 and 69–97%, respectively). The PPV of Thy 5 cytology is 100%. False positive rate (patient with FNA showing malignant, suspicious, or indeterminate cytology, who has a benign macrofollicular adenoma) is 5–7%.
- *Results*—reporting based on RCPath guidelines and classified Thy1–5; most (70%) are benign (Thy2), 5% are malignant (papillary) (Thy5), 10% are indeterminate (Thy3) and can be sub-categorized to Thy3a (lesion uncertain significance) and Thy3f (follicular lesion), 5% suspicious (Thy4) and 10–15% are non-diagnostic (Thy1). Follicular cytology (Thy3) cannot distinguish between adenoma and carcinoma as diagnosis depends on capsule invasion. False negative rate reduced by improved sampling from ultrasound guidance. Thy1 lesions require further investigation or hemi-thyroidectomy.
- *Side-effects*—can cause slight discomfort and minor haematoma. No significant side-effect or seeding effect has been reported.

> **Box 52.4 Ultrasound assessment and selection of nodules for FNAC.**
>
> • Poor evidence/accuracy for size criteria.
> • Morphological criteria superior in accuracy in predicting malignancy.
> • *Benign features*: spongiform, iso or hyper-echoic, egg-shell/peripheral calcification.
> • *Malignant features*: hypo-echoic, microcalcifications, irregular margins, chaotic internal vascularity, shape taller than wide. The presence of more than one feature of malignancy of USS increases diagnostic accuracy from 70% to 90%. The suggestion of extracapsular growth or metastatic lymph nodes requires immediate cytological evaluation [B]. Predictive USS criteria continue to evolve.
> • New techniques such as elastography could be incorporated easily into U classification.
>
> Data sourced from Perros *et al* Guidelines for the management of thyroid cancer (2014) ***Clinical Endocrinology*** 81, Suppl 1

a U1–U5 scoring system for assessing risk of malignancy and guiding FNAC as only for lesions categorized U3 or above unless known risk factors or clinical suspicion (Box 52.4) [B].
• *USS*—indicated in the UK and Europe for all patients with palpable solitary thyroid nodule or suspicious nodule within a multinodular goitre, or as part of the evaluation of neck lymphadenopathy. USS also recommended for all multinodular goitres [C] and incidental nodules on other imaging.
  • *BTA guidance*—all patients with suspected thyroid cancer should have USS neck by an experienced thyroid radiologist. Further evaluation of incidental lesions <1cm not recommended unless known risk factors for thyroid cancer.
  • USS is not indicated as a screening tool for the general population [C].
  • *Findings and accuracy*—see Box 52.4.
• *Radionuclide scanning*—rarely used, only indicated in patients with (a) proven thyrotoxicosis and solitary nodule, (b) proven thyrotoxicosis and dominant nodule in MNG where option of hemi-thyroidectomy.
  • Thyroid FNA is not indicated in such cases [B]. Also indicated in exploring suspected ectopic thyroid tissue, suspected retrosternal goitre, and in iodine-deficient areas (US recommendations) [B, C].
• *Other diagnostic tests*—CT scan, MRI, laryngoscopy, and CXR.

Recommended management

• *FNAC-Thy3f/4/5 or clinically suspicious thyroid nodules*—surgical resection is recommended (see thyroid cancer below) [B].
• *FNAC-Thy2*— 'benign' nodule/s'.
  • *Conservative management (wait and watch)*—if no other indications for surgical resection exist.
  • *Thyroid cysts*—may be cured by aspiration to dryness. Recurrence is common, and may require surgical resection or consideration of percutaneous ethanol injection (PEI) if experience is available [B]. PEI has a low recurrence rate (2–5% over 1y) and can avoid surgical resection where malignancy has been excluded.

Box 52.5 Surgical resection for 'benign' thyroid nodule(s)

- Indications.
  - Clinical suspicion of malignancy.
  - Associated compression symptoms, tracheal compromise on imaging.
  - Cosmetic, discomfort, or anxiety reasons.
  - Growth of nodule/s, especially in retrosternal goitres.
- Recommended approach.
  - *Solitary benign nodule*—lobectomy and isthmusectomy.
  - *Bilateral nodules/multinodular goitre*—total/near total thyroidectomy, never sub-total thyroidectomy.
- *Post-operative complications*—post-op haemorrhage (<1%), recurrent laryngeal nerve injury 1–2% (note detection influenced by post-op laryngoscopy rate) permanent hypoparathyroidism (3–4%)
- *Intra-operative nerve monitoring during thyroid surgery (IONM)*—is used as an adjunct to conventional thyroid surgery by placing electrodes close to the vocal cords. The procedure has no major safety issues, and proven risk reduction when used in re-operative surgery and large (particularly retrosternal) goitres.

  - *Levothyroxine (LT4) suppression therapy*—is not indicated in most cases although the issue remains controversial. LT4 therapy has a clear beneficial effect in iodine deficiency areas (effective reduction of nodule volume), young people diagnosed with 'benign' small thyroid nodule, and in non-functioning nodular goitres [C]. Long-term use is usually required [B] and accurate monitoring to ensure incomplete suppression of thyroid function is essential [C].
- *Surgical resection is indicated in certain cases* (Box 52.5).
  - *Post-operative follow-up.*
  - *Calcium check*—within the first 24h of surgery and subsequently if required.
  - *Calcium replacement*—consider if corrected if calcium falls below 2mmol/L oral calcium (and occasionally activated vitamin D (alphacalcidol) supplementation until calcium level stable. IV calcium gluconate if below 1.8mmol/L or significant symptoms present. Attempted dose reduction must be supervised.
  - *T4 replacement*—should commence prior to being discharged from hospital for all total/near total thyroidectomies.
  - *TSH levels*—should be checked at follow-up around 6wk, including hemi-thyroidectomy as about 15% will require supplementation.
- *Radioiodine therapy for benign disease*—is indicated as in Box 52.6.

Box 52.6 Radioiodine for 'benign' thyroid nodule

Routine use is for definitive treatment of (recurrent) thyrotoxicosis rather than thyroid nodules, specifically small goitres. 'Graves' eye-signs are relative contra-indication.

- Indications for benign nodules.
  - Toxic (autonomous) nodules.
  - High risk for surgery.
- Not recommended.
  - Compressive symptoms.
  - Large nodules that require high dose of radiation.
  - Immediate resolution of thyrotoxicosis is required.

Further reading

British Association of Endocrine Surgeons (2003). Guidelines for the surgical management of endocrine disease. Available from: http://www.baes.info/Pages/BAETS%20Guidelines.pdf.

British Thyroid Association (2006). UK guidelines for the use of thyroid function tests. Available from: http://www.acb.org.uk/docs/default-source/guidelines/TFTguidelinefinal.pdf.

Gharib H, Papini E, Valcavi R et al. (2006). American Association of Clinical Endocrinologists and Associazione Medici Endocrinologi medical guidelines for clinical practice for the diagnosis and management of thyroid nodules. Endocr Pract 12, 63–102.

European Thyroid Association. http://www.eurothyroid.com/guidelines/eta_guidelines.html.

Hegedüs L (2004). Clinical practice. The thyroid nodule. N Engl J Med 351, 1764–71.

Anderson CE, McLaren KM (2003). Best practice in thyroid pathology. J Clin Pathol 56, 401–5.

Jones MK (2001). Management of nodular thyroid disease. The challenge remains identifying which palpable nodules are malignant. BMJ 323, 293–4.

Wass J, Shalet S, eds (2002). Oxford Textbook of Endocrinology and Diabetes. Oxford University Press, Oxford.

Reiners C, Wegscheider K, Schicha H et al. Prevalence of thyroid disorders in the working population of Germany: ultrasonography screening in 96,278 unselected employees. Thyroid 14, 926–32.

National Institute for Health and Clinical Excellence (2008). Intraoperative nerve monitoring during thyroid surgery. Available from: https://www.nice.org.uk/guidance/ipg255.

Thyroid cancer

Basic facts

- *Incidence*—uncommon (top 20 most common cancers for females in the UK). Affects 72.5 per 100,000 females and 1.4 per 100,000 males. The male to female ratio is 1:3. Incidence has been rising slightly in the UK for females.
- Worldwide incidence varies considerably, dependent on use of neck USS. The highest incidence in Europe was reported in Malta (7 times the lowest ranking EU country) and highest rates in the world occur in Northern America (78 per 100,000 females).

Differentiated thyroid cancer

- *Types*—differentiated thyroid cancer: papillary (80%) and follicular (20%). Biologically different cancers, but similar treatment principles.
- *Diagnosis*—usually made preoperatively (suspicious thyroid nodule), rarely intra-operatively (frozen section: NOT for follicular) and post-operatively on definitive histology, particularly incidental (up to 5% benign surgery).
- *Preoperative staging*—thyroid function tests mandatory, CXR, and laryngoscopy recommended prior to surgery. Evaluation of level 2, 3, and 4 lymph nodes using USS is recommended for all thyroid cancer patients [D]. CT (non-contrast) or MRI scans are indicated in patients with extensive or recurrent disease. Staging scintigraphy is not a recommended practice in the UK prior to the first operation.
- *Surgery*—is indicated in almost all cases [B].
  - *Total lobectomy*—is safe and appropriate in early thyroid cancers (cancers <1cm in diameter, no evidence of lymph node involvement (clinically or on USS), no evidence of diseased contralateral lobe, and no distant metastasis).
  - *Total or near total thyroidectomy*— recommended for patients with tumours greater than 4 cm in diameter, or tumours of any size in association with any of the following characteristics: multifocal disease, bilateral disease, extra-thyroidal spread, familial disease, and those with clinically or radiologically involved nodes and / or distant metastases (2-, D).

- *Lymph nodes*—central compartment lymph node (level 6) dissection is recommended for all grossly involved lymph nodes. The use of prophylactic level 6 lymphadenectomy in the UK is controversial but in USA (where radio-iodine used infrequently, it is routine as per the American Thyroid Association guidelines). For other lymph nodal stations, suspicious lymph nodes (clinically or on USS) undergo FNAC. Modified or radical lymph node dissection should be considered in the presence of histologically confirmed regional metastatic cancer following multidisciplinary meeting discussion. (see Box 52.7 & Box 52.8).
- *Post-operative management*—as for benign lesions except that:
  - *Triiodothyronine 20μg tds*—should be commenced post-operatively because of its short half-life prior to a pre-ablation scan if the patient has had a total thyroidectomy. Any residual thyroid tissue is destroyed by radioiodine (see adjuvant treatment). Recombinant human TSH increasingly used to avoid thyroid hormone withdrawal. Long-term TSH suppression using T4 is only recommended for high risk thyroid cancers as concerns about osteoporosis.
  - *Surveillance*—to check for TSH suppression and thyroglobulin estimation is recommended for frankly invasive lesions. Note that thyroglobulin is not of value as a preoperative test as it is produced by normal as well as malignant tissue but is an important monitoring tool after a total thyroidectomy.
- *Staging*—using the TNM pathological classification is recommended.
- *Adjuvant therapy*—radioiodine recommended for the ablation of residual thyroid tissue and treatment of residual or metastatic thyroid cancer. External beam radiotherapy may be indicated in certain cases (metastatic cancers refractory to radioiodine).
- *Recurrent disease*—should be considered for further surgery, radioiodine, or external radiotherapy.
- *Prognosis*—the overall 5y survival rates in England and Wales, corrected for age and sex, is ±20%, being best in younger ages (99% survival rate for patients younger than 40) and worst in the elderly (45% at the age of 70–79).

Box 52.7 Follicular cancer key facts:
- 30% differentiated thyroid cancer
- Middle aged
- 5 yr survival 50%
  Management:
  - <1 cm with minimal capsular invasion : lobectomy
  - Vascular and lymphatic invasion: total thyroidectomy
  - >4 cm: total thyroidectomy +/- level 6, radio-iodine and TSH suppression

When to undertake completion lobectomy?
  - in lLow-risk (females, patients <45 years of age) with ca <2 cm: probably just lobectomy alone and levothyroxine following MDT discussion and informed consent
  - No clear recommendations for other low-risk patients with tumours 2–4 cm in diameter showing minimal capsular invasion
  - Bone mets: radiosensitive

Box 52.8 Papillary cancer key facts
- 60% of DTC
- Under 40
- Best prognosis in adolescents, even with nodal involvement
- Worse in older where there may be follicular variants
- Age is the most important prognostic factor
- Nodal status has remarkably little bearing
- Mets to ipsilateral cervical nodes in 50%
- Often multifocal (30–50% contralateral lobe)
- Remove enlarged nodes which may require lateral dissection
- Consider prophylactic level 6 dissection
- Micro (<1cm) and no nodes: lobectomy alone
- Others :total and radio-iodine ablation post-op

Anaplastic thyroid cancer
- *Diagnosis*—additional diagnostic tests include immunocytochemistry (to differentiate from other types of cancers) and CT/MRI scan for all patients.
- *Treatment*—usually palliative. External radiotherapy may be helpful for symptom relief. Limited resection may occasionally be considered to relieve compression signs and for tumour size over 5cm.
- *Prognosis*—very poor (85% mortality rate in 1y).

Medullary thyroid cancer
- *Incidence*—rare. Occurs as sporadic cancer or as part of familial predisposition (familial MTC or MEN type 2a or 2b).
- *Diagnosis*—additional diagnostic investigations include plasma basal calcitonin and biochemical evaluation to exclude phaeochromocytoma. Other additional investigations include USS for all patients (or CT/MRI), basal calcitonin levels, and genetic screening in suspected familial cases.
- *Treatment*—total thyroidectomy and central compartment (tracheal and paratracheal) lymphadenectomy are recommended for all patients. Neck dissection and hyperparathyroidism should be planned and treated during the first operation based on preoperative investigations. Prophylactic thyroidectomy has a role in familial cases.
- *Prognosis*—the 5y and 10y disease-free survival rates range from 75–95% and 50–65%, respectively.

Thyroid lymphoma
- Rare. Usually presents as rapid onset painful goiter. Associated B symptoms may be present. Risk factor - Hashimotos thyroiditis.
- *Type*—almost always non-Hodgkin's.
- *Diagnosis*—additional diagnostic tests include immunocytochemistry (to differentiate from other types of cancers) using core biopsy (recommended to be performed in theatre).
- *Treatment*—prompt referral to oncologists. Chemotherapy mainstay of treatment Steroids may be very efficient in relieving compression symptoms.
- *Prognosis*—good for early stage lymphomas (50–85% 5y survival rate) and poor for advanced stage lymphomas (15–35% 5y survival rate).

Further reading

British Association of Endocrine Surgeons (2003). Guidelines for the surgical management of endocrine disease. Available from: http://www.baes.info/Pages/BAETS%20Guidelines.pdf.

British Thyroid Association (2006). UK guidelines for the use of thyroid function tests. Available from: http://www.british-thyroid-association.org/info-for-patients/Docs/TFT_ guideline_final_version_July_2006.pdf.

Gharib H, Papini E, Valcavi R et al. (2006). American Association of Clinical Endocrinologists and Associazione Medici Endocrinologi medical guidelines for clinical practice for the diagnosis and management of thyroid nodules. Endocr Pract 12, 63–102.

European Thyroid Association. Available from: http://www.hotthyroidology.com/ebook/ file_info/download1.php?file=_ebook_ht_2008-2009. pdf. Accessed May 2009.

Hegedüs L (2004). Clinical practice. The thyroid nodule. N Engl J Med 351, 1764–71.

Anderson CE, McLaren KM (2003). Best practice in thyroid pathology. J Clin Pathol 56, 401–5.

Jones MK (2001). Management of nodular thyroid disease. The challenge remains identifying which palpable nodules are malignant. BMJ 323, 293–4.

Wass J, Shalet S, eds (2002). Oxford Textbook of Endocrinology and Diabetes. Oxford University Press, Oxford.

Cancer Research UK. Available from: http://info.cancerresearchuk.org/cancerstats/types/thyroid/?a=5441. Accessed May 2009.

National Comprehensive Cancer Network (2009). NCCN clinical practice guidelines in oncology. Available from: http://www.nccn.org/professionals/physician_gls/f_guidelines.asp.

de Groot JW, Plukker JT, Wolffenbuttel BH, Wiggers T, Sluiter WJ, Links TP (2006). Determinants of life expectancy in medullary thyroid cancer: age does not matter. Clin Endocrinol (Oxf) 65, 729–36.

Cancer Research UK (2008). Thyroid cancer survival statistics. Available from: http:// info.cancerresearchuk.org/cancerstats/types/thyroid/survival/.

Further reading

Chapter 53

Surgery for hyperparathyroidism*

Basic facts 520
Recommended investigations 522
Recommended treatment 524
Further reading 526

Key guidelines

- British Association of Endocrine Surgeons (2003). Guidelines for the surgical management of endocrine disease.
- The American Association of Clinical Endocrinologists and the American Association of Endocrine Surgeons (2005). Diagnosis and management of primary hyperparathyroidism.
- National Institute for Health and Clinical Excellence (2014). Minimally invasive video-assisted parathyroidectomy.

* The guidelines on this chapter have been sourced and summarized from different UK, Europe, and international government sources, professional organizations, and medical specialty societies. Leading guidelines have been listed in the further reading section at the end of this chapter.

Basic facts

- *Definition*—hyperparathyroidism (HPT) is abnormal excessive production of parathyroid hormone (PTH) from the parathyroid gland(s), often with resultant hypercalcaemia (Box 53.1).
- *Incidence*—HPT affects 1% of adult population. Incidence increases after the age of 55, and women are more commonly affected
- (3×men).
- *Pathogenesis*—HPT results from solitary parathyroid adenoma (85%) or multiple hyperfunctioning parathyroid glands (including parathyroid hyperplasia, multiple adenomas, and polyclonal hyperfunction) (Box 53.2). Hyperfunctioning parathyroid carcinoma accounts for <1% of cases.
- *Clinical presentation*—over 80% of primary hyperparathyroidism (PHP) in Western countries are found incidentally by routine biochemical tests or on investigation of aetiology of resultant end-organ damage (osteoporosis and renal stones). Symptoms and signs result usually from the combined effect of increased PTH secretion and hypercalcaemia (Box 53.3) but many patients will be asymptomatic.
  - A thorough clinical history usually shows subtle neurobehavioural symptoms (fatigue, weakness, anorexia, mild depression, and mild cognitive or neuromuscular dysfunction) in up to 50% of cases.
  - Symptoms and signs have been immortalized historically by Walter St Goar in the mnemonic '*bones* (bone pain and fractures), *stones* (renal or ureteric stones), *abdominal groans* (pancreatitis, constipation, and peptic ulcer), and *psychiatric moans* (depression and cognitive or neuromuscular dysfunction)'.
  - A detailed family history should be taken to identify potential familial cases, particularly where co-existing phaeochomocytoma or Familial Hypercalcaemic Hypocalciurea (similar biochemical profile but due to reduced renal excretion) is possible.

Box 53.1 Hyperparathyroidism—definitions and classification

- *Primary hyperparathyroidism (PHP)*—the autonomous overproduction of PTH from the parathyroid gland(s), often with resultant hypercalcaemia.
- *Secondary hyperparathyroidism*—the excessive secretion of PTH in response to hypocalcaemia with associated hypertrophy of the parathyroid glands. Most commonly associated with chronic renal failure.
- *Tertiary hyperparathyroidism*—the excessive autonomous calcium-insensitive secretion of PTH after a long period of secondary HPT.

Box 53.2 Parathyroid tumours—molecular biology

- *Activation of oncogenes*—cyclin D1/PRAD1 for sporadic tumours and RET gene for familial tumours.
- *Deactivation of tumour suppression genes*—MEN1 gene for sporadic and familial tumours and HRPT2 gene in familial tumours.
- *Confirmed risk factors.*
  - *History of irradiation to the head and neck (external radiation or atomic bomb)*—dose-dependent effect. High radiation dose (≥12Gy) increases the risk by >50%; low doses (1Gy) increase the risk by 5–10 times (<1% at 35y).
  - *MEN type 1 or 2 syndromes*—PHP is the most common component of MEN1 and represents the initial manifestation of the syndrome in most patients. About 1–2% of all cases of PHP are due to MEN1. MEN2A syndrome is associated with a predisposition to medullary thyroid cancer (90%), phaeochromocytoma (40–50%), and primary parathyroid hyperplasia (10–20%). Parathyroid hyperplasia is not a feature of MEN2B syndrome.

Box 53.3 Clinical manifestations

- *Effect on bone metabolism*—loss of bone mineral density (measured by the dual energy X-ray absorptiometry (DEXA) test), increase in fracture risk (×2–3), distributed variably between cortical sites (mainly long bones), and trabecular sites (mainly vertebrae). Osteitis fibrosa cystica, brown tumours, and subperiosteal bone resorption on the radial aspect of the middle phalanges are found only in patients with prolonged, severe disease.
- *Nephrolithiasis*—occurs in ~15–20% of patients. Only 75% of patients with nephrolithiasis will have HPT.

Recommended investigations

- See Fig. 53.1.
- *Diagnosis*—can be established by demonstrating persistent hypercalcaemia (or serum calcium at the high normal levels) in the presence of elevated (or inappropriately normal) PTH concentrations and elevated urinary calcium excretion.
- *Other laboratory tests*—include measurement of 24h urinary calcium excretion and 25-hydroxyvitamin D for undetermined cases.
- *Differential diagnosis*—should always be reviewed (Box 53.4).
  - The surgeon has the ultimate responsibility to check that other causes of hypercalcaemia have been excluded. In young onset hyperparathyroidism, always exclude phaeochromocytoma pre-op; consider genetic testing. Multiple gland disease more commonly encountered than in older patients, more difficult to treat surgically and has higher risk of recurrence

---

Box 53.4 Differential diagnosis of hypercalcaemia

With associated elevated PTH.
- Primary HPT (sporadic), familial (MEN I and IIA, familial hypercalcaemic hypocalciuria), tertiary HPT (chronic renal failure).

With no associated elevated PTH.
- *Malignancy-related*.
  - *Medications*—e.g. vitamin D intoxication, thiazide, diuretics, lithium, excessive vitamin A.
  - *Miscellaneous*—chronic granulomatous disease, hyperthyroidism, phaeochromocytoma, acromegaly, immobilization, parenteral nutrition, milk alkali syndrome.

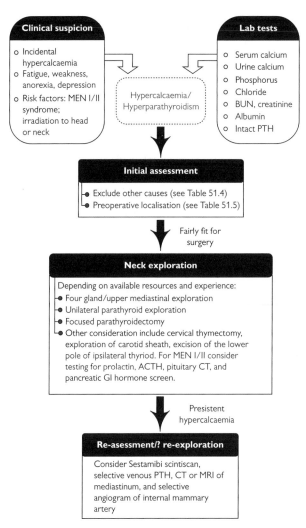

Fig. 53.1 Suggested approach to primary hyperparathyroidism.

Recommended treatment

- See Fig. 53.1.
- *Natural history*—the progress of HPT is usually slow in most patients, if at all. Nevertheless, about 25–60% of untreated asymptomatic patients will develop symptomatic disease during a 10y period.
- *Surgical resection*—the treatment of choice for all symptomatic and asymptomatic patients who are fit for surgery.
  - *Recommendations for asymptomatic patients*—controversial since the recommendations from the NIH consensus conference (2002). Nevertheless, more recent evidence has shown clear benefits of surgical resection as well as significantly reduced risks of operative intervention (see below). Surgery has become the currently recommended approach for all asymptomatic patients who are fit for anaesthesia and surgery by most authorities.
  - *Benefits of early surgical intervention*—include reduced mortality from cardiovascular diseases, improved physical and neuropsychological well-being, decreased risk of kidney stones, improved bone mineral density, and possible decrease of fracture risk. Surgical intervention is possibly more cost-effective than any single hospital admission for a complication of HPT.
  - *Recommendations for technical aspects*—see Box 53.5.
  - *Thoracoscopic excision of mediastinal parathyroid tumours*—should only be performed within a proper trial and clinical governance setting.
  - *Post-operatively*—check serum calcium within the first 24h (and thereafter, if abnormal). Serum calcium should be checked yearly for solitary adenoma patients.
  - *Re-operative parathyroid surgery*—should only be managed within a multidisciplinary setting by a specialist centre with appropriate facilities as cure rate much lower and morbidity higher.
- *Medical management*—has little contribution to the curative management plan. Good hydration, furosemide, oestrogen replacement in post-menopausal women, and bisphosphonate therapy have all some supportive role.
  - *Cinacalcet (an agent which increases the sensitivity of calcium-sensing receptors to extracellular calcium ions, and therefore, inhibits the release of PTH)*—has enough evidence to support its recommendation for the treatment of refractory secondary HPT in patients with end-stage renal disease where surgical excision is contraindicated. Pooled analysis of three largest RCTs (n=1,136) showed that Cinacalcet can reach the target mean PTH levels in <40% of patients (compared to 5% of patients receiving placebo, $p < 0.001$).

Box 53.5 Surgical exploration – technical aspects

- *Preoperative localization*—only required if a 'focused' limited neck exploration is to be performed. No current consensus exists on the specific indications or cost-effectiveness of each localization strategy.
  - There is no substitute for an experienced surgeon with meticulous dissection and haemostasis.
  - Current options include: (1) the 99mTc-sestamibi scanning with the use of a single photon emission CT scan, (2) high resolution USS examination, and (3) intra-operative direct PTH measurement (which can effectively avoid the need for frozen section and confirm cure).
  - Some surgeons use handheld gamma detection devices for radio-guided parathyroidectomy. The combination of 99mTc-sestamibi scanning with USS has a reported combined sensitivity of 94%.
- *Unilateral parathyroid exploration*—can be performed using a collar incision or minimally invasive-type incision. The cure rate following such approach can reach up to 99%.
- *Focused parathyroidectomy (FP)*—can be performed using a small lateral neck incision. This can be performed under local or regional anaesthesia and may be suitable for day case surgery.
  - *Efficiency and risks*—FP can achieve 100% cure rate (defined as normocalcaemia) when combined with intra-operative PTH (iPTH) measurement. The overall complication rate is <1.2% (compared to 3% for open bilateral exploration), the operating time is <30min (compared to >60min for open bilateral exploration),
  - *Thoracoscopic excision of mediastinal parathyroid tumours*—has limited evidence on safety and efficacy, and should ONLY and STRICTLY be used by well-trained surgeons within appropriate clinical governance setting.

Further reading

British Association of Endocrine Surgeons (2003). Guidelines for the surgical management of endocrine disease. Available from: http://www.baes.info/Pages/BAETS%20Guidelines.pdf.

AACE/AAES Task Force on primary hyperparathyroidism (2005). The American Association of Clinical Endocrinologists and the American Association of Endocrine Surgeons position statement on the diagnosis and management of primary hyperparathyroidism. Endocr Pract 11, 49–54.

National Institute for Health and Clinical Excellence (2014) Minimally invasive video-assisted parathyroidectomy.. Available from: https://www.nice.org.uk/guidance/ipg501

The Society of Nuclear Medicine (2004). Procedure guideline for parathyroid scintigraphy. Available from: http://interactive.snm.org/docs/Parathyroid_v3.0.pdf.

National Academy of Clinical Biochemistry (2006). Intraoperative parathyroid hormone. Laboratory medicine practice guidelines: evidence-based practice for point-of-care testing. Available from: http://labmed.ucsf.edu/labmanual/db/resource/IOPTH-CB-Instructions_for_Use.pdf.

Wishart GC (2006). Recent advances in the diagnosis and management of primary hyperparathyroidism (pHPT). Available from: https://www.ncbi.nlm.nih.gov/pubmed/16119109.

Marx SJ (2000). Hyperparathyroid and hypoparathyroid disorders. N Engl J Med 343, 1863–75.

Ruda JM, Hollenbeak CS, Stack BC Jr (2005). A systematic review of the diagnosis and treatment of primary hyperparathyroidism from 1995 to 2003. Otolaryngol Head Neck Surg 132, 359–72.

Hendy GN (2000). Molecular mechanisms of primary hyperparathyroidism. Rev Endocr Metab Disord 1, 297–305.

Silverberg SJ, Bilezikian JP (1996). Evaluation and management of primary hyperparathyroidism. J Clin Endocrinol Metab 81, 2036–40.

Parks J, Coe F, Favus M (1980). Hyperparathyroidism in nephrolithiasis. Arch Intern Med 140, 1479–81.

Tisell LE, Hansson G, Lindberg S, Rangnhult I (1977). Hyperparathyroidism in persons treated with X-rays for tuberculous cervical adenitis. Cancer 40, 846–54.

Schneider AB, Gierlowski TC, Shore–Freedman E, Stovall M, Ron E, Lubin J (1995). Dose-response relationships for radiation-induced hyperparathyroidism. J Clin Endocrinol Metab 80, 254–7.

Brandi ML, Gagel RF, Angeli A et al. (2001). Guidelines for diagnosis and therapy of MEN type 1 and type 2. J Clin Endocrinol Metab 86, 5658–71.

Bilezikian JP, Potts JT Jr (2002). Asymptomatic primary hyperparathyroidism: new issues and new questions—bridging the past with the future. J Bone Miner Res 17 (Suppl 2), N57–67.

Sejean K, Calmus S, Durand Zaleski I et al. (2005). Surgery versus medical follow-up in patients with asymptomatic primary hyperparathyroidism: a decision analysis. Eur J Endocrin 153, 915–27.

Lumachi F, Ermani M, Basso S, Zucchetta P, Borsato N, Favia G (2001). Localization of parathyroid tumours in the minimally invasive era: which technique should be chosen? Population-based analysis of 253 patients undergoing parathyroidectomy and factors affecting parathyroid gland detection. Endocr Relat Cancer 8, 63–9.

Sidhu S, Neill AK, Russell CF (2003). Long-term outcome of unilateral parathyroid exploration for primary hyperparathyroidism due to presumed solitary adenoma. World J Surg 27, 339–42.

Gurnell EM, Thomas SK, McFarlane I et al. (2004). Focused parathyroid surgery with intraoperative parathyroid hormone measurement, as a day case procedure. Br J Surg 91, 78–82.

National Institute for Health and Clinical Excellence (2007). Cinacalcet for the treatment of secondary hyperparathyroidism in patients with end-stage renal disease on maintenance dialysis therapy. Available from: http://www.nice.org.uk/nicemedia/pdf/TA117guidance.pdf.

Hernia

Abdominal wall hernias*

Basic facts 530
Recommended investigations 532
Groin hernias 534
Ventral abdominal wall hernias 538
Further reading 539

Key guidelines

- International Endohernia Society (2014). Guidelines for laparoscopic treatment of ventral and incisional abdominal wall hernias.
- British Hernia Society (2013). Groin hernia guidelines.
- European Hernia Society (2009). Guidelines on the treatment of inguinal hernia in adult patients.

---

* The guidelines on this chapter have been sourced and summarized from different UK, Europe, and international government sources, professional organizations, and medical specialty societies. Leading guidelines have been listed in the further reading section at the end of this chapter.

Basic facts

- *Definition and types*—a hernia is an abnormal protrusion of an organ through a weakness/defect in the body wall that contains it. Classification include groin hernias, ventral abdominal wall hernias (umbilical, femoral), incisional, Spigelian, and lumbar hernias.
- *Incidence*—hernia repair is one of the commonest operations performed by general surgeons worldwide. Inguinal hernias are the commonest type of abdominal wall hernias (~75%). Males are affected 15 times more frequently. Umbilical hernias are second commonest, and affected by pregnancy and truncal obesity. Femoral hernias are third commonest, affecting females more and presenting as emergency in 40% of cases.
- *Pathogenesis*—higher risk in smoking, underlying connective tissue disorders (Ehlers Danlos syndrome, Marfan syndrome), and increased intra-abdominal pressure (obesity, heavy lifting, chronic cough, and chronic straining during defecation and urination). The current notion is that the majority of hernias are a disease of collagen metabolism (reduced ratio of type I to type III collagen).
- *Clinical presentation*—incidental on imaging, asymptomatic lumps, painful lumps or incarcerated or strangulated hernias. *Cough impulse/reducible lump* is often the mainstay in diagnosis in non-emergency setting. *Incarcerated hernias* are irreducible hernias (can present with intestinal obstruction). *Strangulated hernia* occurs when vascular supply to the contents is compromised, resulting in ischaemic and gangrenous tissues (see Box 54.1).

Box 54.1 Groin hernia classification

Direct hernia—the viscera protrude through a weakness in the posterior inguinal wall.
- Anatomically, the hernia base is medial to inferior epigastric vessels. More frequent on the right side (the side where testicle descends last).
- Most are congenital (defective obliteration of the fetal processus vaginalis), commonly associated with increased intra-abdominal pressure (chronic cough, constipation, urinary obstruction, pregnancy, or ascites) and/or reduced muscular tone in the groin area (obesity, cachexia).

Indirect hernia—the viscera pass through the internal inguinal ring. Most common type in males.
- Anatomically, the hernia base is lateral to inferior epigastric vessels, and lie within the spermatic cord.
- Results from a weakness in the floor of the inguinal canal, possibly due to an inborn flaw (commonly), or to 'acquired' defect in the abdominal fibromuscular tissues (straining or heavy lifting have no identifiable relationship).

Femoral hernia—the viscera pass through the empty space at the medial aspect of the femoral canal. Most common type in elderly females.
- Results from a weakness at the entrance of femoral canal, possibly due to a weakness in the pelvic floor muscles (commonly in females due to less bulky musculature, previous childbirth, and atrophy with aging).

Other classifications.
- *Reducible hernias*—contents can be replaced completely.
- *Irreducible/incarcerated hernia*—the contents cannot be reduced at the internal or external ring or the femoral canal.
- *Incarcerated hernia*— ompromised arterial flow to the contents of the hernia sac, resulting in ischaemia and necrosis of the hernia and bowel contents. More common in femoral hernias.
- *Sliding hernia*— ccurs when part of the hernia sac wall is formed by an intra-abdominal viscera, e.g. the colon or the bladder.
- *Richter's hernia*—occurs when part of the bowel wall is trapped and strangulated.
- *Littre's hernia*—occur when the hernia contains Meckel's diverticulum.

Recommended investigations

- Clinical history and examination are the mainstay of treatment.
- Imaging modalities to investigate situations of clinical uncertainty include ultrasound, CT, and MRI. Ultrasound is often the first-line modality, since it is non-invasive, and a dynamic investigation. The use of CT/ MRI is justified in cases involving post traumatic hernias, rare hernias such as Spigelian or lumbar hernias and hernias associated with obesity. CT imaging is recommended in identifying recurrent hernias, and is considered to be superior to clinical examination.

Groin hernias

- The presence of many classification systems for groin hernias corresponds to the lack of acceptance of any single system due to the multiplicity in surgical treatment options for groin hernias.
- The Nyhus classification is the most widely used system, while the European Hernia Society recommends a modified Aachen classification.
- Inguinal hernias are, by far, the commonest groin hernias accounting for as high as 97% of all groin hernias. These are further classified as direct or indirect inguinal hernias according to the relationship of the neck of the hernia sac to the inferior epigastric vessels.
  - Indirect hernias involve the protrusion of the sac through the deep ring, therefore lateral to the inferior epigastric hernias, into the inguinal canal. Therefore, these hernias lie within the spermatic cord, and can extend into the scrotum in males.
  - Direct hernias protrude medial to the inferior epigastric vessels, through Hesselbach's triangle. These hernias do not lie within the cord, but can track along with the cord into the scrotum.
- Femoral hernias arise from the femoral canal, which is bounded superiorly by the inguinal ligament, laterally by the femoral vein and medially by the lacunar ligament. These hernias arise inferior to the inguinal ligament.
- Risk factors for inguinal hernias include smokers, family history of hernias, patent processus vaginalis, collagen disease, abdominal aortic aneurysm, previous appendicectomy (right-sided hernias), prostatectomy, ascites, peritoneal dialysis, long-term heavy work, and COPD.
- Clinical examination is not a reliable method to distinguish between the different groin hernias.
  - Femoral hernias arise below the inguinal ligament.
  - Differentiating between direct and indirect hernias clinically involves the 'occlusion' test, where the hernia sac is reduced, and pressure is applied to the mid-inguinal point (halfway between the anterior superior iliac spine and pubic tubercle), and the patient asked to cough. If the sac is controlled, this is implies the hernia to be indirect in nature, since the pressure is roughly overlying the deep ring.
  - Differentiation of direct and indirect hernias is not considered to be useful since it does not directly affect the management plan.
- *Investigation*.
  - If the diagnosis is unclear, ultrasound is considered to be the first line investigation.
  - MRI should be considered next if ultrasound is inconclusive, and should be done with patient in valsava manoeuvre.
  - Herniography involves the injection of radiopaque contrast into the peritoneal cavity, and can be considered in the presence of local expertise and inconclusive non-invasive imaging.

- *Management of inguinal hernias.*
  - *Natural history*—randomized trials of wait and see policy to hernias vs repair showed a complication rate of 2:1,000/yr in no-repair group, with life-time risk of developing significant pain of 10–15%. The risk of developing a contralateral hernia after unilateral repair is 25% at 10y (BJS 07).
  - Repair of an asymptomatic hernia does not therefore increase the incidence of chronic pain when compared to a wait and see policy. Either treatment option is acceptable with appropriate informed consent. Symptomatic hernias, with pain, are recommended to be surgically repaired. Femoral hernias should be repaired on presentation, including asymptomatic hernias, due to the higher risk of complications.
- *Surgical technique.*
  - *Open mesh repair.*
    —The Lichtenstein 'tension-free' mesh repair is most commonly performed for unilateral inguinal hernias. Alternatively, Shouldice suture layered repair is acceptable. A Cochrane review in 2012 confirmed the Shouldice technique to be the best non-mesh repair technique, though overall recurrence rates were higher compared to mesh repair. (3.6% vs 0.8%)
  - *Laparoscopic repair techniques.*
    —Laparoscopic repair can be performed by either a transabdominal preperitoneal patch plasty (TAPP) or a total extraperitoneal patch plasty (TEP) repair.
    —NICE (2004) report reviewed 37 randomized trials on 5,560 patients with lap vs open hernia repair. Lap repair has less acute and chronic postoperative pain, quicker return to daily activities and work, and fewer wound complications. Recurrence rate is similar, and risk of major vessel, bowel, or bladder injury were similar (except for a slightly higher risk for the TAPP repair). Lap repair took longer to perform and was a more expensive option (without counting the cost of postoperative chronic pain and return to normal activities.
  - Currently, both techniques are regarded as acceptable treatment options with similar outcomes. TEP repairs offer the option of repair under a regional anaesthesia.
  - Commissioning guidance from the Royal College of Surgeons of England in association with the British Hernia Society and the Association of Surgeons of England and Great Britain are outlined in Fig. 54.1.

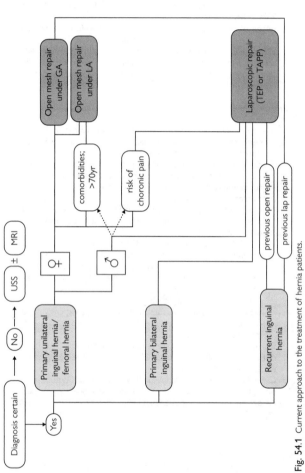

Fig. 54.1 Current approach to the treatment of hernia patients.

Ventral abdominal wall hernias

- *Umbilical and paraumbilical hernias*—congenital hernias arise due to failure of spontaneous closure of umbilical ring where umbilical vessels lie as they pass into the umbilical cord. 80% of these hernias close spontaneously by the age of 2y. Persistent hernias require surgery beyond this age group.

  Risk factors in adults include multiple pregnancies, obesity, cirrhosis with ascites and large abdominal tumours. Paraumbilical and umbilical hernias are five times more likely to obstruct compared to other ventral abdominal wall hernias.
- *Epigastric hernias*—arise from a defect in the linea alba. Male to female ratio of 2–3:1. Predominantly asymptomatic, and most contain perperitoneal fat only.
- *Incisional hernias*—arise from sites of previous incisions. The commonest site is following a midline laparotomy incision (10%). Transverse and paramedian incisions carry a lower risk (7.5% and 2.5% respectively). Prosthetic mesh repairs include onlay, sublay, bridging mesh, and intraperitoneal mesh repairs.
- *Management of ventral abdominal wall hernias*—asymptomatic hernias can be managed conservatively. Indications and factors affecting decision for surgical repair of abdominal wall hernias include symptoms, complications, and comorbidities.
- *Surgical techniques*—use of mesh should be considered in all abdominal wall defects larger than 2cm. The use of suture repairs should be restricted to small hernia defects with no significant risk factors predisposing to hernia formation. Laparoscopic techniques should be ideally limited to hernia defect sizes less than 10cm. A Cochrane review for laparoscopic incisional hernia repairs compared to open repairs demonstrated similar short-term recurrence rates, though reduced wound infections and possibly increased risk of enterotomies in the laparoscopic group.
- *Recurrent hernias*—after previous open hernia surgery, are better managed laparoscopically.
- *Incisional hernia repairs (defects larger than 10cm)*—are best treated with a sublay mesh placement, sublay mesh with a 'sandwich' technique where the hernia sac is used to cover the mesh, and intraperitoneal mesh placement with aponeuroplasty of the anterior fascia.

Further reading

Robert Fitzgibbons Jr, Samuel Cemaj and Thomas H Quinn. Chapter 71 Abdominal Wall hernias. Greenfield's Surgery. Scitentific principles and practice. Fifth edition.

Natalie Dabbas, K Adams, K Pearson, GT Royle. Frequency of abdominal wall hernias: is classical teaching out of date? JRSM Short Rep. 2011 Jan; 2(1): 5

NA Henriksen, DH Yadete, LT Sorensen, MS Agren, LN Jorgensen. Connective tissue alteration in abdominal wall hernia. Br J Surg, 2011 Feb;98(2):210-9

British Hernia society. Groin hernia guidelines, May 2013. www.britishherniasociety.org

Bittner R, Bingener-Casey J, Dietz U, Fabian M, Ferzli GS, Fortelny RH, Kockerling F, Kukleta J, Leblanc K, Lomanto D, Misra MC, Bansal VK, Morales-Conde S, Ramshaw B, Reinpold W, Rim S, Rohr M, Schrittwieser R, Simon Th, Smietanski M, Stechemesser B, Timoney M, Chowbey P.. Guidelines for laparoscopic treatment of ventral and incisional abdominal wall hernias (International Endohernia Society (IEHS) – Part 1. Surg Endosc (2014) 28:2-29

Burcharth J. The epidemiology and risk factors for recurrence after inguinal hernia surgery. Dan Med J. 2014 May;61(5):B4846

Simons MP, Aufenacker T, Bay-Nielson, Bouillot JL, Campanelli G, Conze J, de Lange D, Fortelny R, Heikkinen T, Kingsnorth A, Kukleta J, Morales-Conde S, Nordin P, Schumpelick V, Smedberg S, Smietanski M, Weber G, Miserez M. European Hernia Society guidelines on the treatment of inguinal hernia in adult patients. Hernia (2009) 13:343-403

Scott N, Go PM, Graham P, McCormack K, Ross SJ, Grant AM. Open mesh versus non-mesh for groin hernia repair. Cochrane Database of Systematic Reviews 2001, Issue 3. Art No: CD002197.

Amato B, Moja L, Panico S, Persico G, Rispoli C, Rocco N, Moschetti I. Shoudice technique versus other open techniques for inguinal hernia repair. Cochrane Database of Systemic Reviews 2012, Issue 4, Art No: CD001543

McCormack K, Scott N, Go PM, Ross SJ, Grant A, Colloboration the EU Hernia Trialists. Laparoscopic techniques versus open techniques for inguinal hernia repair. Cochrane Database of Systemic Reviews 2003, Issue 1. Art No:CD001785

Bittner R, Arregui ME, Bisgaard T, Dudai M, Ferzli GS, Fitzgibbons RJ, Fortelny RH, Klinge U, Kockerling F, Kuhry E, Kukleta J, Lomanto D, Misra MC, Montgomery A, Morales-Conde S, Reinpold W, Rosenberg J, Sauerland S, Schug-pab C, Singh J, Timoney M, Weyhe D, Chowbey P. Guidelines for laparoscopic (TAPP) and endoscopic (TEP) treatment of inguinal hernia [International Endohernia Society (IEHS)]. Surg Endosc (2011) 25:2773-2843

Royal College of Surgeons of England, ASGBI and British Hernia Socieety. Commisioning guide 2013. https://www.rcseng.ac.uk/library-and-publications/rcs-publications/docs/hernia-commissioning-guide/

Carlson MA, Ludwig KA, Condon RE. Ventral hernia and other complications of 1,000 nildine incisions. South Med J 1995;88(4):450-453

Sauerland S, Walgenbach M, Habermalz B, Seiler CM, Miserez M. Laparoscopic versus open surgical techniques for ventral or incisional hernia repair. Cochrane database of systemic reviews 2011, Issue 3. Art No: CD007781

Deerenbery EB, Timmermans L, Hogerzeil DP, Slieker JC, Eilers PHC, Jeekel J, Lange JF. A systemic review of the surgical treatment of large incsional hernia. Hernia (2015) 19:89-101

O'Dwyer PJ, Norrie J, Alani A, Walker A, Duffy F, Horgan P. Observation or operation for patients with an asymptomatic inguinal hernia: a randomized clinical trial. Annals of surgery. 2006 Aug 1;244(2):167-73.

Part 14

Skin

Principles of skin malignancies management[*]

Management of Malignant Melanoma *544*
Management of non-melanoma skin malignancies *546*
Further reading *548*

[*] The guidelines on this chapter have been sourced and summarized from different UK, Europe, and international government sources, professional organizations, and medical specialty societies. Leading guidelines have been listed in the further reading section at the end of this chapter.

Management of Malignant Melanoma

Key guidelines
- Cancer Research UK (2015). Skin cancer.
- NICE (2016). Skin cancer.
- NICE (2010). Improving outcome for people with skin tumours.
- British Association of Dermatology (2010). Management for malignant melanoma.

- Melanoma is the second most common cancer in the age group 15–34; More than two young adults in the UK are diagnosed with melanoma every day. People over 65 are more likely to be diagnosed with late-stage malignant melanoma.
- Risk factors include mainly intense, intermittent sun exposure, most frequently on the back in men and legs in women. Individuals, and particularly children, should not get sunburnt [Level I].
- Clinical suspicion should arise in any new mole appearing after the onset of puberty which is changing in shape, colour, or size; long-standing mole which is changing; any mole which has three or more colours or has lost its symmetry; a mole which is itching or bleeding; any new persistent skin lesion especially if growing, pigmented or vascular in appearance; and any new pigmented line or a lesion growing in a nail (esp. with no history of trauma). Certain high-risk patients (atypical moles, giant congenital moles, family history of melanoma, etc.) should be advised on appropriate screening [B].
- *Diagnosis*—is confirmed for any suspected lesion by photographing then excising completely. The axis of excision should be orientated to facilitate possible subsequent wide local excision. The excision biopsy should include the whole tumour with a clinical margin of 2mm of normal skin, and a cuff of fat. Diagnostic shave biopsies should not be performed. The nail should be removed sufficiently for nail matrix to be adequately sampled. Prophylactic excision of naevi in the absence of suspicious features is not recommended [D].
- Pathologic reports should include a minimum dataset (ulceration, thickness, mitotic count, margins, growth phase, infiltration, etc.).
- Melanoma staging should be initially based on histopathology features followed by lymph node and distant location involvement. TNM and AJCC staging systems are adequate. Patients with stage I, II, and IIIA melanoma should not routinely be staged by imaging or other methods as the true-positive pick-up rate is low and the false-positive rate is high [E]. Patients with stage IIIB or IIIC melanoma should be imaged by CT head, chest, abdomen, and pelvis prior to surgery [A]. Patients with stage IV melanoma should be imaged according to clinical need and MDT review. Lactate dehydrogenase should also be measured [A].

- Treatment is by surgical excision. In situ melanoma should have 5mm margins achieved in complete [B]. Melanoma with Breslow thickness of <1mm, 1–2mm, 2–4mm, and >4mm should have 1cm, 1–2cm, 2–3cm, and 3cm clear margins, respectively[A]. Lymph nodes should be sampled using sentinel lymph node biopsy for melanoma stage IB and upwards [A]. There is no role for elective lymph node dissection any more [E]. Nodes clinically suspicious for melanoma should be sampled using fine needle aspiration cytology (FNAC) prior to carrying out formal block dissection [B]. Staging CT scan should be performed beforehand [B]. Appropriate follow-up should be arranged based on melanoma stage [B].
- The treatment of locoregional recurrence in a limb is palliative. Surgical excision, radiochemotherapy, CO_2 laser, or isolated limb infusion or perfusion may be considered [B].

Management of non-melanoma skin malignancies

Key guidelines
- Cancer Research UK (2015). Skin cancer.
- NICE (2016). Skin cancer.
- NICE (2010). Improving outcome for people with skin tumours.
- British Association of Dermatology (2009). Management for squamous cell carcinoma.
- British Association of Dermatology (2008). Management for basal cell carcinoma.

- Cutaneous squamous cell carcinomas (SCCs) are common, arise from the keratinizing cells of epidermis or its appendages, and have a curative rate following local therapy of >90%. SCCs have a higher potential for local recurrence and regional or distant metastases than basal cell carcinomas (BCCs). BCC is a slow-growing, locally invasive malignant epidermal skin tumour predominantly affecting whites. Metastasis is extremely rare.
- Primary risk factor for non-melanoma skin malignancies is UV light exposure. Other risk factors include skin that burns easily and does not tan, light-coloured hair, older age, immunosuppressive treatment, and smoking.
- *Diagnosis*—SCC presents with a wide variety of clinical features (papules, nodules, plaques; smooth, hyperkeratotic, or ulcerative lesions). Skin biopsies are therefore required to confirm the diagnosis. BCC can be diagnosed clinically with confidence by dermatologists. This can be enhanced using good lighting and magnification. Biopsy is indicated only when clinical doubt exists.
- *Low vs high-risk tumours*—affect treatment selection in both SCC and BCC. Factors such as size, site, clarity of margins, histologic subtypes, and failure of treatment define the risk level which correlates strongly with treatment options and outcome.
- *BCC treatment*—topical and non-surgical therapies are advisable for many low-risk BCC lesions. Superficial low-risk BCCs can be treated with excision, electrodesiccation, and curettage (ED&C), or topical 5-fluorouracil or imiquimod. Nodular BCCs can be treated with ED&C or surgical excision. BCCs at high risk for recurrence should be excised using either Mohs surgery or a conventional surgical approach to completely resect the tumour. Radiation therapy is effective for the treatment of BCCs at high risk for recurrence; however, cure rates are lower than Mohs surgery.
- *SCC treatment*—surgical excision is the primary treatment for patients with high-risk cutaneous SCC, using Mohs micrographic surgery or surgical excision with complete circumferential peripheral and deep margin assessment. Adjuvant radiotherapy can also be considered.

SCC with features that suggest a low-risk for recurrence and metastasis are best treated with surgical excision, cryotherapy, electrosurgery, or radiation therapy. Topical chemotherapy (5-fluorouracil or imiquimod) and photodynamic therapy can also be considered in cutaneous SCC in situ radiation therapy is an additional option in older and frail patients.

Further reading

Marsden JR, Newton-Bishop JA, Burrows L, Cook M, Corrie PG, Cox NH, Gore ME, Lorigan P, MacKie R, Nathan P, Peach H. Revised UK guidelines for the management of cutaneous melanoma 2010. British Journal of Dermatology. 2010 Aug 1;163(2):238-56.

British Association of Dermatology (2009) Management for Squamous Cell Carcinoma. http://www.bad.org.uk/shared/get-file.ashx?id=59&itemtype=document

British Association of Dermatology (2008) Management for Basal Cell Carcinoma. http://www.bad.org.uk/shared/get-file.ashx?id=45&itemtype=document

British Association of Dermatology (2010) Management for Malignant Melanoma. http://www.bad.org.uk/shared/get-file.ashx?id=52&itemtype=document

NICE (2016) Skin cancer Available from: https://www.nice.org.uk/guidance/qs130 . Last accessed Sep 2017

Index

Jibawi Surgical 20-03-2018

A

Abbreviations ix-xii
ABCDE approach 148
abdominal aortic aneurysm
    (AAA) 461–8
    basic facts S 462–3
    best medical
        treatment 466
    investigations 464
    risk of AAA rupture 463
    risk factors 463
    screening
        recommendations 464
    surgical
        treatment 466, 467
    symptoms 463
abdominal trauma 156–9
    blunt injuries 156–9
    penetrating injuries 156–9
abdominal wall
    hernias 529–39
    algorithm 536
    basic facts 530
    classification 531
    groin hernias 534–5
    investigations 532
    ventral abdominal wall
        hernias 538
ACE inhibitors 449
achalasia 229–35
    algorithm 233
    basic facts 230
    investigations 232
    treatment 234
ACTH stimulation test,
    contraindications 167
acute kidney injury
    (AKI) 98–101
acute pancreatitis 371–8
admission
    management 41–4
    good practice 42
ALARM symptoms
    achalasia 232
    gastro-oesophageal
        reflux 209–20
    thyroid disease 509
anal fissures 341–8
    basic facts 334
    definitions 343
    patient education 345
    physical examination 343
    secondary causes 343

surgery 346
    treatment 344–6
anaphylactic reaction 93–6
    management 95
anaphylactic shock 145
aneurysm see abdominal
    aortic aneurysm (AAA)
ankle brachial pressure
    index 446
antibiotic
    prophylaxis 169–78
    contraindications 174
    recomm
endations 129, 174
    splenectomy
        patients 436–8
    wound types 171, 175
antibiotics, sepsis and septic
    shock 164, 165, 166
anticoagulation,
    perioperative
    management 137–42
    antiplatelet therapy 141
    new oral (DOACs) 141
        contraindications 449
    recommendations 140–1
antiplatelet therapy 141
    limb ischaemia 449
aorta
    blunt aortic trauma 156–9
    see also abdominal aortic
        aneurysm (AAA)
appendicitis 313–20
    algorithm 317
    basic facts 304
    investigations 316–17
    pregnancy 315
    signs 314, 315
    treatment 318
aprons, 182
ARISCAT risk index,
    postoperative respira-
    tory complications 75
arrhythmias
    risk factors 68
    supraventricular 98–101
aspirin 449
    carotid stenosis 458
    myocardial injury after
        non-cardiac surgery
        (MINS) 86
    perioperative antiplatelet
        therapy 141
    stroke 103
assistance to die 24–5
asthma-like reaction 93

atrial fibrillation (AF) 92–6
    postoperative 87
audit
    clinical governance 36
    consent 54
    day case surgery 49

B

balloon Sengstaken tube
    tamponade 264
Barrett's
    oesophagus 219, 251–8
    basic facts 252
    columnar-lined oesophagus
        (CLO) 252
    investigations 254
basal cell carcinomas
    (BCCs) 546
bedside medicine 19
benign breast tumours 500
    fibroadenoma 500
    phylloides 500
bile duct stones
    (CBDS) 412–13
biliary colic
    clinical features 403
    treatment 407
bladder injuries 156–9
bleeding, preopera-
    tive assessment of
    risk 115–19
    algorithm 118
    clinical 116, 118
    laboratory 117
bleeding tendency 118
blood transfusion 131–5
    fresh frozen plasma
        (FFP) 134
    haemolytic reactions 133
    levels of haemoglobin 131
    platelet transfusions 134
    red cells 132
    risk factors 133
Blumer's shelf 281
blunt abdominal
    trauma 156–9
blunt thoracic trauma 156–9
body mass index (BMI) see
    obesity
Bolant test, negligence 37
botulinum toxin
    injection 344, 345
bowel visualization 327
brain stem death 33, 146
breast abscess 503

breast biopsy 484–5
breast cancer 481–98
   algorithm 487
   basic facts 482
   clinical features 485
   discussion with
      patient 488
   initial staging 486
   investigations and
      diagnosis 484–5
   management 490–4
      adjuvant systemic
         therapy 493–4
      advanced disease 494
      axillary
         management 481–98
      breast
         reconstruction 490
      breast-conserving
         surgery (BCS) 490–2
      ductal carcinoma in situ
         (DCIS) 490–2
   follow-up 494
   lobular carcinoma in situ
      (LCIS) 492–3
   MDT meeting 486
   reporting standards 485
   risk factors 481–98
   see also benign breast
      tumours
breast cysts 500
breast infection 503
breast pain 501
breast tumours,
   benign 500
British Association of Day
   Surgery (BADS) 49
British legal system 28–9
bronchospasm and asthma-
   like reaction 93
bulking agents, endoscopic
   injection 218

C

cancer pain 192, 196
CANET (ARISCAT) risk
   index, postoperative
   respiratory
   complications 75
capacity, patient's 54
carcinoid syndrome 297,
   298, 417
cardiac risk
   factors 68–69
   estimation 69
cardiac risk index (cumulative, Lee index) 69–70
cardiogenic shock 145
cardiovascular failure,
   definitions 145
cardiovascular system

perioperative
   complications 86–90
preoperative
   assessment 68–72
Care Quality Commission
   (CQC) 32, 34–5
carotid artery
   stenosis 453–60
   algorithm 457
   basic facts 454
   carotid duplex scan 456
   investigations 456
   treatment 458–9
carotid endarterectomy
   (CEA) 458–9
catheters 188
cerebrovascular ischaemia,
   cardiac risk factors 69
children 24–5
   2, 4 and 6 rule, periopera-
      tive fasting 82
cholecystectomy,
   laparoscopic 413
cholecystitis, acute 402,
   407, 410
cholesterol, LDL 449
chronic limb ischaemia see
   limb ischaemia
chronic obstructive pul-
   monary disease
   (COPD), preoperative
   assessment 74
chronic pancreatitis 379–86
chronic venous insufficiency
   (CVI) 469–78
   basic facts 470–1
   CEAP classification 471
   investigations 472
   pathophysiology 471
   treatment 474–6
cinacalcet 524
clinical assessment 20
clinical governance 36
cliostazole 448–9
clopidogrel 449, 458
Clostridium difficile infection
   diarrhoea 186, 187, 188
   risk factors 174, 176
coagulopathy 145
   screening 456
   see also anticoagulation,
      perioperative
      management
Cochrane collaboration 3
colonic transit studies 327
colorectal cancer 357–68
   basic facts 358–9
   classification
      (resectable) 363
   CRC by site 360
   familial predisposition 359
   investigations 362

metastasis 417
   algorithm 419
   pathogenesis 358–9
   risk factors 358, 360
   staging 363
   treatment 364–7
      chemo/
         radiotherapy 365
      early rectal cancer 366
      emergency surgery 365
      preoperative
         preparation 365
colour flow duplex
   USS 446–7, 472
columnar-lined oesophagus
   (CLO) 252
   dysplastic CLO 256–7
   malignancy potential 252
   treatment 256–7
   upper GI endoscopy 255
complications see peri-
   operative medical
   complications
compression
   stockings 474–6
confidentiality 34–5
congestive heart failure, risk
   factors 68
consent 51–4
   audit 54
   capacity 54
   good practice 40, 52, 53
   providing sufficient
      information 52
   withholding
      information in 54
constipation in
   adults 323–32
   algorithm 326
   basic facts 324
   causes 325
   diagnostic tests 327
   investigations 326–7
   Rome III criteria 324
   treatment 328–31
continuing professional
   development (CPD) 36
contrast media,
   metformin therapy,
   contraindications 446
coronary syndrome 68
   dual antiplatelet
      therapy 141
   transfusion 132
Courvoisier's sign 389
creatinine, cardiac
   risk 69–70
critically ill patients 143–50
   algorithm 149
   definitions, key 144
   full patient assessment
      148

immediate
   management 148
levels of care 144
organ failure 145
types of shock 145
CT angiography 156–9, 446
cumulative cardiac risk
   index, Lee index 69–70

D

day case surgery 45–50
   audit 49
   British Association of Day
      Surgery (BADS) 49
   discharging patients 48
   patient selection 47
death
   brain stem death 33
   definition 33, 146
   maternal 160
dexamethasone,
   contraindications 167
diabetes, control 449
dietary fibre, food fibre
   contents 329
digital subtraction arteriography (DSA) 446–7
diltiazem, topical 344
discharging patients 22, 43
   criteria 43
   day case surgery 48
   information 43
disciplinary bodies and
   procedures 38–9
distributive shock 145
diverticular disease 333–40
   algorithm 337
   basic facts 334
   definitions 335
   Hinchey classification 335
   investigations 336
   risk factors 335
   treatment 338
diverticulitis, treatment 339
dressing selection, wound
   care 112, 113
driving, DVLA 34–5
dual energy X-ray
   absorptiometry (DEXA)
   test 521
duplex scan (colour flow
   duplex USS) 446–7,
   472

E

echinococcosis 428
emergencies 22
   haemolysis 133
   see also trauma
      management

endocarditis see infective
   endocarditis (IE)
endocrine cancer
   syndromes 295–302
endocrine shock 145
endoluminal
   gastroplication 218
endoscopic injection of
   bulking agents 218
endovenous laser therapy
   (EVLT) 475
epigastric hernias 538
Epstein risk index,
   postoperative respira-
   tory complications 707
equipment, personal
   protection 182
evidence-based
   medicine 3–13
   definition and process 4
   grading of
      recommendations 11
   levels of evidence 10
   research studies 6–7

F

familial hypercalcaemic
   hypocalciurea 520
fasting, perioperative 79–84
   2 and 6 rule 81
   children, 2, 4 and 6 rule 82
   exceptions 83
   higher risk patients 83
fasting, postoperative oral
   intake 83
femoral hernia 531
fibroadenoma, breast 500
fidaxomicin 188
fine needle aspir-
   ation cytology
   (FNAC) 508–10, 514
flail chest 156–9
fluid resuscitation
   pancreatitis 376
   pre-hospital trauma 160
   sepsis 164
food fibre contents 329
foreign bodies,
   ingested 221–7
   algorithm 225
   investigations 224
   management 226
fresh frozen plasma
   (FFP) 134

G

gallstone disease 401–14
   algorithm 408
   basic facts 402
   biliary colic 403, 407

biliary dyskinesia 410
   investigations 404, 412
   management of bile duct
      stones (CBDS) 412–13
   risk factors 403
   treatment 406–7
   USS 404
gastric cancer 279–93
   advanced 281
   basic facts 280
   initial assessment 284
   advanced staging 286
   TNM staging on CT
      scan 285
   TNM staging on
      EUS 287
   investigations 282
   risk factors 280
   treatment 288–90
      cancer resection 289
      chemoradiotherapy 290
      laparoscopic
         gastrectomy 288–90
      lymph node
         dissection 289
      lymph node
         resection 288
gastrinoma 297
gastro-oesophageal
   reflux disease
   (GORD) 209–20
   'ALARM', 211, 212
   algorithm 213
   antireflux surgery, benefits
      and risks 216–17
   basic facts 210
   expert comments 219
   initial approach 212
   management 216–17
   referral 212
   risk factors 210
   Savary–Miller classification
      of reflux disease 215
   secondary
      investigations 214
   symptoms and signs 211
General Medical Council
   (GMC) 38–9
gloves 182
glucagonoma 297
glyceryl trinitrate (GTN),
   topical 344, 345
good surgical practice 17–26
groin hernias 534–5
   classification 531
gynaecomastia 502

H

haemoglobin levels, blood
   transfusion and 131
haemolytic reactionS 133

Haemophilus influenzae 434
type B vaccine 436
haemorrhoid
disease 349–56
basic facts 350
behavioural
modifications 351
classification 351
conservative
management 351, 352
haemorrhoidal artery
ligation 352–5
haemorrhoidectomy
352–5
haemorrhoidopexy
352–5
injection
sclerotherapy 352, 353
pathogenesis 350
rubber band
ligation 352–5
haemothorax 156–9
hand hygiene 180–1
health care-associated
infections
(HCAIs) 180–1
Helicobacter pylori
infection 271
laboratory tests 274
second-line treatment 276
hepatic hydatid disease
(HHD) 428
basic facts 428
investigations 428
treatment 429
hepatobiliary imino-diacetic
acid scintigraphy (HIDA)
scan 410
hepatocellular carcinoma
(HCC) 421–30
algorithm 425
basic facts 422
investigations 424
treatment 426
algorithm 427
herniation, abdominal wall
hernias 529–39
hospital hygiene 180
hypercalcaemia, differential
diagnosis 522
hypercalcaemic
hypocalciurea 520
hyperparathyroidism 519–26
algorithm 523
basic facts 520
clinical manifestations 521
definitions and
classification 521
investigations 522
treatment 524
surgical exploration 525
hypovolaemic shock 145

I

impact factor (IF), research
studies 6–7
incidence, definition 8
incisional hernias 538
infection control 179–89
infection prophylaxis 129,
174
infective endocarditis
(IE) 127–30
basic facts 129
predisposing factors 128
prophylaxis 129
recommendations 129
information, disclosure 34–5
ingestion of foreign
bodies 221–7
injection sclerotherapy 352,
353, 474–6
insulinoma 297
Integrated Care Pathway
(ICP) 46
intermittent claudication
differential diagnosis 445
management 448–50
ischaemic heart disease, risk
factors 68, 69
ischaemic rest pain 445

K

Krukenberg's tumour 281

L

lactational mastitis 503
laser, endovenous laser
therapy (EVLT) 475
laxatives 328–31
legal aspects see medico-
legal aspects
Leser–Trelat sign 281
limb ischaemia 443–52
amputation 446–7
ankle brachial pressure
index 446
clinical features 445
colour flow duplex
USS 446–7
inflow/outflow
procedures 449
risk factor
modification 449
risk factors for PAD 444
lipodermatosclerosis 470
liver injuries 156–9
liver metastasis 415–20
algorithm, synchronous
metastatic colon
cancer 419
basic facts 416

investigations 417
treatment 418
lower limb
ischaemia 443–52

M

McBurney's point 314
macrogols 328–31
magnetic resonance
angiography
(MRA) 446
malaria prophylaxis 438
malignant melanoma 544–5
staging 544–5
malnutrition 200
diagnostic criteria 201
effects 200
screening 202
mastitis
lactational 503
non-lactational 503
medical complications,
perioperative
assessment 85–104
medico-legal aspects 27–40
appearing in court 30
British legal system 28–9
infection control 180–1
Mental Health Act
1983 32
statement 31
melanoma see malignant
melanoma
meningococcal groups A and
B vaccines 436
Mental Health Act 1983 32
mesalazine 338
metastatic disease of
unknown origin 417
metformin therapy,
contraindications 446
methicillin-resistant
Staphylococcus aureus
(MRSA) 184
multidisciplinary team 22
multiple endocrine neoplasia
(MEN) type 1 and 2 296
myocardial infarction,
perioperative 86–90
risk factors 69–70
myocardial infarction,
postoperative 87
myocardial injury after
non-cardiac surgery
(MINS) 86

N

naftidrofuryl 448–9
National Clinical Assessment
Service (NCAS) 38–9

neck, penetrating neck injuries 156–9
negligence 37
Neisseria meningitidis 434
nerve root compression 445
nervous system, perioperative complications 85–104
neuroendocrine tumours (NETs) 295–302
algorithm 301
baseline tests 299
basic facts 296
carcinoid syndrome 296, 298, 417
clinical presentation 297
investigations 298
pathobiology 296
treatment 300
neurofibromatosis type 1 (NF1) 296
neurogenic shock 145
neuropathic pain 197
NHS Modernisation Agency 49
nosocomial infections 180–1
NSAIDs 407
NSQUIP MICA Model 2007, cardiac risk 69–70
number needed to treat (NNT) 8–9
nutritional support 199–206
enteral 204
oral 204
parenteral 205
perioperative 203
preoperative 203
requirements 203

O

obesity 303–10
bariatric surgery 306–9
indications 308
types 308–9
basic facts 304
classification 307
comorbidities 305
preoperative assessment 74
risk factors 307
treatment 306–9
obstructive shock 145
obturator sign 314
odds ratios (OR) 9
oesophageal cancer 237–50
algorithm 241
basic facts 238
chemoradiotherapy 248
endoscopy 240
initial assessment 242
investigations 240

palliative treatment plan 249
pathologic report minimum dataset 247
staging, advanced 244, 245, 247
treatment 246, 265
oesophageal variceal haemorrhage 259–66
basic facts 260
definitions 261
prevention of re-bleeding 266
prophylaxis 262
treatment
active bleeding 264
failure 264
oesophagus
basic facts 230
endoscopic augmentation of LOS using hydrogel implants 218
operative notes 21
standard form 19
oral anticoagulants, direct (DOACs) 141
organ failure 145
osteomyelitis 110

P

pain management 191–8
assessment 192
differential diagnosis 445
neuropathic pain 197
pain transmission—therapeutic implications 192
perioperative pain control 197
postoperative pain 194–6
preoperative assessment 195
types and transmission of pain 192
pancreatic cancer 387–98
algorithm 393
basic facts 388
initial assessment 392
investigations 390, 394
palliative treatment 396–7
risk factors 388
symptoms and signs 389
treatment 396–7
pancreatic injuries 156–9
pancreatitis, acute 371–8
aetiology 372
algorithm 375
basic facts 372–3
possible physical findings 373

severity scoring systems 373
treatment 374
supportive management 376
pancreatitis, chronic 379–86
algorithm 382
basic facts 380
diagnosis 383
investigations 382
pain types 381
risk factors 380
treatment 384–5
parathyroid see hyperparathyroidism
parathyroid tumours 521
paraumbilical hernias 538
penetrating injuries
abdominal 156–9
lower limb arterial 156–9
neck 156–9
penicillin allergy 174
peptic ulcer disease 269–77
algorithm 273
basic facts 270
H. pylori infection 271
investigations 272
treatment 276
perioperative anticoagulation management 137–42
perioperative fasting see fasting
perioperative medical complications 85–104
peripheral arterial disease (PAD) see limb ischaemia
personal protection equipment 182
phylloides tumour 500
plasma B-type natriuretic peptide (BNP) 70–2
platelet transfusions 134
pneumococcal polysaccharide vaccine 436
pneumothorax 156–9
post-splenectomy sepsis (PSS) prevention 433–40
pre- and probiotics 338
pregnancy
appendicitis 315
Kleihauer– Betke analysis 160
trauma management 160
preoperative
assessment 55–78
ASA grades 60
bleeding risk 115–19
cardiovascular system 68–72
general evaluation 58, 59
investigations 62–6
pain 192, 195

preoperative assessment (Contd.)
recommendations: specific surgery and ASA grades 64
respiratory system 74–6
preoperative medication check 81
prevalence 8
professional performance 23
proton pump inhibitors (PPIs), expert comments 219
prucalopride 328–31
pulmonary embolism (PE) 122
pulmonary risk, prediction 74

R

radiofrequency ablation (RFA) 475
radionuclide scanning 509
record keeping 20
recordings 24
rectal cancer see colorectal cancer
red cell blood transfusion 134
red flags, preoperative assessment 59
references 24–5
relative risk (RR) 8
renal failure 145
acute kidney injury (AKI) 98–101
androgen binding 502
cardiac risk factors 69
hypercalcaemia 522
hyperparathyroidism 521
renal support 166
RIFLE classification of ARF 98
TBI 446–7
renal injuries 156–9
renal system, perioperative complications 85–104
research studies 6–7
research question 9–10
scientific paper 12
respiratory complications, postoperative, ARISCAT risk index 74–75
respiratory failure, types 1 and 2 145
respiratory system
anaphylactic reaction 93–6
bronchospasm and asthma-like reaction 93

perioperative complications 85–104
postoperative atelectasis 92
preoperative assessment 74–6
risk reduction strategies 75
risk, relative risk (RR) 8
Rovsing's sign 314

S

safe discharge see discharging patients
safety and quality 23
sclerotherapy, ultrasound-guided foam sclerotherapy 475
sentinel lymph node biopsy 490–1
sepsis and septic shock 145, 161–8
antibiotic use 166
basic facts 152
blood culture 166
definitions 162
MNT plan 164–7
surviving sepsis bundle 164, 165
vasopressors 167
sharps, safe use and disposal 183
shock 145
Sister Mary Joseph's node 281, 389
skin malignancies 543–8
basal cell carcinomas (BCCs) 546
squamous cell carcinomas (SCCs) 546
see also malignant melanoma
smoking
achieving cessation 384, 449
preoperative assessment 74
somatostatin analogues 300
spleen injuries 156–9
spleen, post-splenectomy sepsis (PSS) prevention 433–40
algorithm 437
antibiotic prophylaxis 436–8
basic facts 434
immunization 436
investigations 434
treatment 436–8
squamous cell carcinomas (SCCs) 546

standard operative notes 19
statins 103, 449
statistical analysis 6–7
sensitivity and specificity 9
steroids, good practice 167
stomach and duodenum 269–77
Streptococcus pneumoniae 434
stroke
ABCD score 456
aspirin 449
carotid endarterectomy (CEA) 458–9
clinical presentation 454
clopidogrel 449, 458
definition 454
heparin bridging therapy 139
high-risk 140–1
investigations 456
statins 103, 449
TIA and 454
treatment 102, 103
VTE prophylaxis 125, 139
superficial surgical site infection (SSI) 110
surgery
all types, NICE guidance 62–3
cardiac complication rates 69
type and risk factors 69, 74
surgical site infection (SSI) 170

T

99mTc-sestamibi with USS, hyperparathyroidism 525
thoracic trauma, blunt 156–9
thrombolytic agents, contraindications 87
thyroid cancer 514–16
anaplastic thyroid cancer 516
basic facts 514
differentiated (papillary and follicular) 514–15
lymphoma 516
medullary thyroid cancer 516
papillary, key facts 516
thyroid disease, ALARM factors 509
thyroid nodules 508–13
assessment 509
basic facts 508
histologic classification 509
investigations 508–10

treatment 510–13
  radioiodine 509
  surgical resection 509
toe brachial index
  (TBI) 446–7
transient ischaemic attack
  (TIA) 102, 103, 454
trauma management 151–60
  basic facts 152
  blunt abdominal
    trauma 156–9
  blunt thoracic
    trauma 156–9
  definitions 152
  fluid resuscitation
    pre-hospital 160
  mechanisms 152
  pregnancy 160
  principles 154–5
  special considerations 160
  specific areas/organs 156–9
traumatic brain injury 156–9
Trousseau's sign 389
Trousseau's syndrome 281

U

umbilical hernias 538
urethral injuries 156–9
urinary catheters 188

V

valvular heart disease, risk
  factors 69
vancomycin 188
variceal haemorrhage,
  oesophageal 259–66
varicose veins
  clinical presentation 470
  endovenous laser therapy
    (EVLT) 475
  injection
    sclerotherapy 474–6
  open surgery 475
  radiofrequency ablation
    (RFA) 475
vascular disease 443–52
venous insufficiency
  see chronic venous
    insufficiency
venous thromboembolism
  (VTE) prophylaxis 121–6
  basic facts 122
  current
    recommendations 124
  major risk factors 122
  management 123
  risk assessment 125
venous ulcer 470
  treatment 474–6

VIPoma 297
Virchow's node 281, 389
Virchow's triad 122
visual and audio recordings
  of patients 24

W

WHO Surgical Safety
  Checklist 23
wound care 105–14
  assessment 107
  debridement 109
  dressing selection 112, 113
  infection control 107,
    109–11
  management 108–11
wounds, surgical
  risk factors for developing
    SSIs 171
  risk index for developing
    SSIs 171
  risk of prophylactic
    antibiotics 172
  types 171, 175

Z

Zollinger–Ellison
  syndrome 297